COMPLEMENTARY THERAPIES IN REHABILITATION

HOLISTIC APPROACHES FOR PREVENTION AND WELLNESS

To Nicola —
Show up...
Pay attention...
Tell the truth — live your truth
Let go of the outcome...
Celebrate with me
your victories.

Carol

9/97

COMPLEMENTARY THERAPIES IN REHABILITATION

HOLISTIC APPROACHES FOR PREVENTION AND WELLNESS

Edited by
Carol M. Davis, EdD, PT
Associate Professor
University of Miami School of Medicine
Department of Orthopedics and Rehabilitation
Division of Graduate Programs in Physical Therapy
Coral Gables, Florida

SLACK Incorporated, 6900 Grove Road, Thorofare, NJ 08086

Publisher: John H. Bond
Editorial Director: Amy E. Drummond
Managing Editor: Debra T. Christy
Creative Director: Linda Baker

Cover Art: Jeanne Berg

The artwork in Chapter 8 was created by Jennifer M. Bottomley, PhD, MS, PT.

Jin Shin Do, *Trager*, and *Feldenkrais Method* are registered service marks.

The pronouns *he* and *she* have been used interchangeably throughout this book. This does not indicate gender bias.

Printed in the United States of America

Complementary therapies in rehabilitation: holistic approaches for prevention and wellness/[edited by] Carol M. Davis.
    p. cm.
    Includes bibliographical references and index.
    ISBN 1-55642-281-4
    1. Alternative medicine. 2. Rehabilitation. I. Davis, Carol M. [DNLM: 1. Rehabilitation—methods. 2. Alternative Medicine—methods. 3. Holistic Health. WB 320 C737 1996]
    R733.C656 1996
    615.5—dc2-
    DNLM/DLC
    For Library of Congress   96-44699

Published by: SLACK Incorporated
                    6900 Grove Road
                    Thorofare, NJ 08086 USA
                    Telephone 609-848-1000
                    Fax 609-853-5991

Contact SLACK Incorporated for further information about other books in this field or about the availability of our books from distributors outside the United States.

Last digit is print number: 10 9 8 7 6 5 4 3 2 1

DEDICATION

This text is dedicated to those people who fostered in me my love of physical therapy, and who supported me and encouraged me to strive for excellence in my practice. First:

Geneva R. Johnson, PhD, PT, FAPTA

Dorothy Pinkston, PhD, PT, FAPTA

L. Don Lehmkuhl, PhD, PT, FAPTA

and other members of the faculty at Case Western Reserve University who first described physical therapy for me as a scientifically based specialty in health care that requires the knowledge, skills and compassion of a primary care practitioner. And, one I graduated, they continue to encourage and expect excellence from me as a physical therapist.

My administrators in practice, teaching and research:

Marjorie K. Ionta, PT

Marilyn R. Gossman, PhD, PT, FAPTA

Sherrill R. Hayes, PhD, PT

As a clinician at the Massachusetts General Hospital, and as an academic at the University of Alabama in Birmingham and the University of Miami, I was warmly accepted by each of them at my stage of development as a professional. Then, under their leadership, each supported me and encouraged my individual development in physical therapy, making it possible for me to grow and thrive in my work.

Other significant mentors:

Helen K. Hickey, MEd, PT

Margaret L. More, PhD, PT,

Col. Marilyn Anderson, MA, PT

Ruth B. Purtilo, PhD, PT, FAPTA

Helen K. Saarinen Rahikka, MHSc, BSc (PT), DIP P&OT

Katherine F. Shepard, PhD, PT, FAPTA

Each gave me a very personal nudge at a time in my career when I needed to be assured that the talents that I had to offer physical therapy would, indeed, be important to the profession, and eventually, would be accepted.

My friends and my family who encourage me to continue to understand and refine my destiny as a person as well as a professional, support me when I feel most alone in that process, and invite me to share that learning with them. Especially to:

Susan Doughty

Bill Doughty

Ruth Ouimette

Jamiss Sebert

Patricia Calhoun

Jennifer Bottomley

and Mary Padlack.

To Meryl Cohen, friend and colleague, who constantly reminds me (in the words of A. Arien) to "show up, pay attention, tell my truth, and then let go of the outcome," and who continually encouraged me as we watched it unfold.

Finally, I dedicate this book also to:

Amy E. Drummond, my editor, who walked the long path with me and insisted that this book, which seemed to have a life of its own, would emerge in its own time. All that was required of me was that I put into practice what those named above taught me so well — to never lose the vision, and to do the work each day. If I "chop the wood and carry the water," the rest will take care of itself. It's very nice to have your editor be such a good friend.

Contents

SECTION I: MANUAL THERAPIES

SECTION II: MIND-BODY INTERVENTIONS

SECTION III: MOVEMENT AWARENESS

SECTION IV: TRADITIONAL CHINESE MEDICINE

SECTION V: HERBAL TREATMENT

EXPANDED CONTENTS

CHAPTER 1: PSYCHONEUROIMMUNOLOGY: THE BRIDGE TO THE COEXISTENCE OF TWO PARADIGMS 1
Carol M. Davis, EdD, PT

SECTION I: MANUAL THERAPIES

CHAPTER 2: MYOFASCIAL RELEASE: THE MISSING LINK IN TRADITIONAL TREATMENT 21
John F. Barnes, PT

SECTION II: MIND-BODY INTERVENTIONS

CHAPTER 6: BIOFEEDBACK: CONNECTING THE BODY & MIND 101
Jennifer M. Bottomley, PhD, MS, PT

CHAPTER 7: UNTYING THE KNOT: YOGA AS PHYSICAL THERAPY . .125
Judith Lasater, PhD, PT

CHAPTER 8: T'AI CHI: CHOREOGRAPHY OF BODY & MIND 133
Jennifer M. Bottomley, PhD, MS, PT

SECTION III: MOVEMENT AWARENESS

SECTION IV: TRADITIONAL CHINESE MEDICINE

CHAPTER 12: ACUPUNCTURE IN THE PHYSICAL THERAPY CLINIC . .217
Karen Gordon, PT, AP

CHAPTER 13: POLARITY, REFLEXOLOGY, AND TOUCH FOR HEALTH 235
Mable B. Sharp, PT, MS, CM

CHAPTER 14: JIN SHIN DO 257
Gudrun Heyland Mik, PT, Ulrike Treppmann,PT

CHAPTER 15: SUBTLE ENERGY MANIPULATION AND PHYSICAL THERAPY 267

Peter Selby, PT

SECTION V: HERBAL TREATMENT

CHAPTER 16: INTEGRATING ELEMENTS OF HOMEOPATHY AND PHYSICAL THERAPY: IMPLICATIONS FOR MAINSTREAM THERAPISTS 283

Steve Heinrich, PT

Acknowledgments

This work was made possible with the help of many people. No doubt I will not remember all of them, but at this time, the following especially come to mind.

To those colleagues and students who encouraged me to make this book become real as a resource to those who want help in clearing up the currently muddy waters, special thanks. To:

Sherri Hayes, PhD, PT, who gave me the time and the support to work on this project, even as we prepared our entry level Master's program for reaccreditation.

Neil Spielholz, PhD, PT, for challenging me in such a generous and encouraging way to refine my thinking, especially about research, and about micro bioelectropotentials.

Jay Schleichkorn, PhD, PT, for supporting me as a physical therapist writer, and for all the articles and ads on resources for this particular project.

Charles Recher, PhD, Diane Zuck, MA, PT, Ron Bugaj, MS, PT, David Berger, MA, PT, Gudrun Heyland Mik, PT, Jennifer Bottomley, PhD, PT, Darcy Umphred, PhD, PT, John Barnes, PT, Osa Jackson-Wyatt, PhD, PT, Carolee Winstein, PhD, PT, Mary Lou Galantino, MS, PT, and Frank Wildman, PhD, who encouraged me to carry on with my goal of responsibly integrating holistic approaches into traditional health care.

Leslie Dingley, who cheerfully and rapidly typed my decorative edits of the authors' chapters onto disks so that they could be sent on to the next step of refinement, and who constantly nodded and smiled as I reminded her that one day, this project would, indeed, be completed.

My supporters in the Book Division at SLACK Incorporated:

John Bond, Publisher, who said yes to the idea of this project, and then supported me and made it possible for me to create it in the ways that I believed would make the best contribution.

My editor, Amy E. Drummond, Editorial Director, whose help became so central and invaluable to me that I include her in my dedication.

Debra Clarke, Managing Editor, who worked rapidly to transform the raw material into the final product, always making sure that what appeared on paper was, indeed, what I intended.

Linda Baker, Creative Director at SLACK Incorporated, whose interest in this project resulted in her ability to unearth the cover of this text. We knew it would communicate so much of what we wanted to convey.

And special thanks to Helen K. Hickey, MEd, PT, thanks for being my first mentor (starting back in 1972, and continuing to this day) to pay serious attention to my questions about the links between why we are here on this planet, what we are to do to make the world a better place, and what physical therapy has to do with all of that.

Finally, deep gratitude to the others who are named in the Dedication, who assisted to such a great extent, that the book eventually became dedicated to them.

Contributors

John F. Barnes, PT, is the President and Director of the Myofascial Release Treatment Centers and National Myofascial Release Seminars located in Paoli, Pennsylvania and Sedona, Arizona.

"When I first began teaching, Myofascial Release was viewed as very controversial. It has been rewarding to experience the massive shift in awareness and acceptance of my Myofascial Release Approach. I have had the opportunity of training over 25,000 therapists and physicians. Myofascial Release is now considered to be a highly respected, comprehensive approach that is safe, cost efficient and consistently effective."

David Berger, MA, PT, MFCCI, is a certified Rosen Method Bodywork practitioner, physical therapist and Marriage, Family, Child Counselor intern in private practice in Berkeley, California. He holds master's degrees in physical therapy and in somatic psychology. As a client of Rosen Method, he has experienced profound changes in his own body, feeling tension, anxiety and chronic pain fade away. Rosen Method gave him one way to discover the relationships between his body, beliefs, emotions, and actions. As a practitioner, he has worked with hundreds of clients who develop a deeper understanding of themselves. His work with clients with chronic pain, trauma, abuse histories and relationship issues is broadened by integrating Rosen Method Bodywork, physical therapy, and psychotherapy.

Jennifer M. Bottomley, PhD, MS, PT, has a bachelor's degree in physical therapy from the University of Wisconsin, Madison and an advanced master's degree in physical therapy from the MGH Institute of Health Professionals in Boston, Massachusetts. She has recently completed an intercollegiate doctoral program with a combined degree in Gerontology and Health Science and Service Administration. She has practiced since 1974 in acute care, home care, outpatient clinics, nursing homes, and long-term care facilities. Currently, she works as an independent consultant setting up rehabilitation services in nursing homes and outpatient, home, and community settings in the Northeast. Jennifer is the current vice president of the Section on Geriatrics of the APTA and has served two terms as the treasurer and one term on the Board of Directors for that section. Jennifer is a nationally renowned speaker and educator. She has done clinical research in the areas of nutrition and exercise, foot care in the elderly, wound care, diabetes, and peripheral vascular disease interventions, balance and falls in the Alzheimer's population, T'ai Chi as an alternative exercise form, and social policy development (inclusive of the Managed Care perspective) for the elderly. She has authored numerous chapters and articles in the area of geriatrics. She has co-authored a geriatric text with Carole B. Lewis entitled *Geriatric Physical Therapy: A Clinical Approach*, published by Appleton and Lange Publishers, 1994.

Carol M. Davis, EdD, PT, graduated from Lycoming College in Pennsylvania with a bachelor's degree in biology, and studied physical therapy at Case Western Reserve University (master's degree, 1969). She completed her doctorate in humanistic studies in the School of Education at Boston University in 1982. Following a clinical staff position at the Massachusetts General Hospital, Dr. Davis was appointed Assistant Professor at the University of Alabama in Birmingham, Clinical Assistant Professor with Family and Internal Medicine at the University of Miami School of Medicine (Coordinator of the Fellowship in Clinical Geriatrics), Assistant Professor and co-chair *ad interim* at Sargent College of Boston University, and Associate Professor on physical therapy at the University of Miami School of Medicine where she teaches today. Dr. Davis also serves as Consultant to the Center for Psychosocial Oncology at the University of Miami Hospitals and Clinics and treats patients with the University of Miami Faculty Practice. She regularly conducts postgraduate education workshops in geriatric care, ethics, and teaching attitudes and values. She is the author of *Patient Practitioner Interaction: An Experiential Manual for Developing the Art of Health Care, Second Edition*, published by SLACK Incorporated.

Mary Lou Galantino, MS, PT, is Associate Professor of Physical Therapy at Richard Stockton College of New Jersey. Non-contact therapeutic touch has been incorporated in her clinical practice with patients diagnosed with chronic diseases. She has also developed an alternative/complementary therapies section of the PT curriculum at RSC, where students critically evaluate the research in these various areas. Ms. Galantino's clinical practice at the Garden State Infectious Disease Clinic welcomes the use of complementary therapies. She is completing her doctoral studies in Psychoeducational Processes at Temple University. The focus of her dissertation research is: Blending Traditional and Alternative Strategies for Rehabilitation—Measuring Functional Outcomes and Quality of Life Issues in an AIDS Population.

Karen Gordon, PT, AP, graduated in 1982 with a bachelor's degree in education with a certificate in physical therapy. She served as a staff therapist in the Acute PT Department of Baptist Hospital of Miami, specializing in orthopedics and manual therapy. She then served as Chief of the Acute PT Department from 1984-1991. In 1991, she completed her training in Oriental Medicine and established the Center for Radiant Health, a holistic health private practice incorporating both Western and Oriental medical disciplines.

Steve Heinrich, PT, has been studying the emotional component of pain and recovery for over 18 years. He specializes in craniosacral therapy and myofascial release. He is a senior instructor with Myofascial Release Seminars, and regularly teaches seminars in the Northwest. For more information on this or related subjects, you may contact him in care of SLACK Incorporated.

Osa Jackson-Wyatt, PhD, PT, is Director of Physical Therapy for Natural Ease™ for Daily Living in Rochester, Michigan. She became a physical therapist in 1972, and has a doctorate from the University of Michigan in the specialty area of the human aging process. Dr. Jackson-Wyatt has studied personally with Moshe Feldenkrais and is a certified Practitioner and Assistant Trainer in the Feldenkrais® method. Dr. Jackson-Wyatt lectures around the world on movement, aging, and physical therapy, and is the author of numerous books and articles. Her philosophy is that since the average person only uses 7-9% of his or her movement abilities, it is almost always possible to improve movement skills used in daily life.

Judith Hanson Lasater, PhD, PT, holds a bachelor's degree in physical therapy from the University of California, San Francisco, as well as a doctorate in East-West Psychology from the California Institute of Integral Studies. She is President of the California Yoga Teachers Association, which owns and runs *Yoga Journal* magazine, and has taught yoga since 1971. Additionally, she has taught anatomy, kinesiology, and yoga therapeutics to teachers in the San Francisco Bay Area and travels regularly to teach in almost every state in the U.S. She has also taught in Canada, England, France, Japan, Germany, and twice in Russia, where she was a guest of the Ministry of Health. During her second visit, she directed the production of a video on therapeutic yoga to be used in Russian military hospitals. Ms. Lasater has recently completed her first book for Rodmell Press, Berkeley, California, entitled *Relax and Renew: Restful Yoga for Stressful Times*, which presents the practice and therapeutic aspects of restorative yoga poses.

Guy L. McCormack, MS, OTR, is the chair and associate professor for the Master of Occupational Therapy Program at Samuel Merritt College in Oakland, California. He is an international leader in mind/body medicine, pain management, and therapeutic use of touch. Mr. McCormack received his Bachelor of Science degree in occupational therapy from the University of Puget Sound and his masters of science degree in Allied Health from Ohio State University. Currently, he has qualified for candidacy for his doctorate in human science at Saybrook Institute in San Francisco. Mr. McCormack has given numerous workshops at state and national conferences. He has published extensively in professional journals and textbooks. He is the author of two books, *The Therapeutic Use of Touch* and *Pain Management: A Mind/Body Approach*. He has developed, in collaboration with Positive Images & Wellness, audio- and videotapes in this field.

Mr. McCormack is active in the wellness movement and in integrating alternative or complementary approaches into mainstream healthcare. His expertise is in neuroscience, psychoneuroimmunology, neuromuscular dysfunction, and multicultural systems of healing.

Gudrun Heyland Mik, PT, received her physical therapy education in Heidelberg, Germany, specializing in rehabilitation, neurology, and the treatment of children. In 1983 she studied proprioceptive neuromuscular facilitation in Vallejo, California, and during that experience had her first encounter with Jin Shin Do, which eased the stress of this intensive experience. She took her first Jin Shin Do courses in Berkeley, California, and then continued her studies in Germany. In 1991 she studied Vojta education in Europe. Also during that year, she diverted her health care career to include studies of protestant theology in Bonn. Gudrun has studied Qi Gong Yangsheng with Professor Jiao since 1995. She has a personal interest in the Five Elements theory of nutrition and in Traditional Chinese Medicine.

Peter Selby, PT, is a physical therapist working in Bozeman, Montana. He has spent the past 18 years working in orthopedics and has post-graduate training in osteopathic manual therapy, acupuncture, craniosacral therapy, myofascial release techniques, and osteopathic visceral manipulation. He has also studied Taoist Qi Gong with Mantak Chia and various practitioners in Canada, the United States and China, as well as having studied Western esoteric healing traditions. His special interest is in the integration of the principles of energy medicine into conventional Western practice and thought, and he has spent the past 10 years developing his skills in this area. He has given lectures and demonstrations across the United States and Canada and has presented papers at a variety of international conferences. His chapter presents some of the cornerstones of his insights into Qi Gong and energy medicine as they apply to physical therapy.

Mable B. Sharp, MS, PT, CM, received her Bachelor of Science degree in physical therapy from Wayne State University in Detroit, Michigan. She received her master's degree in Allied Medical Professions Education from The Ohio State University in Columbus, Ohio in 1972. She also has certifications in both basic and therapeutic massage therapy from the International Myomassologist Federation. Until 1991, she was a member of the full-time faculty of the Department of Physical Therapy at Wayne State University, and is currently a practitioner and owner of Health Care Alternatives in Southfield, Michigan. Ms. Sharp's clinical practice encompasses an eclectic approach to patient treatment which utilizes techniques such as traditional physical therapy, reflexology, energy work, craniosacral therapy, and visceral manipulation.

Adrienne R. Stone, PT, became a physical therapist after being captivated by the hearts of children with cerebral palsy during a high school summer work experience. After receiving her Bachelor of Science degree in physical therapy in 1974 and working in acute hospital settings, she began looking for an approach to treatment that would encompass more of the whole person. The *Trager* Approach drew her in and filled that need. Over the years since then, Adrienne has worked closely with Milton Trager, MD. Certified by the Trager Institute as a practitioner since 1982, Adrienne also tutors *Trager* practitioners and students. She teaches *Mentastics* and other classes through the Trager Institute. In addition, Adrienne is a certified practitioner of Rosen Method Bodywork and Movement. Attracted by its gentle yet direct touch and dialogue, she began studying with Marion Rosen, PT, and the Rosen Institute in 1990. Adrienne has benefited significantly both personally and professionally from her experiences with *Trager* and Rosen Method. In her private practice, Adrienne incorporates the benefits of these experiences with her sensitivity of touch, supportive presence, and noninvasive mode. She currently practices in W. Los Angeles and in Pasadena, California.

Jim Zivan Tavrazich, PT, is a physical therapist, certified Rolfer, and Senior Clinician for Henry Ford Health Systems. Mr. Tavrazich has been a physical therapist for 14 years, and a Rolfer for 8 years. He came to Rolfing for help in resolving a chronic somatic pain condition.

"Through my Rolfing process, I discovered the potential of the approach to facilitate healing and well-being, both physical and psychological."

Ulrike Treppmann, PT, was born in 1951 in Wuppertal, Germany. Her physical therapy education took place at Dr. Lubinus School in Kiel. Since 1973, she has specialized in neurological patients. In search of a more holistic aspect, she started her Jin Shin Do education in 1985 and was licensed as a Jin Shin Do teacher in 1990. She began studying Qi Gong Yangsheng with Professor Jiao in 1993. In her own practice, she integrates Western physical therapy and Traditional Chinese Medicine.

Diane Zuck, MA, PT, received her certificate in physical therapy at the University of Pennsylvania in Philadelphia, Pennsylvania, and her master's degree in Movement Sciences from Columbia University in New York. She is a physical therapist in the deaf-blind program at the Perkins School for the Blind in Watertown, Massachusetts, a physical therapy consultant to the May Center for Education and Neurorehabilitation in Randolph, Massachusetts, a school for children with head injury, and a physical therapist with the Hug Center, a pediatric home care agency. Ms. Zuck also maintains a small private practice teaching the Alexander Technique, and is on the faculty at the Alexander Technique Center at Cambridge, Massachusetts. She is currently pursuing coursework and practice in the zero balancing approach and in using a healing touch with animals.

PREFACE

Who knows the exact time that a project that takes over 2 years to complete actually begins? As the "captain of the boat" of the writing and editing of this text, I can remember a few moments that made an unforgettable impression on me, and that inevitably led to the commitment that I made to this task. The first moment was when I was in college 30 years ago, in 1965. My identical twin sister, Susan, closed her eyes at the stimulus of a light bulb lighting, and an obvious change occurred in my EEG reading, as well as in hers, even though my eyes did not close because my light remained off.

Another moment I remember: In my first Myofascial Release course in 1990 when the rhythm I experienced from my partner's cranium (after what seemed like a very long wait) was totally different than any I'd ever experienced before. I was on my way to believing that something really did move under my hands, and that whatever was perceived, it was worth knowing more about. The curiosity I felt about that "unexplainable" perception was very similar to the curiosity that I had about my "unexplainable" experiences with my twin sister.

But even as recently as 5 years ago, it was not easy to discuss my excited discoveries about such perceptions as feeling heat and a "bouncy, full force" (energy?) between my hands, or the benefits of meditating for 20 minutes each morning. Journal articles and texts admonished me that one cannot see or feel energy any more than one can see or feel velocity. All we can experience is the result of energy and velocity. And the mind influencing the body? Well, that may be true, but what does that have to do with science?

Throughout my career, it was important to me to remain loyal to the rigors of empirical science, and yet I was drawn to explore the apparent exceptions to empirical theory, for these exceptions seemed to me to occur in therapeutic innovations that benefited patients in important ways: documented spontaneous remission from large, space-occupying, malignant tumors; tiny premature babies that thrived faster and more fully and went home a week earlier than control babies after receiving loving touch; experimental rabbits that avoided the harmful effects of high cholesterol food after receiving tender affection from a lab assistant; women with breast cancer who survived longer than controls simply by participating in support groups, and so on.

I bought books on quantum physics, I read, I listened carefully, I took a 3-month summer leave and studied and read about the connections between quantum theory and empathy, the subject of my doctoral dissertation. I studied Eastern philosophy and Native American healing practices. I listened to taped interviews of biologists and physicists.

In the early spring of 1991, I began to experience a rather chronic neck pain that, over time, developed into a full blown right upper quadrant syndrome with paresthesia and numbness in my fingers. An MRI ruled out any problem other than poor posture, and stress. Of course, once I finally admitted I had a musculoskeletal problem that was not going to resolve without intervention, I first tried to recover with treatment from all the traditional approaches in physical therapy. I actually made myself rest my neck and back, including submitting to 8 days of bed rest, plus the use of traction, ice, heat, anti-inflammatories, steroid injections, mobilization and exercise.

With no perceivable continuous relief from pain and spasm, I finally tried what I felt would be logical "alternative therapies," one by one, over a period of a year and a half. I sought out physical therapists practicing acupuncture and polarity, and asked them to treat me for the pain and spasm from my cervical nerve impingement. I experienced shiatsu massage for 3 months with no perceived benefit. Then I tried regression therapy, realizing that my pain undoubtedly had a psychological component to it. Many of these treatments require a rather long-term commitment to achieve pain relief and a balancing of the *chi*, or internal energy. At the time, I was in search of a treatment with more immediate relief, and did not give these approaches a fair trial. Finally I asked my yoga instructor if she knew a person practicing Rolfing massage, for I believed that I needed to get my head back on my shoulders once and for all, and someone needed to start at my feet and work up. A neuromuscular therapist who practices a Rolfing-like, deep, connective tissue massage which mechanically and energetically realigns the fascia and soft tissue, finally brought me to long-awaited diminishment of spasm, pain and paresthesia. After fifteen treatments, by successfully realigning my head over my shoulders and my shoulders over my hips, I was habitually standing straighter and feeling free of pain after 2 years.

Over the next few years, I continued my education in Myofascial Release, and I treated patients who reported benefits that surprised them, and me. But I winced each time careless or thoughtless clinicians made claims that seemed self serving ("I've taken craniosacral techniques and I can cure anyone"), and each time a respected colleague reported a perception of damage done to the profession because we were not scientific enough in our treatments or in our research. I recognized that what was required was a more systematic examination of what was happening when alternative therapies were used to complement traditional approaches, and I felt as if I needed to be one part of an effort to clarify and legitimize alternative approaches as "complementary" to traditional physical therapy treatments. But I was lost as to how, specifically, to proceed.

While I took my mini-leave of 3 months and studied holism, quantum theory and empathy in Sedona, Arizona during the summer of 1993, John Barnes, PT, paid one of his visits to the area. We sat on a rock together in the middle of beautiful Oak Creek on the Fourth of July and talked about our profession and about freedom. He pointed to an old shack hanging from the side of the red rock mountain that, over time, had been carved away by the creek around us, and described his vision of transforming that shack into a treatment center that would specialize in the application of Myofascial Release, along with other physical therapy approaches. And he believed that, even if insurance companies would not reimburse for this treatment, patients would willingly pay for it out of pocket.

I told him that my dream was to be courageous enough to publish a text that described how some of our colleagues were quietly studying and successfully using alternative, holistic approaches in their practices. But I lacked the courage to follow through with a proposal to my editor at SLACK Incorporated. As much as I believed in the importance of researching holistic approaches, those which were seated in quantum theory (especially the manual therapies that focus application of energy through the therapists' hands) did not fall into the category of treatments that could be validated by empirical double blind, controlled methods. And I wasn't sure how to begin to validate results.

In late 1993, I submitted an article to *P.T. Magazine* based on my study of touch, empathy, quantum theory and therapeutic presence. It appeared as a theory essay in the September, 1994 issue of the magazine (Vol. 2[9]), devoted to exploring the use of alternative approaches by physical therapists (Solid Objects are Not Solid...and Other Ruminations on Atoms, Energy, and Therapeutic Presence). I received positive feedback on the article, and finally began to feel more courageous about writing the text I had dreamed of, even before we knew exactly how to validate our results. As a result of the other articles in that issue, I now had more contacts of physical therapists actually researching and using alternative therapies.

John Bond, Publisher, and Amy Drummond, Editorial Director, of the Book Division at SLACK Incorporated, routinely take their book authors out to dinner at national conferences. In June of 1994 at the annual conference of the American Physical Therapy Association in Toronto, they took me out to dinner along with Mary Lou Galantino, a physical therapist and another of their authors well known for her writing about the role of physical therapists with patients who are HIV positive. Together Mary Lou and I convinced John and Amy that the book you hold now in your hands was long overdue. We both felt that physical therapists needed to help research and legitimize alternative therapies that complemented our traditional approaches, and that physical and occupational therapists were the best educated rehabilitation professionals to help the public make wise treatment decisions. But first fellow professionals had to be willing to take alternative therapies seriously enough to study them in detail and to become skilled in applying them, and then to develop ways to systematically research their effects.

In the early 1990s, and even still, it seemed as if we were experiencing two ends of a dysfunctional continuum in regard to alternative therapies in rehabilitation. At the conservative end were those clinicians, researchers and educators who would not open their minds to any approach that was not already validated, or validatable, by traditional medical science. At the other end were the laissez faire clinicians who cared less about being accountable for the theory behind their choices and the skillful application of a technique. Their best reason for using an approach was that, "it worked for a colleague who taught me, so I tried it too." And the confusion was further extended in that any list of alternative therapies included so many varieties of systems and approaches, some clearly not complementary to rehabilitation approaches, that professionals tended to dismiss the entire subject as wacky.

Well, as the end of 1996 nears, John Barnes has built his treatment center in Sedona, and it is very successful. Steven Wolf, PhD, PT, FAPTA, respected physical therapist and well-known medical researcher, has led research efforts funded by the National Institute on Aging that show that an alternative therapeutic approach, T'ai Chi, has the potential to improve balance in older people; and other physical therapists are now joining the efforts to help validate therapeutic approaches based on holism and quantum theory. The paradigm is shifting from a linear, hierarchical, reductionistic way of being and of explaining what is observed and real, to a more integrated, holistic, incorporative way of being.

This book is offered to professionals and lay people alike by all of us who were involved in its creation and actualization, as a contribution to help clarify the muddy waters. The authors and I hope to help legitimize treatment approaches that are logically complementary to traditional approaches in rehabilitation. We have found, and document here, that these approaches facilitate wellness and prevention in our patients. Unfortunately, we are not often aware of how this takes place, or we cannot *explain* how this takes place.

Most importantly, by way of this text, we hope to encourage the research necessary to bring these approaches up out of the darkness of suspicion and to stimulate actions needed to assure the safe and effective use of these approaches for our patients, and thus, to help bring order out of the chaos, and encourage the return of true healing to health care.

FOREWORD

Reading this book, its pages, ideas, and therapeutic suggestions will, for many readers, seem as if they are driving around a blind curve and, in fact, might question whether or not their wheels will remain on the road. What we perceive as truth and what we perceive as doubt is just that: our perception. In reality, the curve may not even exist and the car wheels may be locked. People have always resisted change, and Dr. Carol Davis has posed the questions: Are we, as professionals, ready for that change? Are we ready for a paradigm shift? What was questioned 40 years ago as progressive, questionable, and too unconventional is today considered traditional, established, and possibly old-fashioned.

No one questions that efficacy of clinical treatment needs to be established. Yet, research does not discover the truth, it validates it! Similarly, a limited definition of valid, reliable research may lead to paradigm paralysis. Clinical practice using measurable outcomes will guide research, change parameters, define practice, and allow practitioners to change. But when we define research only in terms of traditional experimental designs using a narrow linear model, we become stuck. We will see best what we are supposed to see, and we will fail to see what we feel is in conflict with our belief.

As a researcher, I desire, in fact I live for, answering the question "Why?" As a clinician, I am constantly being confronted with unknowns. At times, my unknowns or encountered mysteries simply cannot be answered using research models commonly accepted as traditional western science. I have the option of rejecting what I know happened or accepting that my research models may not deal with the scope of reality presented within the clinical arena. Dr. Davis has tried to create a stretch or enlargement of today's clinical and research parameters. She has helped to make that blind curve straighter by integrating theory with plausible research explanations. It takes a visionary on the periphery of civilization, not blinded by the city lights, to see the available stars in the sky. Dr. Davis has pointed out many new stars and tried to tie them to a universal interaction. Whether we choose to see a few of her stars, all of them, or new ones we may discover, or if we choose to look at the future while filtering out information that does not match our belief and research understanding, is up to each of us. No one should accept change blindly, nor can the profession accept nontraditional methodology and treatment alternatives without determining efficacy. How we establish efficacy is the query of this book. Dr. Davis has created an opportunity for growth with control and rational analytical thinking, yet suggests change. For that I thank her. Yet, the change can only come from each of us. This is our dilemma. Unknowns create fear, uncertainty, and hesitation. Yet, answers to those unknowns create an excitement that keeps our profession young, growing, and evolving into the future.

Darcy Umphred, PhD, PT

INTRODUCTION

As we approach the end of a decade and the end of a century, the world finds itself in the midst of rapid and substantive changes that perplex many. It is as if the very foundational blueprints of most human processes of interaction have been thrown up in the wind like a deck of cards, and as the cards come back to an order, nothing seems to be the same anymore. Change is predictable, but the magnitude and the depth of changes we are experiencing in technology, economics, ecology, management and business, in science and in the professions of theology, law, medicine, and, indeed, in all of health care, are difficult to keep up with. History reminds us that this magnitude of change often accompanies the final years of a century. In fact, many past centuries faded away amidst the collective terror of the citizens of the world that this would mark the end of time.

This book helps to clarify just one area of this universal movement of substantial change—the changes being made in rehabilitation. Specifically, it focuses on the way rehabilitation professionals view health and illness, and on the choices of treatment for their patients, especially those with chronic illness.

In this text, *medicine* refers to that aspect of health care in our country practiced by physicians and surgeons. *Health care* is that area of care practiced by non-physician professionals and their assistants. Traditional *allopathic*, *reductionistic* or *biomedical* medicine and health care are based on views of reality, substantiated whenever possible by the rigor of scientific research. *Rehabilitation* refers to that aspect of health care where the goal of treatment is to assist the patient to (re)gain the highest and deepest level of independent function possible in society.

Alternative and *complementary therapies*, based on quite different cultural attitudes and beliefs about health, healing and health care than those traditionally accepted, are finding their way into our society as a preferred choice of health care.[1] Nonconventional therapies are being chosen, especially for treatment of chronic illness, as a way of remaining healthy and well, and for preventing disease and decline in overall function—physically, emotionally, mentally and spiritually. This change might be viewed as positive, except that there are very influential and powerful leaders in medicine and health care who believe that diagnosis and treatment must be based on the outcomes of science, thus they are adamantly opposed to any other way of validating health care procedures. They strongly believe that treatment not grounded in science is not only a waste of money, but is potentially dangerous to the lives of those who purchase this care.

CHANGE IN THE PRACTICE OF MEDICINE, HEALTH CARE AND REHABILITATION

CONSUMERS' CHOICES

No one could remain blind to the current reality that massive change is pervading every facet of health care, not only in the United States, but in most Western industrialized countries. Research conducted regularly reports that patients have mixed feelings about the advantages and disadvantages of recent cost-cutting trends, focused primarily on replacing costly fee-for-service payment with pre-paid managed care organizations, or HMOs. One recent national survey[2] reports that, although Americans express concern about the effects that many of the changes in the health care delivery system might have on quality of care, especially the use of non-licensed personnel to carry out activities previously offered by professionals, the greatest factor that influences their choice of health insurance was not reduced cost, but the insurance company's provision of the ability to choose their own health care provider. Forty-seven percent of those polled (1,001 adults) in April, 1996 indicated this primary choice of a preferred provider (followed by choice of hospital for care) was more important than how much they would have to pay for their care.

In the United States stark changes such as the way people gain access to health care have been dictated to health care professionals by those outside of medicine and health care as a way of slowing down the runaway costs of care of the last four decades. These costs are not only the direct costs to the consumer, but to the federal government (and taxpayers) in subsidizing care that cannot otherwise be paid for.

In the early 1980s, diagnostic related groups (DRGs) were introduced as the way of reimbursing hospitals and health care professionals for care given to Medicare patients. The long-established "fee-for-service" payment was eliminated, and soon private health insurance companies dictated how nonhospitalized, essentially "well" patients could gain access to the health care that they were paying for with their insurance. Payment for care from health insurance became allowed only if consumers would join the insurance companies' recommended managed care organizations, and pay a flat fee for all *potentially* needed care within a given period. These new rules often stripped consumers of many of the cherished choices they had previously taken for granted, such as having the "right" to choose their preferred hospital or physician.

PROVIDERS' CHOICES

Of all the changes health professionals have had to adjust to, capitation and managed care may be the one change felt most dramatically among providers of care. Currently, many health care professionals agree that business decisions designed to cut costs by reducing access to needed care have dissolved the ethical ground of those responsibilities which confer upon them their very status as professionals: their ability to choose which facet of medicine or health care they feel drawn to practice, their autonomous ability and responsibility to decide within their practice who should be served, to decide for how long they should be served before discharge, and to decide a just fee for their service. Recently, these age-old, core professional responsibilities have been usurped by business executives who seem to lack both the concern and the ability to make these most important decisions. The foundational ethic of business—*buyer beware*—has subsumed the foundational ethic of health care—*primum non nocere* (above all, do no harm), due primarily to the inability of medicine, health care, and biomedical science to monitor and keep in check the dangerous and outrageously steep rise in cost for services.[3] Unfortunately, among those who suffer most from cost cutting denial of services are patients who would benefit from rehabilitation and preventive care.

POSITIVE CHANGE

The future is not all black. On a brighter note, some managed care organizations, especially those which are not for profit, promote policies that allow the time to include health care professionals in governance and encourage professionals to educate patients about the choices they must make and the relative cost of each choice. These organizations are making substantially more positive contributions to the delivery of care, and are actualizing the brighter and more humanistic aspects of managed care. Unfortunately we read and hear about them far less often than those that act out the darkest side of what was primarily meant to be a positive change for everyone involved in medicine and health care.

In sum, the practice of traditional medicine and health care are "not what they used to be," and although change can be charted throughout the evolution of modern medicine and health care,[4] it seems as if current changes have threatened the very heart of the profession as it has come to be known and believed in.

TRADITIONAL MEDICINE AND HEALTH CARE

It is unarguable that traditional Western medicine responds more effectively than any other health care system in the world to infectious disease, acute illness, and trauma. However, traditional allopathic practitioners have been severely criticized for the past three decades for their inability to respond adequately and compassionately to the needs of the "worried well," those who suffer from chronic illness, the treatment of which makes up 85% of the national health care bill.[5] In addition, articles and editorials abound in newspapers calling for a more individual and humanistic response to patients from doctors and other health care professionals. C. Everett Koop, former Surgeon General and now Senior Scholar at Dartmouth College, lists this poor communication between doctors and patients and the recent trend of the growth of drug-resistant bacteria as his greatest concerns with the current allopathic medical system.[6] Interestingly, he states that appropriate responses to both crises in modern medicine lie in the development of alternative medicine. He specifies that both the holistic approach to care and the use of herbal and botanical substances may help us resolve these failures of scientific medicine.[6] (Actually, herbal and botanical substances make up the basis of current pharmaceuticals, but natural ingredients are mixed with other manufactured ingredients, some of which cause such harmful side effects that they prove to be ineffective.)

These are very uneasy times for patients and medical and health care professionals, and practitioners and patients alike are working to solve the problems. However, surrounding and permeating this problem-solving process in search of cost-effective and reliable treatment is a cultural bias that will not admit any exception to the value of traditional reductionistic science as the way of locating reality within our world culture.

THE ADVENT OF COMPLEMENTARY AND ALTERNATIVE THERAPIES

At the same time that feelings of frustration about the inadequacies of treatment and the loss of choices available within traditional medicine and health care in the United States mount, it was revealed in 1993 that more patients than were estimated are exercising choices about the variety of treatments they prefer for their health and illness, and are willing to pay for these choices, delivered by providers they choose, out of their own pockets.[1] In January of 1993, the *New England Journal of Medicine* reported that, in 1989, "unconventional" treatments were chosen by 34% of 1,539 adults surveyed in a national study. Subjects using unconventional therapies most frequently were "non-black persons from 25-49 years of age who had relatively more education and higher incomes." Care was chosen primarily for chronic conditions, and 72% failed to tell their doctors of their decision. When results were extrapolated to the entire population in the United States, it was determined that the estimated visits (425,000,000) for unconventional therapies in 1989 exceeded the 388 million visits to primary care physicians, and, of the $13.7 billion dollars spent, $10.3 billion, or 75% ,was paid for out-of-pocket.[1]

The impact of the results of this study has been felt on many levels, from those who believed that older people with higher education and higher incomes would view any treatments outside of traditional doctor-approved scientific medicine as quackery and fake, to those who believed that people would be unwilling to pay for medicine and health care out of their pockets. That study, conducted in 1989 and reported in 1993, was, no doubt, soon quite out of date, and most would agree that updated statistics would reflect even larger numbers. Today information about complementary and alternative therapies can be found everywhere, not only on television and radio talk shows and in supermarket tabloids. Indeed, three new peer-reviewed research journals were begun in 1994 and 1995 aimed at facilitating and reporting research.[7-9] The journal *Advances*[10] has been publishing related research from the Institute for the Advancement of Health since 1983, and the *Noetic Sciences Review*[11] from the Institute of Noetic Sciences since 1986.

ALTERNATIVE VERSUS COMPLEMENTARY TO THE TRADITIONAL OR SCIENTIFIC

Readers will come across the terms *complementary* and *alternative* being used seemingly interchangeably. But some authors are examining the confusions that imprecise language adds to the misunderstanding of this rapidly evolving health care system of holistic care. Most favor making as many clear, even if somewhat arbitrary, distinctions as possible when comparing and contrasting "unconventional" or alternative treatments themselves, or conventional (scientifically based) treatments administered in an "unconventional" way, that is, from a holistic rather than a reductionistic theoretical base.

With regard to terminology, in this book the terms *scientific, allopathic, biomedical, traditional, reductionistic,* and *conventional* refer to traditional Western medicine practiced from the theoretical foundations established by the French philosopher René Descartes (1596-1650) in the 17th century, and refined by the great mathematician and physicist Isaac Newton (1642-1727). This theoretical base will be further described later, but Newtonian Cartesian physics primarily is based on the mechanical laws of cause and effect, and utilizes the scientific method proposed by John Dewey to search for that which is "really" real (versus what our five senses may tell us) by proving or disproving a hypothesis, a guess about the cause.

The effect of one and only one variable (cause) is tested in empirical research. The body is reduced, part by part, as much as possible before research is conducted. The common focus of study is one system alone, and only one variable is tested at a time, if at all possible. Thus the term *reductionism:* reducing any interfering systems or contaminating causes (other variables), even the cause of chance or luck, to as cleanly and rigorously as possible ascertain the effect or outcome of the experimental or treatment variable. And reductionists have always been committed to seeking the single most adequate treatment or cure for a disease.

On the other hand, the terms *holistic*, *non-allopathic* (homeopathic, naturopathic, etc.), *nontraditional*, and *unconventional* refer to forms of healing that grew out of non-Western thought, primarily the philosophies of China (Traditional Chinese Medicine, Taoism), India (Ayurveda, Hinduism) and the Eastern parts of the world, as well as out of the spiritual traditions of Native Americans and other cultures. The term *holism* reflects the idea that the mind and body cannot be separated, and that they are, in fact, united in a "whole" that is nurtured by a vital force (ch'i, prana, qi) that circulates throughout the body by way of anatomically elusive pathways or meridians. This vital force maintains balance in the body, ensuring a natural, healthy state and well-being, as long as this force is able to circulate freely.

In the past, *alternative treatments* were those administered from a holistic theoretical perspective as an *alternative* to the prevailing reductionistic science perspective of traditional medicine and health care. Holism's theoretical base emphasizes the importance of the interaction of energy, people and matter to the larger whole (which is always more than the sum of the parts), and in treatment uses to advantage the belief that mind and body cannot be separated. Rather than attempting to locate and treat the one set of symptoms from the one prevailing disease, as is the case with reductionism, holistic practitioners treat the patient's whole mind-body system that is out of balance, a state which therefore "allows" diseases or disorders to develop. This intention on rebalancing the "out-of-balance" vital force frees the mind-body's own natural ability to heal itself, not only eliminating the primary symptoms and the underlying disease, but all other threats to health as well. Thus, holism's aim is to restore natural health and inner balance (homeostasis) and prevent any imbalance which eventually might lead to several nonhealthy states, including depression or a variety of disease states in general. Holism is an integrative, interactive, inseparable description of all matter, and it is based on the theories of quantum or subatomic physics as developed in this century by Einstein, and further refined by David Bohm[12] and others.

Traditional or conventional scientific treatments in medicine and health care are developed and delivered from the highly valued reductionistic perspective, which emphasizes the Newtonian Cartesian importance of hierarchy, and separation of the material (the body, or the physical) from the nonmaterial (the mind, or the mental, emotional, and spiritual) which cannot be seen. This theoretical base has evolved to contemporary times to strive, by way of empirical research and other systematic valid and reliable tools, to find the single best answer to the main problem as it manifests in signs and symptoms of disease.

For the purposes of this text, when either conventional (exercise, massage or manual therapies) or unconventional (alternative) treatments (T'ai Chi, Trager approach, yoga, Rolfing, relaxation techniques) are administered from a *holistic* perspective rather than from a *reductionistic* perspective, *as an extension of, or complementary to,* treatments that are offered in traditional scientific (reductionistic) medicine and health care practice, such as physical and occupational therapy, they are referred to as *complementary* therapies, that is, complementary to traditional scientific, allopathic medical and health care treatments which are based in reductionistic theory.

The most common reason that conventional rehabilitation treatments such as massage, exercise or relaxation techniques are included in the category of alternative or holistic medicine and health care is because, as indicated above, the same treatment can be administered both from a biomedical/reductionist (scientific) world view (eg, massage that mechanistically "pushes" the fluid from the extremities toward the body) or from a holistic world view (eg, massage that "softens" the fascia by way of intentional touch, thereby reinstating a more free flow of ch'i). The treatment may look very similar to the casual observer, but the practitioner will describe different intentions and methods. The relationship to and involvement of the patient may be markedly different in holistic treatment approaches, and the goals of care are less focused on alleviating symptoms and are more focused on removing restrictions to the body's own ability to heal itself.

These two world views of holism and reductionism have some aspects in common, but often conflict and end up competing, not just in medicine and health care. This will be examined more fully below and in Chapter 1.

CREDENTIALS OF CAREGIVERS

Traditional health care and medicine place a high priority on preparation for practice. Often, but not always, holistic therapies are delivered by caregivers who may have earned specific certificates and/or licenses to practice these treatments. Obviously this might offer some form of accountability in knowing how to apply treatment. Sometimes these practitioners have also been educated or licensed in traditional health care practice. For example, some (not all) people practicing massage, teaching exercise and fitness, or prescribing herbal remedies are traditionally licensed massage therapists, physical therapists, physicians, and nurse practitioners. However, the majority of practitioners of alternative therapies are *not* also licensed allopathic medical or health care providers. This presents a problem of practitioner accountability. Licenses, and, indirectly, degrees and certificates signifying learned content, exist to better ensure the public safety. When practitioners cannot produce documentation of their education and/or training and licensure, the public may well be at risk.

CLASSIFICATION

An entirely new health care "industry" has arisen in the United States, and it appears that its growth is more rapid than most would have imagined. Many treatments of this new health care naively are described as "new" or the latest approach when, in fact, the treatment or approach is part of a system of care, of healing, that has been used successfully for thousands of years. Few writers are attempting to clarify any of this confusion as they report each "new" treatment in trade books and newspapers as the "answer" everyone has been waiting for, often the latest cure for cancer or treatment for impotence.

Chiropractic, Ayurveda, Traditional Chinese Medicine, homeopathy, and **naturopathy** are some of the examples found on any given list of complementary or alternative therapies. These practices would best be described as larger health care *systems*, not as specific treatments. On the other hand, examples of alternatives that reflect *approaches* or *styles* of care include **Trager, Feldenkrais, Alexander Technique, yoga, Rolfing,** and **Myofascial Release.** And even more basic, some terms represent specific *techniques or treatments* within approaches that are located in larger systems. For example, the treatment called *auricular acupuncture,* or acupuncture administered on the ear alone, is a technique of the *approach* of **acupuncture** within the health care system of Traditional Chinese Medicine. **Transcendental meditation** and **sesame seed oil massage** are two *techniques* found within the ancient Indian *system* of **Ayurveda.**

WHICH SYSTEM IS THE "RIGHT SYSTEM" OR "BEST SYSTEM" ON WHICH TO BASE TREATMENT?

Neither reductionism nor holism as a theoretical base for care contains all that is needed to answer the medical, health, and prevention problems of people today. Marc

Micozzi, MD, PhD, former Senior Researcher for the National Cancer Institute of the National Institutes of Health, a physician, anthropologist, and epidemiologist, has called for a merging of treatments from both theoretical models, a "final common pathway."[13]

Biomedicine assumes all patients are basically the same, and treatments, designed to combat a single pathologic process, which can be readily repeated producing the same result if the research is valid and reliable.[13] "Complementary medicine assumes that all individuals are different, and the manifestations of disease depend on the unique characteristics of the individual patient." A "constellation" of therapeutic approaches which may vary on a given day, depending on the changing needs of the patient, would integrate both approaches.[14] Complementary health care practitioners who place greater emphasis on the validity of each individual therapeutic experience should be encouraged to develop designed controls for each treatment so that outcomes on the efficacy of a given approach can be determined and shared.

But how possible is it to integrate these two often radically different approaches? Is this problem of fragmentation too large to ever resolve? On a practical level, this text illustrates that integration of the two approaches to care is being practiced every day by physical and occupational therapists, especially when they seem to reach the limits of benefit of allopathic care. The newspapers reporting on complementary therapies very often mention traditionally educated physicians who are also naturopaths or are practicing Aryuveda or acupuncture or using herbal remedies for patients who do not respond well to allopathic measures. Approximately 30 medical schools in the United States, including Harvard, Columbia, Stanford, and Georgetown offer courses in alternative medicine.[15,16]

A SHIFT IN THE PREVIOUSLY UNQUESTIONED REDUCTIONISTIC PARADIGM

This movement in the United States away from the exclusive use of Western biomedicine and health care has been building for several years, and it calls into question foundational ideas about the very nature of commonly accepted definitions of such terms as health, health care, professional care, and medicine. Holism and complementary therapies aimed at prevention and positively influencing or balancing the entire person, their physical, emotional, mental and spiritual aspects, challenges what we have come to hold as sacred in our country. That is the assumption that medicine, based on science and designed to rescue us from inevitable death with the latest technology, or the one specific therapy or drug, is the only "valid" approach to curing problems in the body caused by disease or injury. In fact, discussion about the relative benefits of a reductionistic, linear, hierarchical, approach in contrast to a holistic, nonlinear (network), integrated approach, mirrors discussion within other disciplines such as ecology, religion, psychology, sociology, and leadership management, as well as the philosophy of science. In sum, the people of the world are undergoing such a massive world change in thinking about the nature of what is real and important, that philosophers have identified this movement as a paradigm shift.

The competitive, linear, separated, and hierarchical way of solving problems (mechanistic or Newtonian world view) has resulted in a value system of win-lose, where only one person or idea can "win," or be right, and the rest have to accept that. The rich get richer and the poor are forgotten. Wars settle conflicts, might makes right, and people would rather be right than happy. The ubiquitous index finger raised to signal "we're number one" at televised sports competitions is the dream, indeed, the declaration of many.

Yet there emerges from the sidelines people who would rather be happy than right, who would rather contribute to healing and share, as much as is possible, all of the goods of the community, who see everyone as worthy of and capable of empowerment. These people are those who embrace the holistic principles of the integration, the interconnection and oneness of all people, of all matter. They assert that, until we all come to realize at the deepest levels that cooperation rather than competition results in the inner peace that most yearn for, we will be ignoring the true nature of the reality that science attempts to reveal.

A *paradigm*, first described by Thomas Kuhn in his historic text *The Structure of Scientific Revolutions*,[17] is a pattern of thinking, usually of abstract thinking. The word paradigm more simply refers to unique explanatory models that differ among disciplines. However, paradigm also can refer to a larger explanatory model, one that is culturally determined and is adopted without thought, called a *world view* by anthropologists. Most of what is contained in a world view model or paradigm is "out-of-awareness assumptions that people do not recognize as assumptions, but as 'just the way things are.'"[18,19]

The nature of reality, or of Truth, and beliefs about the right or best way we should go about verifying both, are encased within the world view. An example would be the world view that the sun rises every morning and sets every evening, never even questioned until proven inaccurate when the world was discovered to rotate around the stable sun.

In the mid 1500s, Copernicus suggested that the earth was not the center of the universe, but his ideas were largely rejected until years later. But his idea would not go away because his first suggestion, itself a first approximation at explaining observations that would not fit within the prevailing model of reality, was the beginning of the clearer understanding of what seemed so mysterious. And so it is with the mysterious that keeps tugging at us in health care and medicine. What will explain spontaneous remissions of large, diffuse cancer lesions? What will explain why some people died of bubonic plague, and some who had it, didn't? What will explain why both identical twins with the gene that predicts Alzheimer's disease don't come down with the symptoms at the same time? More adequate theories are always sought to explain the important exceptions not incorporated in the prevailing world view. And the exceptions to the current world view that is based in linear, competitive, win-lose, mechanistic, technological, fragmented, specialist principles are pulling us to reform the inadequacies of our limited explanations.

NEWTONIAN CARTESIAN THEORY VERSUS QUANTUM THEORY

The changes that we are experiencing now, however, transcend so many disciplines that many believe the world view, or cultural *gestalt*, the very way we explain the nature of reality and truth, are coming into question and being "viewed" in a dramatically different way. Many writers in such diverse areas as ecology[20] and management[21] refer to the shift from a Newtonian Cartesian or hierarchical, linear, static, mechanistic, particulate world view to a world view seated within quantum physics. That world view, the foundation of holism, stresses the value of a more nonlinear, egalitarian and integrated view of reality and is interested more in how energy, people, and things interact to better serve the whole.[22]

In quantum theory, all of matter is described not as solid, but as relatively spacious and in constant flux, reflective of the physical nature of the building blocks of matter, subatomic particles, atoms, and molecules.[12] Remember that atoms are made up of a nucleus consisting of positively charged protons and neutron particles that contain no charge. The nucleus of each atom is separated by a relatively vast area of space within which rotate a sufficient number of negatively charged electrons to balance the protons of the nucleus. (The loss of an electron renders the atom unstable, an ion in search of electrons to gain its proper balance, thus a "free-radical.")[23]

The sun and its light composed of photons of energy are the ultimate source of energy on earth, and Einstein's study of the speed of light in relation to matter first suggested quantum theory which, physicists admit, still remains unfinished as an explanatory tool.[23] Quantum theory instructs us to view reality as an integrated holistic system of the seen and unseen, the material and the nonmaterial. Rather than "seeing" a seemingly material static object, such as a table, as fixed or constant in space, we should come to "view" it as an Impressionist artist would paint it, stipled with dots and spaces that flow into each other and seem to form a solid painting. Thus, all of reality, material and nonmaterial, seen and unseen, physical and ethereal, imminent and transcendent, is composed of constantly moving particles that display, at any one time, the characteristics of both particles and waves. And all matter, seen and unseen, all of reality, is dynamic, constantly moving, composed of molecules, atoms, and subatomic particles that constantly emit or consume energy as their electrons fly about, integrate, and separate.[22]

As the foundation for the world view of holism, quantum theory emphasizes that the whole of anything we experience is always more than what we can see or describe, more than just the sum of all the parts. According to physicist David Bohm,[12] "the ultimate nature of all reality is not a collection of separate objects (as it appears to us), but rather it is an indivisible whole that is in perpetual dynamic flux."[22] Mind and matter are simply different aspects of the same flow of movement, or *holomovement*. Reality is constantly moving and is structured in a manner that each portion of the whole contains information about the entire whole. It is impossible and erroneous to separate the material from the nonmaterial and study the material only in the search for reality, as suggested by Descartes and Newton. Arbitrarily making this impossible separation of body from mind has increased the scientific understanding of disease, but has ignored the impact of the psyche on the body. The full cause of, for example, the neurophysiological elevation of the heart rate and blood pressure at the sound of an unexplainable noise in the middle of the night, or the data that confirm that not all of the people exposed die of a virulent infectious disease, has been left ignored or erroneously explained. However, in the early 1900s, before the immune system was identified and described, Claude Bernard, a physiologist studying the intricacies of the liver and the pancreas in helping the body to maintain inner balance, or homeostasis, insisted that germs or microbes were simply the "seeds" which would only cause disease if the "soil," or the internal environment, was too weak to resist.[4]

Human biological reality is both the unseen mind and the material body, and all of the cells of the body "know about" the mind, and the mind "knows about" each cell in the body. The physical body is constantly responding to the unique perceptions, interpretations, and meanings of the mind and emotions (as the rapid heart at the sound of a strange noise in the dark), and the mind and emotions are constantly responding to the state of the physical body (as one feels elated following 45 minutes of invigorating aerobic exercise).

According to anthropologists, the controversy between the Newtonian and quantum world views is made more complicated and difficult to resolve because, as we strive for understanding and a more than adequate, accurate view of reality as we approach the next millennium, singular acceptance of only one of these two powerful paradigms prevails among scientific reductionist researchers. The unparalleled value of reductionism and quantitative analytical science is so ingrained in our world view that many cannot begin to envision its equal coexistence with holism in the search for the explanation of what is real.[18] However, until this coexistence is allowed to happen, there will be an effort to discredit both holistic principles and the complementary therapies that grow out of this theoretical base, which for centuries has served as the foundation of most health care in the world.[4]

CONSTRUCTING REALITY WITHIN A CULTURE

As discussed above, anthropologists claim that the two major means people in society use to make sense of what we experience are reductionism (one right answer or cause for the effect observed), solely preferred by traditional bioscientists, and holism (the relational or integrated), favored by many alternative health care systems and their practitioners. Medical anthropologist Claire Cassidy writes of a recent conference she attended on alternative medicine, where several presenters went into great detail about the "logic of their treatment modalities and their system's use of 'classic' (ancient) texts," whereupon a man stood in the audience and said, "This is all very nice, but what has it got to do with medical progress?"[18] After heated discussion about the logic behind reliance on ancient sources, the conference ended "with a ringing pronouncement from the podium that research is not scientific if it is not replicable. We must get the same answers every time we try, or what we observe as real cannot be trusted as real."[18] This is the current paradigm conflict in action in medicine and health care.

In other words, the only acceptable proof of efficacy for the use of a treatment in traditional, established biomedicine is that which results from research that is quantitative and analytical—the double-blind, randomized, controlled, clinical trial that reduces the chance that the given result is due to something other than the effect of the experimental variable. Reductionism as a method in research refers to the experiment that is carefully designed to eliminate any and all erroneous results due to subjectivity, experimenter bias, and/or placebo or suggestion. The research is so rigorously designed so that the "real" or correct answer or outcome cannot be simply what the researcher (or practitioner) hopes for or expects. In this way, the efficacy of a chosen treatment can be more assured, and the public can be reassured that the treatment they receive has been previously shown, under controlled conditions, to be adequate and safe.

On the other hand, holistic practitioners using quantum theory as the explanatory theory for their world view recognize the inseparable interconnection and flow of all aspects of reality, and would never even attempt to ignore, devalue, or rule out the effects of the mind, feelings, or the relationship of the patient to the researcher or practitioner on the treatment outcome. In fact, the holistic view tries to maximize these forces, especially the placebo effect, or suggestion, to enhance the mind-body's natural ability to heal. In other words, a beneficial treatment outcome for the patient in the moment of care is far more important to health and healing, to rehabilitation, than using only the treatment that matches the standard of care for alleviation of symptoms based on a reductionistic world view.

The holistic practitioner in general, and also in rehabilitation, focuses on the character of the "vital force" or energy or prana or ch'i, and treats the perceived or diagnosed imbalance in that vital force that allowed symptoms to develop in the first place. He or she treats the imbalance as it manifests in that particular treatment session, often by way of applying intrinsic bioelectromagnetic energy during manual therapy techniques such as Non-contact Therapeutic Touch,[24] Myofascial Release,[25] or the Rosen Method.[26]

Double-blind, controlled research that attempts to hide or to "blind" patients, researchers, or practitioners to actual treatment conditions or to inevitable bias in the perception of what is "seen" tries to minimize the reality that this is an impossible thing to do. Most people accept Heisenberg's principle that the observer, "once enculturated in a world view, can never be wholly objective in one's observations: the observer is a part of whatever he or she observes."[18] Reductionist researchers will concede the fact that what is observed is changed by the act of observing, but they proceed, with the greatest attempt to minimize this effect, as if the observer can remain "objective." It is not just near-sighted rigidity that, for the last 150 years or more, has resulted in the conviction that this method, this way of determining reality, is the only valid way to do so. For history reveals that we have, so many times, been led harmfully astray by our five senses and our individual perceptions in our search for the real cause of the observed effect. Ironically, most scientists remain so committed to this one right way that they often display a fervor, and often level sharp criticism at any treatment approach that falls short of validity from the rigor of a well-designed reductionistic study. In fact, Cassidy states, "The determination with which Westerners cling to their cultural preference concerning the power of science approaches a religious fervor."[19]

ADOPTING A WORLD VIEW PARADIGM

How do people come to accept and hold onto, indeed, hold sacred the "correct" way to view what is supposedly "real?" Traditionally, thinking about the foundations of knowledge is the work of philosophers. Many professional researchers and most medical researchers, however, spend comparatively little time studying the philosophy of science. Few people actually could describe much about what assumptions mold their thoughts on research or science. Thus, most people in the Western world, without much critical thought, elevate their idea of what constitutes science: the quantitative scientific method, as either the only valid scientific research method, or, without question, the highest and supreme way to search for the nature of reality.[19] Ironically, the founder of reductionism, René Descartes, attempted to raise the level of inquiry of his day out of the mystical and religious and into observable cause and effect by mandating that, only that which can be seen, the physical or material, could be studied. Science has focused on developing modern technology to greatly expand previously unseen matter into that which can be seen by sophisticated microscopes, telescopes, and electronic imaging so that it will fall into the category of the material, but until recently comparatively less attempt has been made to "see" other seemingly nonmaterial essences, for example, the mind or the energy fields of the body.[27]

The fact that Cartesian hierarchy commands that which cannot be verified by science is not trusted to be real, or contributing to knowledge of the truth, may help to explain the elitist hierarchy that can be observed in medicine that, at times, is observed not only between practitioners of traditional medicine versus alternative medicine, but even within the specialties of traditional medicine. Cardiologists and neurologists often are perceived to command more power than psychiatrists, physicians of the mind. Finally, most harmful to the coexistence of the two paradigms is the belief that those not seeking a singular reality are considered not scientific and therefore are not trustworthy.

Anthropologists maintain that, "everyone has beliefs, and all realities are constructed; the facts of science are as culturally contextualized as those of law, theology, or social manners."[18] Medicine may emphasize science as its way of justifying practice, but as scientific as biomedicine claims to be, the common view is that medicine is an "art based on a science" that is, according to anthropologist Cassidy, created and maintained more by paradigmatic preferences than by the rules of science.[18] Perhaps subconsciously the fact that medicine is based on simply a preferred way of "coming to know what is true" is responsible both for an insecure insistence that it is the only way, as well as for the concern that another way will be dangerous and cannot be trusted not to cause great harm and a waste of precious time. Or, more critically, is it the result of countless examples where people have trusted nonscientific, fraudulent treatments that have resulted in loss of life, and loss of precious time in which the results of science could have reversed the fateful outcome? Likely both may be true. Obviously, what is needed then is a way of verifying the safety and legitimacy of treatment methods that can assure the public that they will not be victims of harm, and that this treatment satisfies their current need for care in a cost-effective and previously tested way.

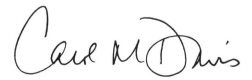

REFERENCES

1. Eisenberg DM, Kessler RC, et al. Unconventional medicine in the United States. *N Engl J Med.* 1993;328:245-252.

2. American Nurses Association. National survey reveals concerns about cost-cutting trends in patient care. *Healthcare Review.* 1996;5:5.

3. Pellegrino ED. What is a profession? *J Allied Health.* 1983;12(3):168-176.

4. Institute of Noetic Sciences, Poole W. *Heart of Healing.* Atlanta, Ga: Turner Publications, Inc; 1993.

5. Bergner P, Kail K. The U.S. health care cost crisis: a crisis of chronic disease. *American Association of Naturopathic Physicians.* 1992;September.

6. Koop CE. Foreword—the art and science of medicine. In: Micozzi MS, ed. *Fundamentals of Complementary and Alternative Medicine.* New York, NY: Churchill Livingstone; 1996.

7. *Journal of Consciousness Studies/Controversies in Science and the Humanities.* Thorverton, United Kingdom: Imprint Academic; 1994.

8. *Journal of Alternative and Complementary Medicine/Research on Paradigm, Practice and Policy.* New York, NY: Mary Ann Liebert, Inc.

9. *Alternative Therapies in Health and Medicine.* Aliso Viejo, Calif.

10. *Advances.* New York, NY: Institute for the Advancement of Health; 1996.

11. *Noetic Sciences Review.* Sausalito, Calif: Institute of Noetic Sciences.

12. Bohm D. *Wholeness and the Implicate Order.* Routledge and Kegan Paul; 1980.

13. Micozzi MS. Preference. In: Micozzi MS, ed. *Fundamentals of Complementary and Alternative Medicine.* New York, NY: Churchill Livingstone; 1996.

14. Berger D. Each patient is a miniature research project. *PT Magazine.* 1994;2(9):75.

15. Brown-Besley MW, Pyvus B. Alternative healthcare: effective treatment or quackery? *Healthcare Review, Northern New England.* 1996;9(5):1.

16. Daly D. Alternative medicine courses taught in U.S. medical schools. *J Alt Compl Med.* 1995;1(1):111.

17. Kuhn TS. *The Structure of Scientific Revolutions.* 2nd ed. Chicago, Ill: University of Chicago Press; 1970.

18. Cassidy CM. Social science theory and methods in the study of alternative and complementary medicine. *J Alt Compl Med.* 1995;1(1):19-40.

19. Cassidy CM. Cultural context of complimentary and alternative medicine. In: Micozzi MS, ed. *Fundamentals of Complementary and Alternative Medicine.* New York, NY: Churchill Livingstone; 1996.

20. Capra F. *The Turning Point/Science Society and the Rising Culture.* New York, NY: Simon and Schuster; 1982.

21. Wheatley MJ. *Leadership and the New Science.* San Francisco, Calif: Berrett-Koehler Publishers, Inc.; 1992.

22. Keepin W, Bohm D. A life of dialogue between science and spirit. *Noetic Sciences Review.* 1994;30:10-16.

23. Sharme H. *Freedom from Disease*. Toronto, Canada: Veda Publishing; 1993.

24. Kreiger D. *The Therapeutic Touch: How to Use Your Hands to Help and Heal*. Englewood Cliffs, NJ: Prentice-Hall; 1979.

25. Barnes J. *Myofascial Release*. Paoli, Pa: Pain and Stress Control Center; 1991.

26. Mayland E. *Rosen Method: An Approach to Wholeness and Well-Being Through the Body*. 1991.

27. Harman W. The scientific exploration of consciousness: towards an adequate epistemology. *J Consciousness Studies*. 1994;1(1):140-148.

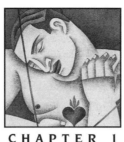

CHAPTER 1

PSYCHONEURO-IMMUNOLOGY
THE BRIDGE TO THE COEXISTENCE
OF TWO PARADIGMS

Carol M. Davis, EdD, PT

INTRODUCTION

In 1971, Herbert Benson and colleagues published results of research that seemed to point toward a mind-body link, and coined the term "relaxation response."[1,2] At the same time, Robert Ader and Nicholas Cohen were researching the phenomenon of anticipatory nausea resulting from the effects of chemotherapy on patients.[3] Patients began to become sick just thinking about the drugs, long before they took them. They were aware of Pavlov's dogs salivating to the sound of the bell (research published in 1928),[4] and that was really all that they were looking for—a laboratory model to confirm that similar conditioning was what was happening also to their patients. They gave rats cyclophosphamide along with saccharine-sweetened water. Then, when they took away the chemotherapy and gave the sweetened water alone, they looked to see if the rats vomited. When they did, they indeed had their laboratory model of "learning" by conditioning that seemed to be occurring in Ader's patients.

Ader realized, however, that the chemotherapy not only caused nausea in patients, it also depressed their immune systems, lowering patients' resistance to infectious disease. What he did not anticipate is that, when the rats were given the sweetened water alone, not only did they develop nausea, the rats also "learned" by conditioning to depress their immune systems. This biochemical result seemed to provide powerful evidence, using reductionistic research methods, that the mind and the body are not able to be separated.[5] Somehow the mind (which is thought still to reside in the nervous system), "told" the immune system to become suppressed in the absence of the chemotherapeutic immune suppressive agent.

Interestingly, Ader and Cohen make the point in the second edition of their landmark text,[3] that the effects on conditioning were observed and reported as early as 1896 by Mackenzie,[6] who provoked an allergic response in a patient with asthma by showing the patient an artificial rose. Later, Osler repeated this observation. But science had no theory that would substantiate such a response, for the mind "had no influence on the body." Anyone can see how valuable a contribution they made by publishing their results, no matter what the prevailing theory of science would accept or reject.

Subsequent research over the last 20 years has demonstrated, again with rigorous science, that there is a continuous dialogue between the mind and the nervous and immune systems which suggests that the emotions can affect the immune system in both positive and negative ways. With his results, Ader coined a term to describe a new basic science of mind/body medicine, health care, and research: *psychoneuroimmunology* (PNI),[3] psycho (from the mind or psyche), neuro (via the brain or neurons), immunology (to the immune system).

Two pathways of communication have been identified between the mind and the body: the autonomic nervous system (sympathetic and parasympathetic) and the non-adrenergic non-cholinergic nerves (NANC). Felten[7] maintains that these pathways innervate bone marrow, thymus, spleen, and mucosal surfaces where immune cells develop, mature and encounter foreign substances. "Each [of the two nerve systems] communicates with the immune cells directly through the release of chemical messages which range from adrenaline, noradrenaline, and acetylcholine to small proteins called neuropeptides...and cause an inflammatory or anti-inflammatory effect on the immune system."[7]

This foundational challenge to Cartesian separatist thought opened the way for reductionistic methods to be used to verify holistic principles, and the beginning of an important bridge was formed which may span the seemingly uncrossable void to link reductionism and holism into coexistence.

APPLICATION OF PNI TO CLINICAL MEDICINE

With regard to the initial studies that tested the application of PNI to patient care, in 1991, the *New England Journal of Medicine* reported that rates of both respiratory infection and clinical colds increase in a dose-response manner with the increase in degree of psychological stress.[8] In 1992, David Spiegel, a psychiatrist at Stanford Medical School, published his research conducted in 1989 that suggested that breast cancer patients randomly placed in weekly support groups lived markedly longer than control patients assigned only to regular care.[9] These studies have been followed by countless more,[3] and now research departments in the nation's major medical centers that are investigating hypotheses based on the science of PNI compete successfully for NIH grants. Among the most important to rehabilitation is the research which investigates the effects of massage[10] and exercise[11] on the immune systems of those with chronic and fatal diseases such as HIV and AIDS.

At the encouragement of Senator Thomas Harkin, a congressional mandate created the Office of Alternative Medicine in 1992 to investigate and approve proposals for research on alternative methods of healing. Although roadblocks and criticisms from the prevailing science bias against alternative approaches made the initial 2 years of this office quite difficult,[12] the Office seems to be establishing itself at last. Scientists at NIH did not want to add possible "legitimacy by association" to researchers who had no formal education in reductionistic methods. They felt that practitioners of holistic approaches were using their association with NIH to promote illegitimate research, but in the end they realized that they had no choice but to accept the congressional mandate.[12]

In spite of the fact that proposals seldom could be reviewed for the usual NIH standards of the quality of the principle investigator's "track record," nor for "scientific merit," in 1996 the Office awarded selected research centers a total of $9,744,535 in grant funds. In a rather critical article found in the June 18, 1996 *New York Times*,[12] the following institutions were listed as recipients:

1. The University of Virginia School of Nursing (use of magnets to relieve pain)
2. Kessler Institute for Rehabilitation (use of Chinese herbs with neurological problems including stroke)
3. Columbia University (Chinese medicine and women's health)
4. University of Texas Health Science Center at Houston (alternative cancer therapies)
5. Beth Israel Hospital in Boston (conventional therapy for low back pain versus acupuncture and massage)

6. Minneapolis Medical Research Foundation (alternative therapies for addiction)
7. Bastyr University in Seattle (survey of 1500-2000 people with AIDS to determine alternative therapy use and results)
8. University of Maryland School of Medicine (alternative medicine effects on bone and muscle pain)
9. University of California—Davis (survey alternative practitioners, including Native Americans, on use of therapies to treat patients with asthma)
10. Stanford University (alternative therapies such as massage and the use of support groups to enhance the quality of life of older people)[12]

Interactions between the mind or psyche and the neural and immune systems have been shown to have relevance in a broad range of diseases, such as cancer and arthritis, viral infections such as HIV, and other autoimmune diseases, but knowledge of just how these systems interact is still not conclusive.

Black's recent study, reported in December 1995 in *Scientific American*,[13] reveals how the brain and the immune system

> interact via hormones, neurotransmitters, and cytokines traveling through blood and nerves. This bidirectional chemical communication is regulated by corticotropin releasing factor, which is stimulated by thoughts and emotions or immune activation to affect the hypothalamic-pituitary-adrenal axis. Stress, in particular, compromises immunity. Stressful life events have been linked with susceptibility to infection, reactivation of herpesvirus, and with cancer and HIV progression. Effects on depression, as well as other clinical aspects, are also under study.[13]

The positive effects of exercise, massage and therapeutic touch, and manual therapies on the immune system securely places both alternative therapies and PNI research in rehabilitation.[10,11] These therapies are listed among the "alternative therapies" in the *Chantilly Report of the National Institutes of Health*[14] and are placed in categories as follows:

1. Mind-body interventions—psychotherapy, support groups, meditation, imagery, hypnosis, biofeedback, dance and music therapies, art therapy, prayer, and mental healing.
2. Bioelectromagnetics application to medicine—thermal applications of nonionizing radiation: radio frequency (RF) hyperthermia, laser and RF surgery, and RF diathermy. Nonthermal applications of nonionizing radiation for bone repair, nerve stimulation, wound healing, etc.
3. Alternative systems of medical practice—70-90% of all health care worldwide. Popular health care, community-based health care, professionalized health care, traditional oriental medicine (including acupuncture, Ayurveda), homeopathy,

anthroposophically extended medicine (elements of naturopathy plus homeopathy), naturopathic medicine.

4. Manual healing methods—touch and manipulation, osteopathy, chiropractic, massage therapy, biofield therapeutics (healing touch, therapeutic touch and SHEN therapy).

5. Pharmacological and biological treatments—drugs and vaccines not yet accepted in mainstream medicine (antineoplastons, cartilage products, EDTA, immunoaugmentive therapy, 714-X, Coley's toxins, MTH-68, neural therapy, apitherapy, iscador, biologically guided chemotherapy).

6. Herbal medicine—folk remedies that rely on botanical knowledge of the effects of herbs on the body.

7. Diet and nutrition in the prevention and treatment of chronic disease—perhaps the best-known example is Dean Ornish's program for heart disease that emphasizes nutrition, yoga, meditation, and guided imagery or visualization, as well as exercise.

THE INTEGRATION OF REDUCTIONISM WITH HOLISM

It appears from the most recent literature that holistic practices and reductionistic medicine and health care finally are coming together, and many holistic practices do lend themselves to verification with reductionistic methods, but some clearly do not. Meanwhile, the public and health care professionals are continuing to explore the benefits of complementary and alternative therapies. Most important, because of the reductionistic results revealed by PNI, biomedical research is finding it more difficult to ignore the mind-body connection.

While research is being conducted, and these two explanatory paradigms struggle to coexist, nurses and physical and occupational therapists are utilizing various complementary therapies in their practices and are experiencing what they and their patients describe as success, even when traditional approaches such as exercise and mobilization have not helped. This text was created to help reveal the variety of efforts in this area. The chapters in this text may make it more difficult for those who would dismiss complementary therapies out-of-hand as nonscientific and not appropriate for professionals to use because their results cannot be duplicated in controlled studies.

The accepted belief among holistic practitioners with regard to interrater reliability is that holistic methods have the intention to affect not just one system, but all body systems by influencing the patient's vital life force in a positive way through the manipulation of the body's energy system. In spite of numerous studies, the very existence of body energy is still questioned by most reductionists.[15] However, holistic practitioners believe that once the bioelectromagnetic field is altered by one therapist, another therapist with his or her own energy field will not be able to locate the same energy field response from the patient, as it has already been affected by the first researcher.[16]

But that does not mean we should ignore the need to understand and test alternative approaches to help make them complementary in rehabilitation. The most common complaints of those who chose "nonconventional" therapies in Eisenberg's 1990 study[17] were chronic conditions often treated in outpatient physical therapy departments, such as musculoskeletal pain, headache, arthritis, and back pain, as well as insomnia, depression, and anxiety, which often accompany chronic musculoskeletal conditions.

Just as Dr. Mackenzie reported the inexplicable finding of his patient's allergic response to an artificial rose in 1895,[6] practitioners must continually document and publish systematic observations of methods, clinical decision making, the patient's descriptions of the effects of treatment, and subsequent outcomes when alternative and complementary therapies are used.

PROFESSIONALS BEST SUITED TO TRANSFORM ALTERNATIVE THERAPIES INTO COMPLEMENTARY THERAPIES

Clearly, doctorally and post-doctorally prepared scientists, rehabilitation professionals, psychologists, physicians, and exercise physiologists are most adequately prepared to conduct the scientific studies that will go a long way to allow us to offer the greatest number of safe and tested alternatives to the greatest number of patients at the most reasonable cost. Then we will be working toward a truly sustainable health care system.[1] However, many post-baccalaureate prepared health professional clinicians and teachers also have the appropriate educational background suited to conduct systematic studies and tests, to prepare in-depth case studies, and contribute to a central data bank designed to report the outcomes and adequacy of those therapies not easily explored by controlled reductionist research.

Likewise, most professional level health practitioners are well educated in the theoretical foundations and the art of treatment, and can rather easily expand their knowledge and art to utilize alternative therapies and make them complementary for their work. For example, psychologists, art and music therapists, and ministers, priests, and rabbis are well positioned to apply selected appropriate mind-body interventions listed above in the *NIH Chantilly Report*.[14] Physical and occupational therapists, as well as nurses and massage therapists, are, or should be, well educated to perform alternative massage methods. As this text illustrates, physical therapists can rather easily extend their traditional education in touch and exercise to incorporate the approaches of therapeutic touch and other touch therapies such as Jin Shin Do, Rolfing, Qi Gong, and the Rosen Method. Physical therapists often are well suited to have interest and desire to undertake the years of training required to develop the art and skill needed to be certified as Feldenkrais and Alexander practitioners. Indeed, many have done this, as well as have taken necessary training to apply the Trager Approach, T'ai Chi, and so on.

Some physical therapists have also extended their professional education to be qualified to conduct research on alternative therapies.[18] For example, at Emory University, Steven Wolf, PhD, PT, FAPTA, was awarded a National Institute on Aging FICSIT (Frailty and Injuries: Cooperative Studies of Intervention Techniques) grant to study the effects of T'ai Chi on balance in older people.[18] As the authors of this text reveal, even more physical and occupational therapists have studied specific alternative approaches in order to make them complementary to their practice. Mind-body approaches such as yoga, T'ai Chi, and those aspects of Traditional Chinese Medicine, acupuncture, acupressure, polarity, reflexology, and Touch for Health, which are proposed to act to "balance" the vital energy and assist in pain control and in the prevention of disease, are all being practiced by physical therapists.

Exercise, along with diet, nutrition, and herbal medicine, and improved medications that mimic the body's own immune system defenses, have become the foundation of the treatment plans that turn what once were rapidly fatal diseases, such as AIDS, into chronic diseases that one can live many years with.[11] Physical therapists seem best prepared to prescribe exercise for ill persons whose disease has affected many systems. In contrast, exercise physiologists and sports medicine personnel have entered the exercise area with an emphasis on exercise prescription for prevention and wellness.

THERAPEUTIC PRESENCE—HOLISTIC PRINCIPLES IN ACTION

Embracing a new theory of care that is diametrically opposed to the system that we are trying to reform carries many risks. For example, believing that all illness is metaphor and that we are all 100% in control of our health is as absurd as believing we are passive victims of germs and our genetic heritage and there's nothing we can do except follow the physician's orders.[19] Even before being validated, even against the advice of some medical scientists, alternative therapies are being integrated with conventional therapies routinely as complementary to facilitate healing, and the valuable aspects of holism cited above are being applied universally in health care. If people have consistently reported, over a long period of time, that a treatment works to help relieve symptoms, thus they feel better and their symptoms are indeed relieved, then this outcome measure of personal anecdote should be considered one type of evidence of efficacy, whether or not the treatment fits the qualifications of accepted research design.[20]

Just as this text illustrates, based on the teachings of such ancient practices as Traditional Chinese Medicine and Aryuveda, and based on the recordings kept by more recent systems of thought such as homeopathy and naturopathy, the alternative approaches based on holism are being applied with increasing frequency as complementary to conventional practice.

HOLISTIC APPLICATION OF TRADITIONAL AND COMPLEMENTARY TREATMENTS

Psychoneuroimmunology has helped to show that healing is facilitated not only by the alternative approach itself, but also by way of the principles of therapeutic presence, or the holistic nature of *how health professionals are with their patients*. The characteristics of one who uses *oneself* as a therapeutic agent with the patient reflect the philosophy of holism.[21] Cancer surgeon and holistic physician Bernie Siegel points out continually how important the doctor-patient relationship is to the recovery from cancer.[22]

John Carmody, a marathon athlete recovering from leg surgery for his incurable multiple myeloma, writes in the journal *Second Opinion*[23] that the first of his two postoperative physical therapists responded to his fatigue from surgery and two crushed lumbar vertebrae with great insensitivity, "You just have to push through the pain...it's mainly a question of your will to get better." He goes into rather lengthy detail documenting her callousness and indifference to him, not only to his weakness, but to his fear of never being able to walk again. For example, her response to his request for help in positioning his hands and feet to get up off the bed to use his walker was, "It doesn't matter. Just get on with it. Push off the bed and start walking." Finally, he responded to her continual insinuations that he was a rather clumsy coward with an outburst, an attack on her to "back off," accusing her of patronizing him and showing a severe lack of sympathy for his unique situation as a patient. He was an athlete with pain from his treatment for incurable cancer, but more than that, he was a productive writer, and a person able and willing to benefit from needed instruction. Yet she never seemed to relate to those unique characteristics in him. She treated him as if he were a "thing," a noncompliant complainer.

When this therapist was replaced by a second clinician, his perceptions of the first therapist's insensitivity and nastiness were confirmed. His second physical therapist acknowledged his pain, and instructed him to breathe through it as a way to assist relaxation and pain control. She took the time to show him where he should place his hands to take his weight as he rose from the bed to begin walking with the walker. She spoke to him gently and encouragingly, and conveyed optimism, telling him she knew he could do this, it would just take time. This gentle and personal approach got him over his hopeless hump, and soon he progressed, first to using crutches and, eventually, to a welcome discharge home.

At home, as he exercised he heard the voice of the second therapist encouraging him and, as he felt stronger, he added swimming and other challenges for increasing his strength and function. She had facilitated hope, and he was motivated to recover because she had spoken to him, connected with him in his uniqueness, and had believed in him and encouraged him by her very presence.[23] The positive effects of compassion on the patient's healing response illustrate PNI, no matter whether the treatment employed is traditional or complementary.

What are the roots of compassion? What allows some of us on some days to be able to extend ourselves to our fellow humans who happen to be our patients, but not on others? What forces interfere with the capacity to respond with sympathy or empathy to patients? And why is it important to be able to be therapeutically present? Isn't just satisfying our contract to "teach and fix" enough?[24]

Therapeutic presence is the capacity to, at the least, sympathize with patients, or enter into "fellow feeling," and interact from the space of genuinely shared emotion.[25] This demands that professionals feel with their patients and respond to them in a way that acknowledges the "feeling with," the interconnection.[26] Biomedical ethicists suggest that our moral obligation as health care professionals mandates that patients, as people, should never feel dehumanized or treated as "things" separate from the human race.[27] According to our Codes of Ethics and to the writings of medical ethicists, we are morally obliged to act in certain ways that reflect what it means to be professional, to respond to fellow human beings who place trust in us because of their vulnerability in times of need.[27,28]

In other words, part of medical and health care education should be devoted to developing self-awareness of the behaviors that we bring with us into our professional education that interfere with communicating interest in and rapport with our patients. These behaviors are based on the appropriate values and attitudes of the mature healing professional so that competent practitioners can know how to display morally responsible caring to patients, even on days when their lives are out of balance and stressful. Patients deserve to be responded to, not only with proficient knowledge, but with well-advised care and compassion, suited to the uniqueness of each person and his or her problem.[21,27,28]

The Crossing Over in Empathy—Holistic Integration

Therapeutic presence describes a connection with patients that is based on the principles of holism, of interconnectedness, that makes an uncomfortable wall, a separateness, impossible. In contrast to sympathy, empathy is a unique interaction that actually involves the experience of "crossing over" into a "shared moment of meaning" that is deeply felt, and makes it impossible not to experience the impact of one's actions on the patient, both negative and positive.[24,29] And anyone, health professional or patient, who has experienced the emotional "at-oneness" felt with the crossing-over moment in empathy, where one is so identified with the other that, for a brief millisecond, you forget that the other is separate from you, has experienced the interconnectedness of holism.[24] Sympathy is not, as many would believe, harmful for patients.[25,26] Indeed, it is encouraging and helpful for patients to feel as if a health care professional has walked with them on their journey for a while, and that the feelings shared were more than simply acknowledged, they were "fellow feelings" resulting from a strong bond or connection. Pity *is* harmful in that pity is sympathy with a feeling of being worthier than the one pitied, and so it distances the patient with a "poor you" attitude that again depersonalizes the patient.[24,26]

Therapeutic presence, or using one's self to make a warm and encouraging connection with the patient, is based on the important acknowledgment that the mind and feelings of the patient are inseparably linked with the patient's physical body, and that the patient's feelings and emotions and beliefs are just as critical in patient recovery as exercise, medications, and rest.[21]

Carmody comments from the patient's perspective:

> [R]easonable patients—the majority—know full well that medicine is fallible, uncertain, and very human. What healers risk in meeting their patients as their equals in humanity is little compared to what they stand to gain. For both the efficacy of their treatments and their growth as human beings, health care professionals will be wise to take down as many barriers as they can, give away as many distancing privileges as possible. [Health professionals] who have been sustaining me are alike in their ability to create a sense of "we." We patients and healers are sharing a joint venture, even a joint (somewhat macabre) adventure. This sharing can make us free. I feel free to ask about any problem and express any emotion, positive or negative. They, I hope, feel free to speak truthfully, to be playful or somber as the moment dictates. In a word, we have all become friends, and also joint apprentices to a basal truth: All of us are simply people. Our lives are short. None of us has ever seen God, let alone been mistaken for God.[23]

This interconnectedness stands in sharp contrast to the rigid boundaries of allopathic medicine where health care workers are taught to work "on" patients. I am not suggesting that the important boundaries that must exist between patient and therapist to insure therapeutic objectivity be dissolved. Many have written on the dangers of the miscommunications that can be harmful to therapist/patient effectiveness when helper/helpee boundaries are ignored.[24] Patients should never feel obligated to help their practitioners, nor, as Carmody felt, should they ever feel as if their helpers are concerned only with the physical, with their leg, blood count, or urine output. Patients have the right to believe that their health care practitioner is concerned about them as unique human beings with special rights, patients' rights, always acknowledging the inextricable interaction of mind and body. The meaning that a patient attributes to his or her experience of illness or injury has very much to do with his or her past history and very personal hopes for the future. To ignore this in patient care is to ignore the uniqueness of the person, and risk the necessary cooperation of the patient for the goals which are set for care. To ignore this is to fail to maximize the positive effects of the mind on the body.

Patients need professionals to be clearly worthy of their trust, both in the knowledge and skill they bring to their problem, and trustworthy in the relationship that is formed.[28] What Carmody asks for, and what holism suggests, is that the professional recognize the importance of patient autonomy. Autonomy is the moral responsibility that professionals do all possible so that the patient can remain in charge of his or her own problem. With this in mind, the most relevant perspective, for both patient and professional, is to acknowledge that they both need each other, not only to be able to fulfill their unique missions, but also in order to grow, develop, and change. In this way, patients take on a more equal status in the interaction, practitioners consult with them at every choice point, and always follow the moral tenets of informed consent. This important moral attitude serves to lift self-esteem and help patients to feel autonomous and adult in a culture that can be very unfamiliar and frightening. This preservation of one's self esteem can be an important mind/body advantage in the healing process of the patient, and in preserving the quality of the moments that practitioners spend with their patients.

APPLYING HOLISTIC PRINCIPLES IN HEALTH CARE

Whether employing traditional or complementary therapies, *The Heart of Healing*[1] suggests that there are several ways in which medicine and health care can change to reflect therapeutic presence, the compassionate use of one's self as a partner to the patient in the process of examination and treatment, which actualizes the finest ideals of holistic practice. What is suggested is that health care should reflect the following changes:

1. <u>A commitment to treat people, not diseases</u>. Instead of asking, "What is wrong with this person, and how can it be fixed?" we will ask, "Who is this [unique] person, and how can he or she be helped to achieve maximum health?" Depending on the nature of the problem, once evaluated carefully, patients might be better served by a psychotherapist, a physical therapist, a bodyworker, or biofeedback for chronic headache.

2. <u>A reassessment of the appropriate use of technology</u>. Twenty-eight percent of the $70 billion spent by Medicare in 1985 went to people during their last year of life, and 30% of that $70 billion was spent during the last month of life alone.

3. <u>A new openness to complementary therapies</u>. The survey published by Eisenberg and associates1[17] seemed to show that patients who were educated chose carefully the benefits and risks of trying "nonconventional" therapies. Unfortunately, an editorial in the same issue of the January, 1993 *New England Journal of Medicine*, deprecated many of the alternative treatments Americans had chosen. "Many of the relaxation techniques, massage therapies, special diets, and self-help groups could be considered to be lifestyle choices more than therapeutic interventions," the editorial stated. Other therapies were singled out as being "patently unscientific," including chiropractic, herbal medicine, homeopathy, and acupuncture—although the editorial did grant that such therapies are sometimes recommended by, or even delivered by, physicians.[1] At the very least, since the mid 1980s research in PNI has strongly concluded that lifestyle choices *are* therapeutic interventions.

4. <u>A new view of prevention</u>. Even though more Americans are exercising than ever, and more Americans have quit smoking than ever, prevention still lags behind in insurance reimbursement, and in money for health care.

   Money for infant, child, and maternal health programs for the poor dropped steadily in the 1980s. This drop in funding has led to higher rates of prematurity and related developmental disorders, such as cerebral palsy and mental retardation. The savings gained in cutting money for prenatal programs is dwarfed by the costs of caring for the premature babies.[1]

The new health care system should be directed not only toward preventing disease and integrating alternative approaches that help the body to heal itself, it should also be concerned about the whole, the world community, and preventing social conditions that foster disease and poor health.

INTEGRATIVE MEDICINE

No system of medicine or health care has all of the answers. Conventional or Western medicine and health care do some things very well. "But conventional medicine manages crises so well that it tends to treat every condition as if it *were* a crisis."[30] Andrew Weil, a graduate of Harvard Medical School, has developed a new medical school residency curriculum at the University of Arizona that teaches what he terms *Integrative Medicine*. He maintains that if we would apply allopathic medicine only to crisis cases, then money would be saved and harm would not be done to the body's own ability to heal in the attempt to eliminate symptoms of a disease. He suggests that:

> Allopathic medicine and health care are appropriate for approximately 10-20% of all health problems, and that for the other 80-90%, where there is no emergency and where there is no need for strong measures, there is time to experiment with other methods, alternative therapies which are cheaper, safer, and ultimately more effective because they work with the body's healing mechanisms rather than working against them.[30]

Weil's new 2-year fellowship for family and internal medicine physicians has the main goal to, "emphasize the body's own healing system and healing potential so that doctors and patients will work from the premise that people can get better, that the body can heal itself, and that we should explore all available methods and ideas out there that can facilitate the process."[30] The fellowship begins with a course in the philosophy of science, "to train doctors to know what science is, what are its appropriate uses, and how to interpret scientific research." The next didactic area of study is the history of medicine, including Traditional Chinese Medicine and Ayruvedic medicine, placing a great emphasis on mind/body interactions. Fellows will also be instructed in the spirituality of medicine, emphasizing experiences of death and dying, and the birthing process. Finally, they will be required to master the universally useful approaches of interactive guided imagery, successful for stress-related illness, and the techniques of two of the following three alternative health care systems: osteopathic manipulation, medical acupuncture, and homeopathy.

Eventually nurses and other practitioners will be invited into the program, and a long-term goal is to develop an Integrative Medical Clinic, devoted to patient care and research on patient outcomes. Patients will be matched for age and condition, one will be followed by the conventional medical clinic, the other by the Integrative Medical Clinic. In this way, Weil hopes to collect the data that will start to turn around the resistance for funding of alternative therapies and therapy for prevention from insurance agencies and other funding sources. Fellows were due to be accepted in June 1996 at the University of Arizona, Tucson.[30]

Because health care and medicine occupy a central place in our culture, Weil hopes that the changes in the care of people will spill over into other social systems and professions, and that the principles of holism will begin to be viewed as preferable to the current linear and fragmented way that we interact with one another in society and in the world.

CONCLUSION

Healing and medical care once were synonymous in medicine, even in the United States, but are no longer.[1] The focus of medicine and health care in the 20th century has been on correct diagnosis of symptoms and on curing symptoms with the one best "magic bullet" available. High technology and reductionistic science have served us well in crisis medicine and in the cure of infectious disease. As we come to the final years of the 20th century, and to the end of the first millennium of the common era, we may remember that one of the definitions of *millennium* is "a thousand years of peace and prosperity."[31] Current information, indeed, much more now than the wake-up call of the 1991 data from Eisenberg's study,[17] have forecasted that consumers will find a way to be served by a health care system that returns the emphasis of care to the whole body's ability to heal itself, even as they receive the benefits of allopathic medicine.[12] Weil comments that this is one of the true benefits of capitalism. Neither consumers nor providers in business are bound by an ideology. Where the market goes, business goes, and consumers are helping to drive a rapidly changing health care system "market."[30]

What seems necessary is a form of medicine and health care that combines the best of allopathic medical care and holistic treatment. This text is offered as support for part of the beginning of this paradigmatic shift. The shift is indeed occurring, with or without cooperation, and it would be good for health care practitioners, researchers, and teachers to be aware of how this shift is affecting their practice, and what research and credentialling methods are needed to help insure the safety of patients.

When people are ready to acknowledge that it is far more important to link who we are in health care and what we do with healing and service, with doing the good for fellow members of our community, rather than with just being part of a business whose job is to correctly diagnose a disease based on symptoms and then treat that disease alone, we will begin moving into our rightful place in society as health professionals.[1]

When medical scientists agree to be flexible about what constitutes acceptable rigor or merit in research, and minimize their suspicion of alternative approaches because these approaches appear to allow the body to heal itself by influencing all systems for the good (thus these approaches fail to fit the criteria of rigorous science),[32] then we will see an even greater advancement of a health care system that more adequately meets the needs of citizens at less cost.

What is being asked for, indeed, demanded by many, is health care based on the principles of holism that emphasize healing over curing, and that is safe, supported by systematic research whenever possible, and that is less costly and toxic. This new health care will bring to the world the safest, most cost-effective, and most flexible system possible both for prevention and healing. And then what it means to help someone, really help a person, will become clear to many of us for the first time.

REFERENCES

1. Institute of Noetic Sciences, Poole W. *The Heart of Healing.* Atlanta, Ga: Turner Publications, Inc; 1993.
2. Wallace RK, Benson H, Wilson AF. A wakeful hypometabolic physiologic state. *American Journal of Physiology.* 1971;221(3):795-799.
3. Ader R, Cohen N. The influence of conditioning on immune responses. In: Ader R, Felten DL, Cohen N, eds. *Psychoneuroimmunology.* 2nd ed. San Diego, Calif: Academic Press; 1991:611-646.
4. Pavlov IP. *Lectures on Conditioned Reflexes.* New York, NY: Liveright; 1928.
5. Ader R, Cohen N, Felten D. Psychoneuroimmunology: interactions between the nervous system and the immune system. *Lancet.* 1995;345:99-103.
6. Mackenzie JN. The production of so-called "nose cold" by means of an artificial rose. *American Journal of Medical Science.* 1895;91:45-57.
7. Felten SY, Felten DL, Olschowka JA. Noradrenergic and peptide innervation of lymphoid organs. *Chem Immunol.* 1992;52:25-48.
8. Cohen S, Tyrrell DAJ, Smith AP. Psychological stress and susceptibility to the common cold. *N Engl J Med.* 1991;325:606-611.
9. Speigel D. *Science News.* 1992;317(19):141.
10. Galantino ML, McCormack GL. Pain management. In: Galantino ML. *Clinical Assessment and Treatment of HIV/Rehabilitation of a Chronic Illness.* Thorofare, NJ: SLACK Incorporated; 1992:104-114.
11. LaPerriere A, Antoni M, Fletcher MA, Schneiderman N. Exercise and health maintenance in HIV. In: Galantino ML. *Clinical Assessment and Treatment of HIV/ Rehabilitation of a Chronic Illness.* Thorofare, NJ: SLACK Incorporated; 1992:65-76.
12. Kolata G. In quests outside mainstream, medical projects rewrite the rules. *New York Times National.* 1996;CXLV(50, 462):A1,14.
13. Black PH. Psychoneuroimmunology: brain and immunity. *Scientific American.* 1995:16-25.
14. Alternative Medicine: Expanding Medical Horizons. The Chantilly/Virginia workshop report on alternative medical systems and practices in the United States to the National Institutes of

Health. September 14-16, 1992.

15. Rubik B. Energy medicine and the unifying concept of information. *Alternative Therapies in Health and Medicine.* 1995;1:34-36.

16. Hanten WP, et al. Craniosacral rhythm: examination of interexaminer and intraexaminer reliability of palpation and relationships between the rhythm and cardiac and respiratory rates of the subject and examiner. *Phys Ther.* 1996;76(5):S5.

17. Eisenberg DM, Kessler RC, et al. Unconventional medicine in the United States. *N Engl J Med.* 1993;328:245-252.

18. Reynolds J. Profiles in alternatives. *PT Magazine.* 1994;2(9):52-59.

19. Borysenko J. The best medicine. *New Age Journal.* 1990;47:102-103.

20. Cassidy CM. Cultural context of complementary and alternative medicine. In: Micozzi MS, ed. *Fundamentals of Complementary and Alternative Medicine.* New York, NY: Churchill Livingstone; 1996.

21. Davis CM. *Patient Practitioner Interaction/An Experiential Manual for Developing the Art of Health Care.* 2nd ed. Thorofare, NJ: SLACK Incorporated; 1994.

22. Seigel B. *Love, Medicine and Miracles.* New York, NY: Harper and Row; 1986.

23. Carmody J. The case: bad care, good care, and spiritual preservation. *Second Opinion.* 1994;20(1):35-39.

24. Davis CM. What is empathy and can empathy be taught? *Phys Ther.* 1990;70(11):707-715.

25. Schleler M. *The Nature of Sympathy.* Hamden, Conn: Anchor Books; 1970.

26. Wyschogrod E. Empathy and sympathy as tactile encounter. *J Med Phil.* 1981;6(1):25-34.

27. May WF. *The Physician as Healer/Images of the Healer in Medical Ethics.* Philadelphia, Pa: Westminster Press; 1983.

28. Pellegrino ED. What is a profession? *J Allied Health.* 1983;12(3):168-176.

29. Stein E. *On the Problem of Empathy.* 2nd ed. The Hague, Netherlands: Martinus Nijhoff/Dr. W Junk; 1970.

30. Weil A. The body's healing systems/the future of medical education. *J Alt Comp Ther.* 1995;1(1):305-309.

31. *Webster's II/New Riverside Dictionary.* Boston, Mass: Houghton Mifflin Co; 1984.

32. Harris S. How should treatments be critiqued for scientific merit? *Phys Ther.* 1996;76(2):175-181.

33. Spielholtz N. To the editor: critiquing treatments for scientific merit. *Phys Ther.* June 1996;76(6):666.

SECTION I

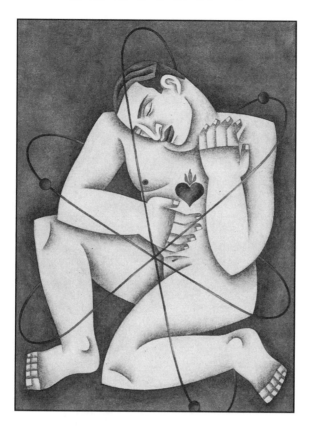

MANUAL
THERAPIES

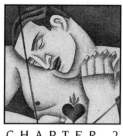

CHAPTER 2

MYOFASCIAL RELEASE
THE MISSING LINK IN
TRADITIONAL TREATMENT

John F. Barnes, PT

INTRODUCTION

Myofascial release is a whole-body, hands-on approach for the evaluation and treatment of the human structure. Its focus is the fascial system. Physical trauma, an inflammatory or infectious process, or structural imbalance from dental malocclusion, osseous restriction, leg length discrepancy, and pelvic rotation all may create inappropriate fascial strain.

Fascia, an embryologic tissue, reorganizes along the lines of tension imposed on the body, adding support to misalignment and contracting to protect the individual from further trauma (real or imagined). This has the potential to alter organ and tissue physiology significantly. Fascial strains can slowly tighten, causing the body to lose its physiologic adaptive capacity. Over time, the tightness spreads like a pull in a sweater or stocking. Flexibility and spontaneity of movement are lost, setting the body up for more trauma, pain, and limitation of movement. These powerful fascial restrictions begin to pull the body out of its three-dimensional alignment with the vertical gravitation axis, causing biomechanically inefficient, highly energy-consuming movement and posture.

Janet Travell's detailed description of the myofascial element[1] has taught us that there is no such thing as the muscle we have identified in traditional anatomy and physiology. Every muscle of the body is surrounded by a smooth fascial sheath, every muscular fascicle is surrounded by fascia, every fibril is surrounded by fascia, and every microfibril down to the cellular level is surrounded by fascia. Therefore, it is the fascia that ultimately determines the length and function of its muscular component, and muscle becomes an inseparable component of fascia. The implications of this important fact have been largely ignored in Western or traditional health care.

FASCIA

The fascia is a tough connective tissue that spreads throughout the body in a three-dimensional web from head to foot functionally without interruption. It has been estimated that if every structure of the body except the fascia were removed, the body would retain its shape. As described by Scott,[2] the fascia serves a major purpose in that it permits the body to retain its normal shape and thus maintain the vital organs in their correct positions. It also allows the body to resist mechanical stresses, both internally and externally. Fascia has maintained its general structure and purposes over the millennia. These functions are evident in the earliest stages of multicelled organisms, in which two or more cells were able to stay in contact, communicate, and resist the forces of the environment through the connective tissue.[2]

Fascia covers the muscles, bones, nerves, organs, and vessels down to the cellular level. Therefore, malfunction of the system due to trauma, poor posture, or inflammation can bind down the fascia, resulting in abnormal pressure on any or all of these body components. It is through that process that this binding down, or restriction, may result in many of the poor or temporary results achieved by conventional medical, dental, and therapeutic treatments.[3]

As Travell[1] has explained, restrictions of the fascia can create pain or malfunction throughout the body, sometimes with bizarre side effects and seemingly unrelated symptoms that do not always follow dermatomal zones. It is thought that an extremely high percentage of people suffering with pain, loss of motion, or both, may have fascial restriction problems. Most of these conditions go undiagnosed, however, as many of the standard tests, such as radiographs, myelograms, computerized tomographic scans, and electromyograms, do not show the fascia. If we can't see it, we can't look for restriction with our eyes.

Touching patients with skilled hands, however, can be one of the most potent ways of locating fascial restrictions and effecting positive change. Touching patients through mobilization, massage, and various forms of exercise and movement therapy, coupled with the gentle, refined touch of myofascial release and the sophisticated movement therapy called myofascial unwinding, creates a sensorimotor interplay. This experience of contact and movement is the very experience we need to reprogram our biocomputer, the mind-body, the basis for learning any new skill. Those practicing myofascial release use the skin and fascia as a handle or lever to create new options for enhanced function and movement of every structure of the body. Myofascial release helps remove the straitjacket of pressure caused by restricted fascia, eliminating symptoms such as stiffness, pain, and spasm. Then, through its influence on the neuromuscular and skeletal systems, it creates the opportunity for patients to "learn" new enhanced movement patterns. Manipulation and myofascial release both are highly effective treatments when they are accomplished with skilled hands and mind. They are designed to be used together to enhance the total effect. Joint manipulation is specific, attempting to improve the motion and function of a particular joint. Myofascial release, however, is a whole-body approach designed to discover and rectify the fascial restrictions that may have caused the effect or symptoms.

DISCOVERING FASCIAL RESTRICTIONS

The skin has many ways of perceiving the universe. It is the largest organ of the body, covering approximately 18 square feet and weighing about 8 pounds, that is, 6% to 8% of total body weight.[4,5] It has about 640,000 sensory receptors that are connected to the spinal cord by over half a million nerve fibers. The tactile fibers vary from 7 to 135 per square centimeter.[4-6]

The tactile surface of the skin is the interface not only between the body and our world, it is the interface between the mind's thought process and our physical existence.[6] This is also the interface by which therapists can facilitate incredible changes in the patient through the amazing plasticity of the central nervous system and the brain. Embryologically, both the skin and the nervous system are produced by ectoderm. When considering the connection of mind and body, we might ask, is the skin the outer surface of the brain or is the brain the deepest layer of the skin?[6,7]

Touch by itself can be powerfully therapeutic.[4] It can also serve as a powerful diagnostic tool, by itself and through its role in proprioception. In general, of all the senses, the proprioceptive sense is least understood by most people, thus it is seldom consciously used. However, when this sense is developed through the awareness and use of the more holistic right brain, rather than the logical left brain "knowing," proprioceptive input opens up vistas of untapped intuitive potential for clinicians in both evaluation and treatment. The development of our proprioceptive sense also allows us to detect the quality and quantity of the often unnoticed very fine motion that is inherent in our bodies. As I developed and refined this approach, I discovered that when we quiet our mind and body, and gently touch the patient with both hands, for example, on the dorsum of the feet, our proprioceptive senses help us in our evaluation by feeding us information as if our hands were moving like a mirror image to the patient's movement, thus detecting the subtle motions occurring in the patient's body that we cannot see or feel any other way. This activity, when practiced and refined, allows us to discover fascial restrictions and feel when they release. The informed touch of myofascial release also allows us to feel the motion that will take the patients' bodies into the three-dimensional position necessary for more total structural release, or, as for many, for bringing disassociated memories to a conscious level, as I will discuss later.

MYOFASCIAL RELEASE: THE BLENDING OF THE CURRENT AND THE EMERGING EXPLANATORY PARADIGMS

A paradigm is a theoretical model that provides a way of describing, believing, and understanding what we consider to be real.[8] A paradigm "shift" changes our models of reality, our concepts, and logic, and thus it can create anxiety, fear, and anger in those persons deeply entrenched in the status quo. For others, it represents an opportunity for growth. Fear paralyzes some, while for others it provides the stimulus and motivation to move to higher and deeper levels of understanding, awareness, and achievement. The current paradigm or theory that Western medicine is based on (reductionism) is becoming less and less adequate as it fails to explain such common phenomena as spontaneous remission of tumors, how the mind and emotions affect the physiology of the body, extrasensory perception, and other observed and documented occurrences.

The current paradigm that drives medicine and health care therapy and research springs from the centuries-old either/or logic of Aristotle. In it, everything is isolated, individual, and separate. There is "no middle ground," there are no shades of gray. This kind of thinking makes one theory wrong because another is right, or one person wrong because another is right.[9] Such thinking is exclusionary; it does not acknowledge connectedness among individuals or allow for the possibility of the coexistence of explanatory models.

Based on the logic of Aristotle, the universe, as perceived by Isaac Newton and Rene Descartes, is a giant machine that functions precisely, logically, sequentially, and correctly. This model of classic physics, which is the basis of our current paradigm, is informed by reductionistic research which carefully allows for only one correct solution to a problem. In the field of medical science, theory based on this model and its research have reduced human illness to the "biochemistry of disease," completely losing sight of the fact that the disease or dysfunction is part of a whole person. That this model "has reached its limits and has crossed into absurdity" is obvious.[9] The emerging explanatory paradigm (holism) places priority on describing connectedness, relativity, complexity, multiple possibilities, and a nonlinear mind-body unity. The practice of myofascial release has to do with wholeness, connectedness (connective tissue), the wave and particle theory of atoms, and the subatomic realm of quantum physics.

As outlined in Chapter 1, quantum physics, in part, describes the awareness and facilitation of interwoven, nonlinear systems in the universe where the whole is greater than, and makes sense of, the parts.[10,11] This theory contrasts reductionism, where the parts make sense of the whole, because the whole is nothing more than the total of all the parts.[10]

This paradigm shift requires a change of perspective and represents a "breakthrough in science. It connects living biological systems to physics and shows nature to be much more than just mechanical. The whole universe is alive and participating."[9]

Traditionally, medical education teaches that emotions are totally separate from the structure of the body. The body is essentially a machine, and when a part breaks down it is to be medicated or surgically altered, or have some form of therapy directed at it and it alone. For years, this Cartesian viewpoint or model has been accepted as true, and patients were treated accordingly, even though logic and our experience tells us it could not be true.

Myofascial release is a logical expansion of the very roots of the health professions. It incorporates quantum theory into practice but it does not necessitate the dismantling of traditional health care or physical therapy. Rather, myofascial release represents a powerfully effective addition of a series of concepts and techniques that enhance and mesh with our traditional medical, dental, and therapeutic training.

A CLOSE EXAMINATION OF THE ANATOMY AND PHYSIOLOGY OF FASCIA

The fascia generally is classified as *superficial*, or lying directly below the dermis; *deep*, surrounding and infusing with muscle, bone, nerves, blood vessels, and organs to the cellular level, or *deepest*, the dura of the craniosacral system, encasing the central nervous system and the brain.

At the cellular level, fascia creates the interstitial spaces. It has extremely important functions in support, protection, separation, cellular respiration, elimination, metabolism, and fluid and lymphatic flow. It can have a profound influence on cellular health and the immune system. Therefore, trauma or malfunction of the fascia can set up the environment for poor cellular efficiency, necrosis, disease, pain, and dysfunction throughout the body.[12]

MOLECULAR STRUCTURE OF FASCIA

Connective tissue is composed of collagen, elastin, and the polysaccharide gel complex, or ground substance.[13] These form a three-dimensional, interdependent system of strength, support, elasticity, and cushion.

Collagen is a protein consisting of three polypeptide chains that line up to form fibrils in such a way as to ensure that there are no weak points that could give way under tension. Collagen fibers thus contribute strength to fascial tissue and guard against overextension.

Elastin, another protein, is intrinsically rubber-like. Its fibers are laid down in parallel with an excess length of collagen fibers in places where elasticity is required, such as skin and arteries. This combination absorbs tensile forces. Tendons, specialized for pulling, mainly contain these elastocollagenous fibers.

The polysaccharide gel complex, mainly composed of hyaluronic acid and proteoglycans, fills the spaces between fibers. Hyaluronic acid is a highly viscous substance that lubricates the collagen, elastin, and muscle fibers, allowing them to slide over each other with minimal friction. Proteoglycans are peptide chains that form the gel of the ground substance. This gel is extremely hydrophilic, allowing it to absorb the compressive forces of movement. Cartilage, which acts as a shock absorber, contains much water-rich gel.

As long as the forces are not too great, the gel of the ground substance is designed to absorb shock and disperse it throughout the body. If fascia is restricted at the time of trauma, the forces cannot be dispersed properly and areas of the body are then subjected to an intolerable impact, and injury results. Injurious forces do not have to be enormous; a person who lacks sufficient "give" can be severely injured by minor forces.[3,13]

Realizing this, we can explain the sports and performance injuries that recur despite extensive therapy, strengthening, and flexibility programs. An athlete with fascial restrictions will not efficiently absorb the shocks of continued activity. Thus, the body absorbs too much pressure in too small an area, and during performance the body keeps "breaking down."

This same effect takes place over time from the microtrauma of discrepancies of leg length due to weight bearing on a continuously torsioned pelvis. Each step sends imbalanced forces throughout the body, which then tries to compensate through muscular spasm and fascial restrictions, ultimately producing symptoms.

Myofascial release techniques are performed to reduce these symptoms of pain, spasm, and malalignment. In addition to increasing range of motion, the enormous pressure of the fascial restrictions is eliminated from pain-sensitive structures, alleviating symptoms, restoring the normal quantity and quality of motion, and restoring the body's ability to absorb shock without compensatory injury.

THE FUNCTIONS OF FASCIA

The fascia, as mentioned earlier, is particularly significant in supporting and providing cohesion to the body structures; thus, its functions are varied and complex. Functional, biomechanically efficient movements depend on intact, properly distributed fascia. Fascia creates a plexus to support and stabilize, thus enchancing the body's postural balance. Appropriately, loose fascia permits movement between adjacent structures, which are free of friction due to the presence of bursal sacs. In addition, loose tissue contains a fluid that serves as a transport medium for cellular elements of other tissues, blood and lymph. In this manner, fascia also supports a nutritive function.[14]

Fat is stored in the superficial fascia. This layer also provides a covering that helps conserve body heat. The deep fascia is an ensheathing layer. It maintains physiologic limb contour and enhances venous and lymphatic circulation. In combination with intermuscular septa and interosseous membranes, the deep fascia provides additional surface area for muscle attachment.[14]

Structurally, the planes in connective tissue allow passage of infectious and inflammatory processes. The presence in the tissue of histiocytes, however, offers a defense against bacteria. These phagocytes also remove debris and foreign matter from fascia. In addition, connective tissue neutralizes or detoxifies both endogenous (produced under physiologic conditions) and exogenous (introduced from outside the body) toxins. Finally, its fibroplastic qualities permit fascia to assist in healing injuries by depositing collagenous fibers by way of scar tissue.[14]

MYOFASCIAL RELEASE EFFECT ON COLLAGEN

Collagen comes from the ancient Greek word that means "glue-producer." The feeling one perceives during myofascial release treatment is rather like stretching glue. The therapist follows this sensation with sensitive hands as it twists and turns, barrier through barrier, until an increased range of motion is accomplished.

A therapist cannot mechanically overstretch the collagenous aspect of the fascia. Although we are as yet unable to prove it, the improvements seen after myofascial release are probably due to a stretching of the elastic component, a shearing of the cross-links that can develop at the nodal points of the fascia, and a change in the viscosity of the ground substance from a more solid to a gel state. This change in viscosity increases the production of hyaluronic acid and increases the glide of the fascial tissue. Also observed regularly is what appears to be a positive effect on the spindle cells, the Golgi tendon organs of the musculotendinous component, and the tone of the peripheral, autonomic, and central nervous systems.[3]

Thus, to separate fascia from its influence on muscle and their influence on each other is impossible. In other words, we have been evaluating and treating an illusion. Reality demands that we consider both muscle and fascia as inexorably linked as one, understanding their integrated characteristics and then using this new information to inform our evaluation and treatments. My experience has shown that medicine, modalities, muscle energy techniques, mobilization, manipulation, temporomandibular joint appliances, massage, and flexibility and exercise programs affect only the muscular and the elastic components of the fascial system. Only myofascial release affects the total fascial system. This is why it is important to add myofascial release techniques to our current treatment regimens. Otherwise, we are only treating part of the problem and part of the patient. The inclusion of myofascial release allows the conscientious health professional to offer patients a truly comprehensive approach.

MYOFASCIAL RELEASE TECHNIQUES

The myofascial skeletal system, with its combined ability to provide both compressive forces by hydrostatic pressure and tensile strength, creates a space truss system that realistically replaces the post and lintel or lever model.[3] Pierce[15] refers to this principle of natural construction as "minimal inventory/maximum diversity." In the spine, post or columnar loading as support of the body has only limited use. In certain species, in certain positions, and when it converts to a lever, it is highly energy consuming and an unlikely support system in nature. D'Arcy Thompson[16] suggests that trusses can be a model for structural support in vertebrates. Trusses have clear advantages over post and lintel construction as a structural support system for biologic tissue. Trusses have flexible, even frictionless, hinges with no coupled moments about the joint, and the support elements are in tension and compression only, with no bending moments. Loads applied at any one point are distributed about the truss as tension or compression, rather than local loading as levers, as in post and lintel construction. There are no levers in a truss. The truss, being fully triangulated, is inherently stable and cannot be deformed without producing large deformations of the individual members, even with frictionless hinges. Only trusses are inherently stable with freely moving hinges. Any structure that has freely moving hinges and is structurally stable is a truss. Vertebrates, having stable structural configurations, in spite of essentially frictionless hinges, must therefore be constructed as trusses. The tension elements of the body—the soft tissues, muscles, ligaments, and connective tissue—have largely been ignored as supporting members of the body frame and have been viewed only as the stabilizers or motors. In loading a truss, the elements that are in tension could be replaced by flexible materials such as ropes, wire, or muscles or other soft tissues.

It is imperative that our structures have the ability to respond appropriately to our gravitational field as it plunges down through us. Ideally, we should be balanced around the vertical axis of this constant gravity; otherwise, imbalance almost always shortens the body and increases the expenditure of energy. Myofascial release, along with therapeutic exercise and movement therapy, improves the vertical alignment and lengthens the body, providing more space for the proper functioning of osseous structures, nerves, blood vessels, and organs.

Due to an injury to the lumbosacral area, patients have been known to experience distant symptoms such as occipital headaches, upper cervical pain and dysfunction, feelings of tightness around the thoracic area, lumbosacral pain, and tightness and lack of flexibility in the posterior aspect of the lower extremity. It is this author's belief that, during traumatization or with the development of a structural imbalance, a proprioceptive memory pattern of pain is established in the central nervous system. Beyond the localized pain response from injured nerves, these reflex patterns remain to perpetuate the pain during and beyond healing of the injured tissue, similar to the experience of phantom limb pain. Also in operation is the psychosomatic mode of adaption, which is part of Selye's general adaption syndrome.[17]

If fascia has tightened and is creating symptoms *distant* from the injury, all of the appropriate traditional localized treatments will produce poor or temporary results because the imbalance and excessive pressure from the myofascial tightness remain untreated. Myofascial release techniques are therefore performed *in conjunction with* specific symptomatic treatment. It is believed and observed that the gentle tractioning forces applied to the fascial restrictions will elicit heat from a vasomotor response that increases blood flow to the affected area, which will enhance lymphatic drainage of toxic metabolic wastes, realign fascial planes, and most importantly, reset the soft tissue proprioceptive sensory mechanism. This last activity seems to reprogram the central nervous system, enabling the patient to perform a normal functional range of motion without eliciting the previous pain patterns.[18]

The goal of myofascial release is to remove fascial restrictions and restore the body's equilibrium. When the structure has been returned to a balanced state, it is realigned with gravity. When these aims have been accomplished, the body's inherent ability to self-correct returns, thus restoring optimum function and performance with the least amount of energy expenditure. A more ideal environment to enhance the effectiveness of concomitant symptomatic therapy is also created.

The therapist is taught to find the cause of symptoms by evaluating the fascial system. Visually analyzing the structure of the human frame, palpating the tissue texture of the various fascial layers, and observing the symmetry, rate, quality, and intensity of the craniosacral rhythm make up this evolution process. The technique requires continuous reevaluation during treatment, including observation of vasomotor responses and their location as they occur after a particular restriction has been released. This provides instantaneous and accurate information, enabling the therapist to proceed intelligently and logically from one treatment session to the next, to the ultimate resolution of the patient's pain and dysfunction. Detailed systematic documentation of this information will assist us in compiling the data for further qualitative research needed to explain and predict patient outcomes.

When the location of the fascial restriction is determined, gentle pressure is applied in its direction. It is hypothesized that this has the effect of pulling the elastocollagenous fibers straight. When hand or palm pressure is first applied to the elastocollagenous complex, the elastic component is engaged, resulting in a "springy" feel. The elastic component is slowly stretched until the hands stop at what feels like a firm barrier. This is the collagenous component. This barrier cannot be forced; it is too strong. Instead, the therapist continues to apply gentle sustained pressure, and soon the firm barrier will yield to the previous melting or springy feel as it stretches further.

This yielding phenomenon is related to viscous flow; that is, a low load (gentle pressure) applied slowly will allow a viscous medium to flow to a greater extent than a high load (quickly applied) pressure.[19] The viscosity of the ground substance has an effect on the collagen, since it is believed that the viscous medium that makes up the ground substance controls the ease with which collagen fibers rearrange themselves.[19] As this rearranging occurs, the collagenous barrier releases, producing a change in tissue length.

It is important to keep in mind the properties of fascial tissue. Viscoelasticity "causes it to resist a suddenly applied force over time. *Creep* is the progressive deformation of soft tissues due to constant low loading over time. *Hysteresis* is the property whereby the work done in deforming a material causes heat and hence energy loss."[20] The therapist follows the motion of the tissue, barrier to barrier, until freedom is felt. The Arndt-Schultz law also explains how the gentle, sustained pressure of myofascial release can produce such consistent changes and improvements. The law states that "weak stimuli increase physiologic activity and very strong stimuli inhibit or abolish activity."[21]

The development of one's tactile and proprioceptive senses enhances the "feel" necessary for the successful completion of these techniques. We were all born with the ability to feel the releases and the direction in which the tissue seems to move from barrier to barrier. When first learning myofascial release, students perform the techniques mechanically. With a little practice, they discover the feel and move to a more artful or higher level of achievement.

No prior knowledge of mobilization or manipulation is required to learn the concept and techniques of myofascial release. The procedures should be combined with neuromuscular technique (muscle energy), joint mobilization, and manipulation by skilled practitioners. However, since it is usually fascial restrictions that created the osseous restrictions in the first place, releasing the fascia first is often the desired order of treatment.

The biomechanical, bioelectrical, and neurophysiological effects of myofascial release represent an evolutionary leap for our professions and our patients. This is a total approach incorporating a physiologic system that, when included with traditional therapy, medicine, or dentistry, acts as a catalyst and yields impressive, clinically reproducible results.[3]

MYOFASCIAL CRANIAL TECHNIQUES

Application of myofascial release to the cranium is most effective when light pressure is used. Once you have learned to "read the body," more pressure may be indicated at times. Practitioners are taught to start lightly on the mechanical level. Through time and experience, their awareness and sensitivity increases to the point where treatment on the head or body flows in a dynamic fashion.

DIRECT AND INDIRECT CRANIAL TECHNIQUES

Many people performing cranial therapy use what I term a "direct technique." Although I started this way, trial and error finally taught me that an indirect technique is usually far more productive for lasting results. It is nontraumatic and extremely effective.

With the direct technique, the therapist aligns each cranial bone according to how it appears in an anatomy book. This is a logical solution. The problem with direct technique is that it does not pay attention to the fascial system.

It is the fascial system, firmly attached to the cranial bones by the endosteum, that determines the three-dimensional position of the cranial bones and, eventually, their function. Indirect technique uses the fascial system as a handle or lever to realign the cranial bones, or other osseous structures, into their correct physiological position so that they achieve maximum function. This technique avoids the guesswork of mimicking pictures of anatomic structures or the need to use the arbitrary statistical average approach. Rather, it is truly physiologic therapy that allows the body to self-correct.

A helpful way of viewing the differences between traditional direct and myofascial indirect cranial techniques is to imagine a screen door with a stuck latch. Direct technique is the equivalent of trying to pull forcefully against the latch to get the door open. If we use force in treatment, the body's protective mechanism responds by pulling back. If we then tug a little harder, the body pulls back to an even greater degree. Indirect technique is the equivalent of gently closing the stuck screen door a little more and then opening it. It will almost always open easily and nontraumatically. Applying this concept to the body or head, one exaggerates the lesion (shuts the screen door a little more) and then decompresses (unlatches the screen door).

My experience has shown that while a direct technique is excellent as a last resort or finishing technique, especially when the dysfunction is primarily an osseous restriction, it is usually most effective to start with an indirect technique. Therefore, myofascial cranial techniques start with compression—exaggeration of the lesion—followed by decompression. It seems that when we compress lightly and follow the body part three-dimensionally where it wants to go (the direction of ease), we will reach the exact position where the body must be in order to release itself.

A still point, or a feeling of complete stillness that results from shutting down of the craniosacral rhythm, occurs at that position. "The craniosacral system is characterized by rhythmic, mobile activity which persists through life." "It is distinctly different from the physiological motions which are related to breathing, and different from cardiovascular activity as well." "The normal rate of craniosacral rhythm in humans is between 6 and 12 cycles per minute."[22]

During the still point, a reorganization of the neuromuscular system occurs and the holding or bracing patterns change.[3] A new balance or reference point is found and a positive therapeutic event involving structural, emotional, and intellectual improvement occurs. This change or release then allows us to decompress. As with other forms of myofascial release, we allow our hands to follow where the tissue wants to go, barrier to barrier, until all is released and balanced.

I believe that confusion about what techniques (direct or indirect) to use has arisen because we were taught to differentiate between flexion and extension, side-bending and rotational lesions, and how to correct them mechanically. The problem with this lies in the realization that, in vivo, there is no such thing as a strictly flexion or extension lesion, or a strictly side-bending or rotational lesion. These are simply linear labels of the most predominant part of the lesion. Although they are convenient teaching tools, they are illusions. In life, all lesions are three-dimensional, having a component of either flexion or extension, side-bending, and rotation. No machine or person is intelligent enough to figure out what degree of any of these dimensions is necessary to find the exact position for the body to release. Only the wisdom of the body's self-correcting mechanism can do this. Quieting the mind and following where the fascia or the body wants to go naturally (as in myofascial unwinding) will take the therapist exactly into the degree of flexion or extension, side-bending and rotation that the individual needs, barrier to barrier, until the individual is released and balanced.

Cranial therapy is by nature gentle and thus has virtually no serious side effects. Because of its potent influence on intracranial fluid dynamics, however, the following are considered definite contraindications:

1. Acute intracranial hemorrhage: therapy may prolong the duration of hemorrhage by interrupting clot formation.
2. Intracranial aneurysm: treatment may induce leak or rupture.
3. Herniation of the medulla oblongata: a life-threatening condition.
4. Recent skull fracture: the techniques are best avoided.
5. Acute systemic infections: therapy is generally avoided; however, cranial compression and a distraction-induced still point may help reduce fever.

MYOFASCIAL UNWINDING: THE BODY REMEMBERS

To ask how the mind communicates with the body or how the body communicates with the mind assumes that the two are separate entities. The research of Eccles and Popper confirms this.[23] Recent research[24] and my experience with myofascia have shown me that they seem to respond as a single unit or two sides of the same coin. Mind and body act as if they are different aspects of the same spectrum, immutably joined, inseparable, connected, influencing, and intercommunicating constantly. Myofascial release techniques and myofascial unwinding seem to allow for the complete communication of mind with body and body with mind which is necessary for healing. I believe that the body remembers everything that ever happened to it, and Hameroff's research indicates that the theory of *quantum coherence* points toward the storing of meaningful memory in the microtubules, cylindrical protein polymers that we find in the fascia of cells.[24] Mind-body awareness and healing are often linked to the concept of "state-dependent" memory, learning, and behavior, also called deja vu.[17] We have all experienced this, for example, when a certain smell or the sound of a particular piece of music creates a flashback phenomenon, producing a visual, sensorimotor replay of a past event or an important episode in our lives with such vividness that it is as if it were happening at that moment. Based on the work of Hameroff and colleagues[24] and my experience, I would like to expand this theory to include position-dependent memory, learning, and behavior, with the structural position being the missing component in Selye's state-dependent theory as it is currently described.[25]

My experience has shown that during periods of trauma, people form subconscious indelible imprints of the experience that have high levels of emotional content. The body can hold information below the conscious level, as a protective mechanism, so that memories tend to become dissociated or amnesiac. This is called memory dissociation, or reversible amnesia. The memories are state (or position) dependent and can therefore be retrieved when the person is in a particular state (or position). This information is not available in the normal conscious state, and the body's protective mechanisms keep us away from the positions that our mind-body awareness construes as painful or traumatic.

It has been demonstrated consistently that when a myofascial release technique takes the tissue to a significant position, or when myofascial unwinding allows a body part to assume a significant position three-dimensionally in space, the tissue not only changes and improves, but memories, associated emotional states, and belief systems rise to the conscious level. This awareness, through the positional reproduction of a past event or trauma, allows the individual to grasp the previously hidden information that may be creating or maintaining symptoms or behavior that deter improvement. With the repressed and stored information now at the conscious level, the individual is in a position to learn which holding or bracing patterns have been impeding progress and why. The release of the tissue with its stored emotions and hidden information creates an environment for change.

Recent neurobiologic research into the nature of neuronal activity during a specific mental event remains inconclusive.[26] But Taylor[27] suggested that content inherent in consciousness may only be relevant when compared to previous memory. The meaning of an input is given by the degree of overlap such an input has to past inputs. Korb[28] has written about how inputs can have meaning, and I refer the reader to that research.

Selye's classic work[17,25] is concerned with the phenomenon of state-dependent memory, learning, and behavior, the general class of learning that takes place in all complex organisms that have a cerebral cortex and a limbic-hypothalamic system. Pavlovian and Skinnerian conditioning are specific varieties of state-dependent memory and learning.[17]

Memory and learning in all higher organisms take place by way of two internal responses:

1. A memory trace forms on the molecular-cellular-synaptic level.[29,30]
2. There is an involvement of the amygdala and hippocampus of the limbic-hypothalamic system in processing and encoding the memory; recall of the specific memory trace may be located elsewhere in the brain.[6,31]

The limbic-hypothalamic system is the central core to Selye's general adaption syndrome. The neurobiology of the three stages of the syndrome, the alarm reaction, the stage of resistance, and the stage of exhaustion, help explain the observed outcomes of myofascial release and myofascial unwinding, and illustrate the mind-body integration.

The hormones that are responsible for the retention of memory, epinephrine and norepinephrine, are released during the alarm stage just before the trauma by the activation of the sympathetic branch of the autonomic nervous system. The state or position the person is in *at the moment of trauma* is encoded into the system as the person progresses into the second stage, the stage of resistance. At that point, the system adapts and develops subconscious strategies to protect itself from further trauma, fear, or memories by avoiding those three-dimensional positions the body is in at the time of the insult. The emotions also communicate this mind-body information by way of the neuropeptides. This creates a vicious cycle of interplay among the endocrine, immune, and autonomic neuromyofascial systems and the neuropeptides.

If this cycle continues for too long, the person enters the third, or exhaustion stage, in which the body's defense mechanisms expend enormous amounts of energy, thereby depleting one's reserve and perpetuating or enlarging the symptom complex.

Selye[17] frequently described this type of resistance as being "stuck in a groove," something we have all experienced. When something familiar happens we react subconsciously in a habitual pattern before we can consciously be aware of it to control it. For example, if you were injured in a car accident, every time you see a car coming too fast you tighten and brace against the possible impact. People replay these incidents and the automatic, habitual bracing patterns associated with them subconsciously, until these hidden memories and learned behaviors are brought to the surface. Myofascial unwinding helps bring this information to a conscious level, allowing patients to reexperience it and let go, if they choose.

How is it that normal bodily movements or daily activities do not reproduce these memories, emotions, and outdated beliefs? I believe that these positions represent fear, pain, or trauma. In an attempt to protect oneself from further injury, it seems as if the subconscious does not allow the body to move into positions that reenact the microevents and important microcognitions essential for lasting mind-body change. The body then develops further strategies or patterns to protect itself. These subconscious holding patterns eventually form specific muscular tone or tension patterns, and the fascial component then tightens into these habitual positions of strain as a compensation to support the misalignment that results. Therefore, the repeated postural and traumatic insults of a lifetime, combined with the tensions of emotional and psychologic origin, seem to result in tense, contracted, bunched, and fatigued fibrous tissue.

A discrete area of the body may become so altered by its efforts to compensate and adapt to stress that structural and, eventually, pathologic changes become apparent. Researchers have shown that the type of stress involved can be entirely physical, such as the repetitive postural strain developed by a typist, dentist, or hairdresser, or purely psychic, such as the muscle tightening associated with chronic repressed anger.[14]

More often that not a combination of mental and physical stresses alters the neuromyofascial and skeletal structures, creating a visible, identifiable physical change, which, itself, generates further stress, such as pain, joint restriction, general discomfort, and fatigue. A chronic stress pattern produces long-term muscular contraction, which, if prolonged, can cause energy loss, mechanical inefficiency, pain, cardiovascular pathology, and hypertension.[14]

THERAPIST TECHNIQUE REQUIRED TO FACILITATE RELEASE

Working in reverse, myofascial release and myofascial unwinding release the fascial tissue restrictions, thereby altering the habitual muscular response and allowing the positional, reversible amnesia to surface, producing emotions and beliefs that are the cause of the holding patterns and ultimate symptoms. In order to allow this spontaneous motion to proceed without interference, it is important for the therapist to quiet his or her mind and feel the subtle inherent motions in the patient. Quietly following the tissue (myofascial release) or body part (myofascial unwinding) three-dimensionally along the direction of ease, the therapists guides the patient's movement into the significant restrictions or positions. With myofascial unwinding, the therapist eliminates gravity from the system, unloading the structure to allow the body's gravity-oriented righting reflexes and protective responses to temporarily suspend their influence. The body is then free to move into positions that allow repressed state or position-dependent physiologic or flashback phenomena to recur. As this happens within the safe environment of a treatment session, the patient can facilitate the body's own inherent self-correcting mechanism to obtain improvement.

When a significant position is attained, the craniosacral rhythm, when palpated, is felt to shut down into a still point. During this still point, a reversible amnesia surfaces, replaying all the meaningful physiologic responses, memories, and emotional states that occurred during a past traumatic event. Rossi describes this dissociation, or reversible amnesia, as a "double-conscious state."[32] In other words, what is experienced and remembered at the time of the original incident or trauma, *and the meaning attached to it*, is dependent on the psychophysiologic state of the individual at the time that the experience took place.[24] The resulting dissociation, or block, between the conscious and subconscious minds may be the major source of many poor or temporary traditional physical therapy outcomes.[32]

Myofascial release and myofascial unwinding bring the tissue or support the body part into a position eliminating gravity as the patient moves spontaneously. This allows the individual to be more fully aware of his or her divided consciousness. Reactivating the original conditions and the resultant physiologic responses by influencing the fascia to release results in a flashback phenomenon, which brings the repressed memory to conscious awareness and then allows the patient to have the choice to change. No longer do patients habitually find themselves holding or stiffening to protect themselves from future pain or trauma. Genuine release of fear and emotion takes place simultaneously with physical fascial release and physiologic release of the associated stress hormones.

As a result of observing the outcomes of many patients who have benefited from myofascial release and unwinding, I have concluded that the myofascial release approach is more than just an assemblage of techniques. Instead, it helps create a whole-body awareness, allowing the health professional to facilitate more than just structural change, but also growth and the possibility for a more total resolution of restrictions, emotions, and belief systems that may impede patient progress physically, emotionally, and cognitively. Thus, this treatment is holistic in nature, and complements traditional physical therapy based on reductionism.

FASCIA AND THE OLD AND NEW EXPLANATORY PARADIGMS

Clinical evidence has demonstrated that restrictions in the fascial system are of considerable importance in relieving pain and restoring function.[3] Myofascial release becomes vitally important when we realize that these restrictions can exert tremendous tensile forces on the neuromuscular-skeletal systems and other pain-sensitive structures, creating the very symptoms that we have been trying to eliminate.[33]

The prevailing view of the skeleton is that it is a group of bones. The vertebrae are "stacked" one on top of the other, the rest of the bones are "hitched on" somehow, and the whole mechanism is moved by the muscles that attach to the bones. Because the function of the fascial system largely has been ignored or misunderstood, we have developed an erroneous view of how our bodies truly function. We also have developed techniques to treat this misunderstood or "fictional" body. When these techniques do not achieve our desired outcomes, we tend to blame the patient for having a poor attitude or for not complying.

TENSEGRITY

What is really happening in our bodies can be best explained by the term "tensegrity," coined by the architectural genius Buckminster Fuller, as interpreted by Deane Juhan.[6] Juhan noted that the vertical position of the skeleton is dependent on tensional forces generated by the fascia, the tone and contractility of the muscular components, and the hydrostatic pressure exerted by fascial compartments. The osseous structures (bones) act as rigid beams whose position and motion are determined by the guy wires (myofascial elements) attached to them. The integrity of a tensegrity unit depends on the *tensional force of these guy wires*, not on the compressional strength or stable balance of the rigid beams. It is the relationship among the fascia, muscles, and osseous structures that constitutes the tensegrity units of the body.[6,34]

There is not a single horizontal surface anywhere in the skeleton that provides a stable base for anything to be stacked upon it. The design of our bodies was not conceived by a stone mason. Weight applied to any bone would cause it to slide right off its joints if it were not for the tensional balances that hold it in place and control its pivoting. Like the beams in a simple tensegrity structure, our bones act more as "spacers" than as compressional members; more weight is actually borne by the connective system of cables than by the bony beams.[6]

From this viewpoint, one can readily appreciate how crucial it is for the fascial "cables" to be of the proper length throughout the system. An abnormally tight cable in the lumbar area will negatively affect the entire balance of the spine and cranium. Conversely, increased or imbalanced tension in the upper regions of the body will produce compensatory tensions throughout the lower aspects of the structure, adversely affecting proper alignment.[6] This more accurate view of the body necessitates an understanding of the function of the fascial system and requires a total reversal of perspective.

As I developed this myofascial release approach, it became obvious that more than muscles and fascia responded; the whole body was involved. Treating a musculoskeletal symptom in isolation was no longer possible. During myofascial release, the body did not react like an inert machine, but rather was responsive, almost plastic or moldable under the therapist's hands. The tissues seemed to hold a consciousness, or thoughts of their own.[24,27] As releases occurred, patients reported memories or emotions emerging that were connected to past events or traumas. As their fascial systems changed and the memories or emotions surfaced, patients felt better and their symptoms improved, even though they previously were unresponsive to all other forms of traditional care that were tried. Current research about the possible role of fascia in the phenomenon of the mind-body connection is being conducted by Taylor[27] and others.

As noted, the traditional or Western focus of medical and therapeutic education and treatment was symptoms. The word *symptom*, derived from Greek, means "sign" or "signal." Symptoms are not the actual problem, however, but signs of the problem, and treating the symptom does not necessarily affect the cause or source of the signaling. Modern physiology suggests that symptoms are the body's adaptive responses to stress, imbalance, or infection. Viewed this way, effective therapy must facilitate a return to balance,[3] not just relieve symptoms. All of the holistic complementary therapies are based on this belief.

To discover the cause of the imbalance that is creating the distant effect (symptoms), we use the principles of both traditional mechanistic therapy and the newer, more general theory of the nonlinear whole-body. We treat the interconnecting system through relieving restrictions in the three-dimensional network of fascia utilizing a mind-body approach. The two viewpoints, together with their techniques, dovetail comprehensively to maximize our ability to promote healing. For example, we may begin with myofascial releases around the shoulder and neck and then move to traditional shoulder mobilization. For those interested in understanding both the Cartesian theory and the emerging "new" quantum theory, Rupert Sheldrake's *The Presence of the Past* is an excellent resource, as well as Micozzi's new text, *Fundamentals of Complementary and Alternative Medicine*.

The exponents of these two viewpoints have continued to argue, each claiming to be right while the other is wrong. It is possible that many of their explanations are both "right," and simply represent different perspectives of the whole picture. In a practical sense, treating specific symptoms complements the more general whole-body myofascial release approach. The latter, the mechanistic and specific, highlights where the former, the holistic, might be most appropriately utilized, thereby making mobilization and exercise regimens even more effective. In other words, both traditional physical therapy and myofascial release are parts of the whole and they can be used together to enhance the result. Treating both the cause and effect of symptoms often produces more lasting improvement.

However helpful the specific mechanistic approach is, it is obviously time for us to change our erroneous and misleading view of the human as a machine. The medical, dental, and physical and occupational therapy professions are all based on Newtonian physics, which is 300 years old, and was proven to be totally inadequate more than 50 years ago. Yet the very foundation of our scientific training is based on this inadequate information. When a theory is created out of an inaccurate belief, many other assumptions based on the fundamental inaccurate belief also will be incorrect, leading us to misunderstand how our bodies actually function in vivo.

Too many health professionals have become captivated by the obvious, the symptom, paying no attention to the possible cause—fascial restrictions. We have missed something so fundamental because the model we were taught and believed in, based on Newton and Descartes, was incomplete. Not only was the fascia of the body ignored, it separated what we could see, the physical or the material, from what we could not see, nonmaterialistic feelings and emotions, and dictated that only the materialistic should be of concern. However, both a) scientific and b) anecdotal information have emerged stating that by including the fascial system in evaluating patients, we can treat the cause of the symptoms nontraumatically with consistently effective and permanent results.[3]

APPLICATION OF MIND-BODY THEORIES TO TRADITIONAL PHYSICAL THERAPY

An important component of the theory behind the mind-body connection is the ability for people to transmit natural bioelectrical currents along the endogenous electromagnetic fields of the three-dimensional network of the fascial system of another person. Medical applications of *exogenous* bioelectromagnetics (like x-ray) are very common. *Endogenous* bioelectromagnetic fields, natural within all living beings, have only more recently been studied.[35]

Increasingly, medical researchers and experienced health professionals are beginning to view the body as a self-correcting mechanism with bioelectric healing systems. According to one author,[36] while some scientists are starting to explore the body's sensitivity to electromagnetic energy, those of the old school still choose to ignore the matter because it upsets their long-held theories. Such an attitude is unwarranted, however, and also may be unhealthy. It is known that electromagnetic fields "trigger the release of stress hormones...(and) can affect such processes as bone growth, communication among brain cells and even the activity of white cells."[36]

Becker and Seldon[37] found naturally occurring direct-current signals that they called "the current of injury" (COI). These signals are thought to be transmitted by the sheaths of Schwann and glial cells that surround their neurons. Others, however, consider the body's healing currents to use the microcapillary systems. In this theory, the bioelectric circuits are turned on when membrane conductivity closes down, and the electric flow then takes the path of least resistance through the blood stream.[38] The mechanism has not been determined, but clearly, the body sends endogenous electromagnetic energy wherever its healing effects are required.[37]

When we use traditional physical therapy electromagnetic devices (exogenous), it is not clear if the body interprets the energy of many of our modalities and of our sometimes abrupt manual techniques as intrusive, and therefore resists our efforts.[37] If this is the case, the body would likely recognize such resistance as important to its survival. Many therapeutic efforts to heal have, in fact, caused patients discomfort. This may begin to show why endogenous microcurrents and the gentle, sustained pressures used in myofascial release produce results when conventional modalities and other hands-on techniques have failed. If the body does not view these as intrusive, it is not compelled to resist. Instead, the techniques are accepted as assistive, and as allowing the organism's self-corrective mechanisms to be facilitated.

This is not to say that conventional modalities, exercises, and hands-on techniques are not valuable; certainly they are. It means that to treat the body comprehensively, the approaches must be combined, as they enhance each other in a complementary fashion and produce consistent results.

Copper wire is a well-known conductor of electricity. If copper wire becomes twisted or crushed, it loses its ability to conduct energy properly. It is thought that fascia may act like copper wire when it becomes restricted through trauma, inflammatory processes, or poor posture over time. Then its ability to conduct the body's bioelectricity seems to be diminished, setting up structural compensations and ultimately, symptoms or restrictions of motion.

The diminution of our fascial system's ability to conduct energy may be due to melanin.[39] Melanin is present in copious quantities in the fascia, and neuromelanin is present in the neural structures and brain, which are encased by fascia all the way down to the cellular level. Melanin has superior conducting properties at room temperature and is synthesized in mast cells, also found in the fascia, which influence the immune system. As a superconductor, melanin may regulate firing of nerve cells. It seems centrally involved in the control of all physiologic and psychologic activity.[39]

The neuromelanin-neuroglial system is the major site of mental organization.[39] The nervous system is made up principally of glial cells. These cells have electrical properties that appear to be responsible for the piezoelectric phenomenon. Piezoelectric behavior is an inherent property of bone and other mineralized and nonmineralized connective tissues. Compressional stress has been suggested to create minute quantities of electrical current flow.[37]

Myofascial release can restore the fascia's integrity and proper alignment and, similar to the copper wire effect, can enhance the transmission of our important healing bioelectrical currents. Just like untwisting a copper wire, myofascial release techniques seem to restore the fascia's ability to conduct bioelectricity, thus creating the environment for enhanced healing. Release techniques also can structurally eliminate the enormous pressures that fascial restrictions exert on nerves, blood vessels, and muscles.

FASCIAL "MEMORY"

Another observed patient response from myofascial release techniques also is explained more thoroughly within the mind-body paradigm. Recent evidence and my experience have demonstrated that embedded in our structure, particularly the fascial system, lie memories of past events or trauma.[3] These stored emotions can produce lessons in literal or symbolic form from which the patient can discover blocks that may have been hindering his or her healing process. By using effective communication skills, the therapist often can facilitate the efforts of a psychiatrist or psychologist well-trained in counseling, and help the patient discover the sources of blockage preventing full recovery.

It appears that not only the myofascial element, but also every cell of the body has a consciousness that stores memories and emotions.

> ...Research findings (suggest) that the mind and body act on each other in often remarkable ways. With the help of sophisticated new laboratory tools, investigators are demonstrating that emotional states can translate into altered responses in the immune system, the complex array of organs, glands and cells that comprises the body's principal mechanism for repelling invaders. The implications of this loop are unsettling. To experts in the field of psychoneuroimmunology, the immune system seems to behave almost as if it had a brain of its own. This is creating a revolution in medicine, in the way we view physiology. More than that, it is raising profound and tantalizing questions about the nature of behavior—about the essence of what we are.[9]

The new field of psychoneuroimmunology stems from the three classic areas of neuroscience, endocrinology, and immunology. Scientists have discovered a neuropeptide bidirectional network of communication between our body and mind by way of the emotions.[40]

Neuropeptides are information carriers composed of 50 to 60 chemical substances and their corresponding receptors, making or preventing something from happening.

> Receptors are not fixed: they have been accurately described as looking like lily pads that have floated up from the depth of the cell. Like lily pads, their roots sink downward, reaching the cell's nucleus, where the DNA sits. DNA deals in many, many kinds of messages, potentially an infinite number. Therefore, it makes new receptors and floats them up to the cell wall constantly. There is no fixed number of receptors, no fixed arrangement on the cell wall, and probably no limit to what they are tuned in to. A cell wall can be as barren of lily pads as a pond in winter, or as crammed as one in full flower in June.[41]

The neuropeptides are the key to the biochemistry of the emotions that are not just in the brain, but also in the cells of the entire body. In other words, the mind is not confined to the brain. We are an integrated totality, a mind-body network of information flowing throughout every system and cell of the body.

A network, like a web or fish net, is different from a hierarchic structure which has one top place. Theoretically, you can plug into a network at any given point and get to any other point. By viewing the three-dimensional fascial system as a network, we can begin to appreciate how releasing the tissue at any one point in the body affects other areas, such as the spindle cells of the muscles, the Golgi tendon organs, the circulatory system, the lymphatic system, the body's organs, and the position and function of the osseous structures. By way of the hormonal and neuropeptide systems, information is then sent to the peripheral, autonomic, and central nervous systems to allow physical and emotional change and reduce pain, thus improving the quantity and quality of motion.

Remember that the discovery of invisible bacteria that transmitted disease, and the discovery of penicillin, were important turning points in Western medicine. Both were greatly resisted as being impossible to be true. The paradigm shift that is now occurring due to the understanding and awareness of the importance of quantum theory to how we view the mind-body, and the discovery of the inseparability of the mind from the body resulting in the network of communication within the mind-body concept, are creating yet another revolution.

It has been demonstrated over and over that when a fascial barrier is engaged in myofascial release or when a person reaches a significant position during myofascial unwinding, the tissue releases and a memory or emotion surfaces. This electrophysical event produces a positive change and improvement in the patient. Myofascial release and myofascial unwinding are not linear but result in a whole-body effect, capable of producing a wide variety of physical, emotional, and mental effects.

The fascial and neuropeptide systems have thus turned our view of how our bodies function upside down and inside out. This is good news, for our old view of the body as a mindless machine was embarrassingly inadequate. While advances in medicine, surgery, and electronics have accomplished marvelous things, much more can be done. A better understanding of the fascial system that surrounds and influences every other system and cell of the body, and how cells can communicate with the brain and central nervous system and vice versa, allows us to see the enormous value of myofascial release in positively affecting the whole person.

Thus we have a physiologic basis for emotions, and emotions and structure cannot be separated, no matter how hard we might try. The improvements in emotional tone and structure have been demonstrated consistently for years with the various forms of myofascial release.[3]

SUMMARY AND CONCLUSIONS

Myofascial release techniques were discovered and are performed acknowledging that the existing view of the body as a machine is totally incorrect, and acknowledging that the fascia cannot be separated from each and every cell and structure that it surrounds. This approach starts with the belief that one must influence the patient's fascial restrictions in order to obtain and secure permanent recovery from the causes of pain and paresthesia secondary to postural or structural malalignments.

Fascia is not accessed by traditional mechanical methods such as joint mobilization or traditional stretching methods. Fascia, instead, responds to the intentional application of endogenous bioelectromagnetic energy fields from within the therapist, through the palms and fingers of the therapist's hands to soften the molecular structure of the fascia, facilitating a yielding or release of its barriers or restrictions.

The mind seems to store memories and experiences in restricted fascia, for upon the release of restrictions, patients commonly become transported back to an injurious experience and with similar emotion, relate the experience in detail. Once the trauma is completely experienced and the fascial restrictions have given way, healing can commence.

Traditional Western medical theory based on the philosophies of Isaac Newton and Rene Descartes cannot explain these observed patient experiences and outcomes. However, the emerging new explanatory theory of mind-body holism, based on quantum theory of the behavior and characteristics of atoms and molecules, offers explanations for these and many other "unexplainable" outcomes.

Myofascial release is not offered to replace traditional physical therapy techniques, but to supplement them as a complementary approach in evaluating and treating patients with pain, restriction of motion, and structural symptoms. Success in the application of these techniques requires therapists to keep an open mind regarding holism and mind-body theory, and to develop themselves personally in such a way that their manual techniques and their attitudes and priorities in care reflect a centered, creative, artful attention to the patient's description of the problems and to the feedback they receive from the patient's mind-body as they apply their treatment. Touch must be applied with focused awareness and the conscious purpose to mechanically and bioenergetically release fascial restrictions and thus facilitate the reorganization of the mind-body neuromuscular system.

Our goals are to learn from each patient; to teach by example; and to remain attentive, creatively focused, sensitive, nonjudgmental, supportive, and compassionate in accepting the patient's story as authentic and treatable. And then we must document our results in detail to start building a database from which we can publish our outcomes so that all may benefit.

Myofascial release offers a beginning into a new world of evaluation and care that is intelligent, based on sound theories, humane in its holistic approach, and effective when traditional mechanistic approaches to care have failed. The organization and publication of systematic and thorough documentation of qualitative and quantitative data is encouraged so we can share results with one another for the good of all patients.

REFERENCES

1. Travell J. *Myofascial Pain and Dysfunction*. Baltimore, Md: Williams & Wilkins; 1983.

2. Scott J. Molecules that keep you in shape. *New Scientist*. 1986;111:49-53.

3. Barnes JF. *Myofascial Release: The Search for Excellence*. Paoli, Pa: MFR Seminars; 1990.

4. Montague A. *Touching: The Human Significance of the Skin*. New York, NY: Harper & Row; 1971:4.

5. Barnes JF. The significance of touch. *Physical Therapy Forum*. May 1988;7:10.

6. Juhan D. *Job's Body*. Barrytown, NY: Station Hill Press; 1987.

7. Netter FH. *The CIBA Collection of Medical Illustrations: Nervous Systems*. West Caldwell, NJ: CIBA; 1983:197.

8. Kuhn TS. *The Structure of Scientific Revolutions*. Chicago, Ill: University of Chicago Press; 1970.

9. Kurtz R. *Body Centered Psychotherapy: The Hakomi Therapy*. Ashland, Ore: The Hakomi Institute; 1988.

10. Bohm D. *Causality and Chance in Modern Physics*. Philadelphia, Pa: University of Pennsylvania Press; 1957.

11. Bohm D. *The Special Theory of Relativity*. Boston, Mass; Addison Wesley; 1988.

12. Page L. *Academy of Applied Osteopathy Yearbook*. 1952:85-90.

13. Hall D. The aging of connective tissue exp. *Gerontology*. 1968;3:77-89.

14. Chaitow L. *Neuro-Muscular Technique—A Practitioner's Guide to Soft Tissue Mobilization*. New York, NY: Thorsons; 1985:13-15.

15. Pierce P. *Structure in Nature as a Strategy for Design*. Cambridge, Mass: MIT Press; 1978:xii-xvii.

16. Thomson D. *On Growth and Form*. London, England: Cambridge University Press; 1965.

17. Selye H. *The Stress of Life*. New York, NY: McGraw-Hill; 1976.

18. Barnes JF, Smith G. The body is a self-correcting mechanism. *Physical Therapy Forum*. July 1987;27.

19. Jenkins DHR. *Ligament Injuries and Their Treatment*. Rockville, Md: Aspen Publications; 1985.

20. Twomley L, Taylor J. Flexion, creep, dysfunction and hysteresis in the lumbar vertebral columns. *Spine*. July 1982;2:116-122.

21. *Dorland's Medical Directory*. 26th ed. Philadelphia, Pa: W.B. Saunders; 1985.

22. Upledger J, Vredevoogd J. *Craniosacral Therapy*. Seattle, Wash: Eastland Press; 1983:6.

23. Popper KR, Eccles JC. *The Self and its Brain*. Berlin, Germany: Springer; 1977.

24. Hameroff SR. Quantum coherence in microtubules: a neural basis for emergent consciousness. *J Consciousness Studies*. Summer 1994;1(1):91-118.

25. Selye H. History and present status of the stress concept. In: Goldberger L, Breznitz S, eds. *Handbook of Stress*. New York, NY: Macmillan; 1982:7-20.

26. Searle JR. Minds, brains and programs. *Behavioral and Brain Sciences*. 1980;3:417-424.

27. Taylor JG. Towards a neural network model of the mind. *Neural Network World*. 1992;6:797-812.

28. Korb KB. Stage effects in the Cartesian theater: a review of Daniel Dermetts' "Consciousness Explained." *Psyche*. Dec 1993;1(1).

29. Hawkins R, Kandel E. Steps toward a cell-biological alphabet for elementary forms of learning. In: Lynch G, McCaugh J, Weinberger N, eds. *Neurobiology of Learning and Memory*. New York, NY: Guilford Press; 1991:384-404.

30. Rosenzweig M, Bennett E. Basic processes and modulatory influences in the stages of memory formation. In: Lynch G, McCaugh J, Weinberger N, eds. *Neurobiology of Learning and Memory*. New York, NY: Guilford Press; 1984:263-288.

31. Siegel B. *Love, Medicine and Miracles*. New York, NY: Harper & Row; 1986.

32. Rossi EL. From mind to molecule: a state-dependent memory, learning, and behavior theory of mind-body healing. *Advance*. April 1987;2:46-60.

33. Klebe RS, Caldwell H, Milani S. Cells transmit spatial information by orienting collagen fibers. *Matrix*. 1989;9:451-458.

34. Ingber DE, Folkman J. Tension and comprehension as basic detriments of cell form and function: utilization of a cellular tensegrity mechanism.

35. *Alternative Medicine: Expanding Medical Horizons, Report to the NIH on Alternative Medical Systems of Practices in the United States*. Pittsburgh, PA: US Government Printing Office,

Superintendent of Documents; 1992:48-50.

36. Cowley G. An electromagnetic storm. *Newsweek*. July 1989:77.

37. Becker RO, Seldon G. *The Body Electric: Electromagnetism and the Foundation of the Life*. New York, NY: William Morrow; 1985.

38. Picker RI. Microcurrent therapy: "jump-starting" healing with bioelectricity. *Physical Therapy Forum*. July 1989;27.

39. Barr F. Special issue: melanin as key organizing molecule. *Brain/Mind Bull.* August 1983;12(13):1.

40. Ader R. *Psychoneuroimmunology*. New York, NY: Academic Press; 1981.

41. Chopra D. *Quantum Healing: Exploring the Frontiers of Mind/Body Medicine*. New York, NY: Bantam Books; 1989.

SUGGESTED READINGS

Sheldrake R. *The Presence of the Past*. New York, NY: Times Books; 1994.

Micozzi MS, ed. *Fundamentals of Complementary and Alternative Medicine*. New York, NY: Churchill Livingstone; 1996.

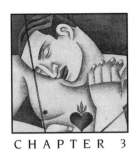

CHAPTER 3

ROSEN METHOD BODYWORK

David Berger, MA, PT, MFCCI

INTRODUCTION

Rosen Method Bodywork® is a form of hands-on, nonintrusive somatic bodywork, the goal of which is physical relaxation and emotional awareness to assist and facilitate a client's innate healing capacities. In Rosen Method Bodywork, a client will learn how to relax her barriers, or muscular holding and tension, so she can again move more freely and easily with fewer symptoms, allowing her full range of possibilities for movement and expression in life to come forth. As in most somatic practices, the client's experience from within her body, instead of the practitioner's observations and perceptions, are of primary importance.[1] As Marion Rosen, PT, founder of Rosen Method, states, "We meet people cloak to cloak and not essence to essence. Our work is about helping a client change from who she thinks she is into who she really is."[2]

With Rosen Method, a client learns she can remove her cloak of holding or tension and allow her true self to emerge. When a client relaxes and feels free to express emotions without inhibiting herself, her body can use all of its resources in the healing process. It may need to heal from a musculoskeletal dysfunction, chronic pain or illness, emotional trauma, or other problems. Rosen Method Bodywork can facilitate a person's own healing processes to work more efficiently and effectively. This chapter is written in the language of Rosen Method instead of being translated into physical therapy terminology. This way the reader can appreciate the milieu of the work and not just the theory and technique. When appropriate, such as in the case studies, physical therapy terminology is added for clarity and precision.

There has been no research of Rosen Method Bodywork using a reductionistic scientific model. Phenomenological and anecdotal evidence of clients' changing somatic and life experience, however, is abundant and will be used in the form of case studies to augment this chapter. These may help stimulate future reductionist methodogical studies.

MARION ROSEN, PT: FOUNDER OF ROSEN METHOD BODYWORK

Marion Rosen, PT, was born in Nurenberg, Germany in 1914 into a moderately affluent Jewish family. During her teenage years in Germany, the political environment in Germany began to change. After Hitler came to power, she realized she would have to leave Germany soon and knew she would have to earn a living for herself. She had a talent for languages and tried to become a translator. However, since she was Jewish (although raised Lutheran) she was not allowed to go to university.

During her late teens, Rosen was introduced to Lucy Heyer, a masseuse, dancer, and student of Carl Jung, who also did relaxation work and work with the breath. Heyer had studied with Elsa Gindler, a woman considered by many to be an originator and master of somatic practices that utilize the breath, the body, and awareness. Heyer was also the wife of a Jungian analyst and psychiatrist. The Heyers were treating clients with massage, breath work, and relaxation concurrently with psychoanalysis for clients, and found that clients improved much faster than with analysis only.

Heyer took Rosen as a student. They treated Dr. Heyer's clients in silence using massage and work with the breath. This was Rosen's introduction to the power of touch and the ability of the human body to heal. Some clients she treated would begin to cry during the treatment, many would lose their pain, and others would just feel better. However, only the analyst talked with the clients.

Rosen studied with Heyer for 2 years. She then fled Germany for Sweden to wait for a visa to the United States. She did not know anyone in Sweden, but managed to find her way to a dance studio where she massaged and watched the dancers. She treated a dance teacher who had sprained her ankle, and after only three treatments, all the pain was gone. This so impressed the teacher that she invited Marion to spend as much time at the studio as she wanted. She took great advantage of this opportunity, although she never got to dance, a love of hers from childhood.

Rosen also studied physical therapy in Sweden, completing what was to be her first formal training in physical therapy. Her visa to the United States finally came through and she started her journey to America. Although her original intention was to travel to New York to study with Karen Horney, a Jungian analyst using similar bodywork in her practice, she had to travel west because of the war. Alone at 24 years old, she settled in Berkeley, California and worked the evening physical therapy shift with injured shipyard workers.

Rosen's next endeavor was to go to the Mayo Clinic physical therapy program as an advanced student; she completed her courses in 6 months. Although she returned to her orginal physical therapy position after studying at the Mayo Clinic, she soon grew tired of having such limited time to treat patients (she was treating up to 40 patients a day). She and a colleague started their own private practice in the mid-1940s in Oakland, California, and she continued in the same office for 30 years. As her reputation grew, physicians referred patients with the simple order to "do what you think is best" instead of the more common specific orders. Many of the patients referred to Rosen were among the most challenging to the physicians, and educational for her.

As Elaine Mayland, a senior Rosen Method teacher, notes:

> Patients who came to her with problems with physical origins taught Marion the potential of the body to heal itself. They taught her a great deal about the nature of the will to be well as a factor in maintaining body movement and health. She noticed that patients who talked with her about the events of their lives at the time of their accident or injury were the ones who recovered most quickly. She became convinced of the connection between mind and body and became increasingly successful in treating patients with psychosomatic illnesses—those developing with origins in emotional stress and withholding.[3]

An important development in Rosen's life came in the 1970s in a workshop with Werner Erhard entitled "Mind Dynamics." She was introduced to his work by a client whose musculoskeletal symptoms suddenly improved after taking the workshop. This training helped deepen her understanding of the mind-body connection, and she realized that she knew more than she ever admitted to herself or to clients. It was after this that the verbal part of her work took form in her clinical practice. She began talking to clients about their lives, listening to their words and bodies and responding with care and genuineness when they spoke their truth. Prior to this, as an apprentice with Lucy Heyer, only the psychiatrist spoke with clients. As a masseuse, she never spoke with clients about their conditions or lives. She now realized she had something to teach, and so began her career of teaching Rosen Method Bodywork.

She has taught her work since the late 1970s and continues to teach students and treat clients today at the age of 82. Her work is presently taught throughout the United States, Canada, and Europe, and there is a school in Russia. The Rosen Institute in Berkeley, California certifies schools around the world to teach Rosen Method Bodywork.

THEORY: NORMAL FUNCTION AND THE DEVELOPMENT OF BARRIERS OR DYSFUNCTION

An infant is born into the world with the possibility of moving freely and without tension. As she breathes, her entire body moves with her breath. As she develops, she naturally figures out how to move in a multitude of ways. She cries without inhibition, screams without a second thought, laughs with joy, and expresses a full range of other emotions with ease. Her somatic brilliance is unequaled: Without cognitive, rational education she knows how to suck, and learns to express herself, roll, creep, walk, and jump. She figures out who her caregivers are, what is safe to do and what is not. She learns how to speak, understand language, and develop concepts.

With the socialization process a child undergoes in order to learn how to succeed in her culture comes a narrowing of possibilities for movement, ease, and expression. A child learns how to move in certain ways; how to express herself in ways that are acceptable to her parents, family, school, and religion; and how to adapt herself to her culture.[4] These ways are often different and more limited than an infant's natural instincts. Muscular effort is required to modify, inhibit, and narrow a natural range of expression and feeling. This limits movement possibilities and a full range of musculoskeletal functions. Often, disease and illness eventually result from somatic vulnerabilities due to limited movement patterns.

This muscular effort becomes chronic tension patterns, or patterns of holding, resulting in barriers to the natural essence, or self, of the person. These patterns, used in a limited number of ways over many years, can result in physical dysfunction and symptoms often treated by physical therapists because the person cannot use her body parts the way they were meant to be used (Figure 3-1).

If a child is taught, for example, that it is wrong, in fact frowned upon, to cry when she

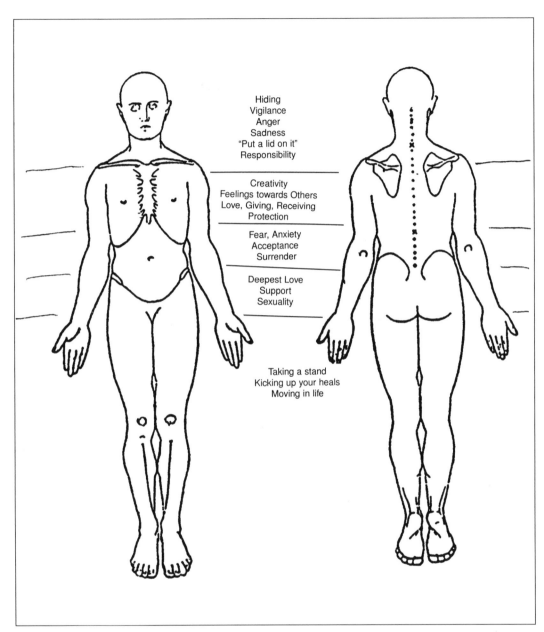

Figure 3-1. Rosen Method Bodywork General Body Map.

feels sad or scared, she will learn how to hold down her tears. This requires the tensing of anterior neck musculature. While she learns how to do this as a child, she may forget how to cry and, as an adult, maintain her tension patterns even though she may not remember why she was not allowed to cry as a child. Inhibiting herself requires physical tension, or holding. Repression is the muscular act of inhibition, and can result in forgetting the actual event (in this case, not being allowed to cry as a child) that led to the act of repression or inhibition of free expression.[5]

Marion Rosen's conclusion that a child's inhibition of emotional expression results in barriers to her true essence was the result of different aspects of her life. First, working with thousands of clients over many decades gave her insight into the role of expression and emotional freedom in the healing process. Another aspect was spending time with her daughter, from whom she learned about the development of the body, movement, the psyche, and emotions. She also learned a great deal about "the effects of child rearing practices upon the free and natural movement of the body"[3] and the expressive abilities of a child. Finally, her own experiences growing up in Germany and the journey she underwent to come to the United States also affected her work.

Rosen's was not a unique theory, but was arrived at independently from other practitioners. During the 1930s Wilhelm Reich, once a student and prodigy of Sigmund Freud, first described how the body tightens, condenses, and compresses as a byproduct of socialization. "Armor" is what Reich called the tightened musculature which forms a person's posture. "Character Structure" is how he defined the resultant personality traits. Reich called this physical act of holding in "repression," and defined repression as a bodily or biological function.[5] Rosen calls this holding a barrier to the person under the holding. Many contemporary somatic practices, often noted under the umbrella profession of Somatics, are based on aspects or refined versions of Reich's original theories and seek to help clients experience themselves more clearly from within. They are often practiced by body-oriented psychotherapists and bodyworkers.

TECHNIQUE

The technique of Rosen Method Bodywork is quite simple. The various parts of the technique, including the touch, the verbal part of the work, and the breath will all be described in detail.

GENERAL GUIDELINES

Rosen Method is practiced in one-on-one sessions with a client. Often clients come for relief of physical symptoms, but may also come for their own personal development, as an adjunct to psychotherapy or for spiritual growth. A practitioner will talk with a new client, usually on the telephone but also during the first session, about why she is coming for bodywork and what she hopes to receive or accomplish from the work. This is often done while the client is sitting up, but may also be done while the client is lying on a treat-ment table. Prior to treatment, the practitioner will do a body reading to acquire somatic information about the client.

Usually, a client wears only her underwear and is draped appropriately to respect her privacy. Many times, however, a practitioner will ask a client to leave on whatever clothes she needs to feel comfortable and safe. He may suggest that shorts and a tee shirt or bathing suit top be worn. A client first lies prone on the treatment table with a pillow under her lower legs only. If she has cervical or other musculoskeletal problems, other pil-lows and towels can be used to reduce the tension in these areas. A face cradle is usually not used so a practitioner can see a client's face during the session. Pregnant women can be treated in sidelying. After about 30 minutes or so of treatment, a client is asked to turn over and lie supine for the remainder of the 50- to 60-minute treatment session. While supine, the pillow is moved beneath her knees. Near the end of a session, a practitioner will usually tell the client, "I'm going to stop in a minute or two," so a client has time to prepare for ending. After the session is over, a client may stay on the table for a few min-utes before getting up, dressing, and leaving. There is often no or little dialogue after the session so a client can remain in the state of awareness from the session without having to jump back into a left brain, rational, intellectual milieu too quickly.

Clients usually come for sessions once weekly, but that will vary depending upon a client's financial situation, reasons for coming, scheduling, etc. The duration of treatment depends upon the client's needs. Sometimes only one session is needed; other times a client may come for many years. If Rosen Method is part of the physical therapy treatment, the client will come for the duration of physical therapy and the work can be integrated into the physical therapy treatment program. Prior to treatment, a physical therapy eval-uation is done in addition to a Rosen body reading. Some physical therapy clients contin-ue to come for Rosen Method after their physical symptoms are alleviated because they realize how much they are receiving and healing as a result of the work and are willing to pay for it themselves. According to Marion Rosen, "They get rid of the symptoms. From then on it is up to them to go further, to want to stay well and do more. Rosen Method goes a step further than physical therapy."[2]

As one client said:

> I started to understand my chronic physical pain as a calling card. After years of trying to get it fixed, I saw it was a door opening for me to understand myself more fully, if only I would walk through it and not try to obliterate it. Even though my pain is often gone now, I continue to come for Rosen sessions because I want to understand my deeper self more clearly. Rosen Method has helped me understand myself and develop a new relationship with my body.

TOUCH: MORE THAN SKIN DEEP

The quality of touch used by a Rosen Practitioner is specific, noninvasive, and very sensitive. The practitioner meets the client's muscle tension with equal pressure, neither too lightly nor too forcefully. The touch might be deep or superficial, depending upon the type, depth, and location of holding, but the quality does not change. By meeting the holding equally instead of doing something to it by manipulating and trying to change it, the muscle has the opportunity to relax and stop holding as it is ready. Gentle, sometimes imperceptible movement of the muscle gives the client's body a subtle reminder of what it is like to move, something many clients have forgotten during all the years of holding.

A Rosen Practitioner has no predetermined agenda for a client. Nothing is done to make something happen in a particular way. The client's own pace of relaxation and letting down of barriers is respected, honored, and followed. In this way a client is the leader, and the practitioner, while a facilitator, is at the same time a follower, allowing the internal wisdom of the body to guide the therapy. This is imperative because people do not change until they are ready for change; a body or muscle will not relax until it is ready; a barrier needed for many years will not release until the person "underneath" is ready. A Rosen Practitioner trusts the internal wisdom of the body to help the client heal and improve in function.

A Rosen Practitioner's hands are touching much more deeply than the skin and muscle. He is touching the person, the self doing the holding and creating the barrier. As one Rosen teacher described it, "You touch the soul of the client when you work."[6] The very essence of a client's being or self is touched, allowing the person on the other side of the barrier to come forth.

Through his hands, a practitioner can feel many things. The temperature, texture, and quality of the skin are the first elements sensed. The degree and distribution of tension, or muscle holding, can be felt. The direction of holding is also important, as it gives a practitioner information about what the client does not allow and cannot do functionally. One of the most important elements a practitioner can feel is a client's breath—its distribution or lack thereof, its depth, its fullness or incompleteness, its rhythm.

A client who had tried various kinds of therapies to ease her pain from an L5, S1 disc bulge after a lifting injury 1 year earlier described the touch as follows:

> I've been worked on a lot by massage therapists, my bones have been moved by physical therapists and chiropractors, I've tried biofeedback, meditation and medication. It all helped, but something was always missing. With Rosen Method, even though it doesn't feel like much is being done during a treatment, I feel so relaxed afterward and my pain is gone. It feels like I've been seen and accepted for who I am and my body takes a sigh of relief.

BREATH

"Through my hands I talk to the body and the breath gives me the answer."[2] The breath is one of the most focused-on aspects of the body in Rosen Method. Although the practitioner is constantly observing the client's breath, he very rarely discusses it with the client and never asks her to breathe a certain way. This would only engage a client's conscious, rational mind and inhibit her automatic, natural, wave-like breath which appears when a client is deeply relaxed. Helping a client rediscover this breath is one goal of Rosen Method.

The breath is the guide to the unconscious since it is innervated by both the voluntary and autonomic nervous systems. With a natural, full, relaxed breath a deep wave of movement moves through the entire body. While in prone and supine, a client's breath is observable from head to knees. When a baby breathes, its entire body moves with the breath, or the breath moves through the entire body. As a child grows older and is socialized, the breath becomes limited. It is in these areas of holding that the practitioner focuses his treatment to facilitate relaxation, allowing breath to move into them. This, then, can help a client find new possibilities for movement and function in her life.

The diaphragm is the primary muscle of respiration. With its attachment circumferentially, joining the lower and upper halves of the body, it is the most important muscle in the body. When swinging freely and fully, the diaphragm gives a free 24-hour massage to many internal organs which lie adjacent to it. When it is held with anxiety or fear, constriction takes place and circulation and organ function can be compromised, respiratory capacity decreased, and well-being diminished.

The diaphragm is worked on during most Rosen sessions, and is contacted in the lower thoracic area while a client is prone and along the bottom of the rib cage while a client is supine. Indirectly, it can be treated by working in the areas of the vagus nerve in the neck. The movement of the diaphragm and the client's breathing are used by the practitioner as a guide to the client's internal unconscious process. As the held breath changes and the diaphragm relaxes, gurgling and other abdominal sounds may be heard. More of the body begins to move with the breath, and the practitioner uses this as an indication that the client is moving from a more held, repressed, or dissociated mode into a more relaxed mode where what was held in the unconscious may have a chance to surface into consciousness. While a practitioner, or even the client, may not be aware of what is happening on this level, a practitioner understands that whatever is going on for the client at this time is important. He may or may not say anything but always is respectful of its importance emotionally for a client. "This is when a client contacts her essence; this is when the healing happens."[2]

This change will usually happen every session, but not necessarily. One physical therapy client who came for 3 months of treatment for a cervical sprain/strain injury from a motor vehicle accident continued for over a year of Rosen Bodywork after her acute pain eased. Her original signs of cervical pain radiating into her left shoulder and symptoms of C3,4,5 rotational dysfunctions cleared with soft tissue work, muscle energy technique, myofacial release, and a strengthening/stabilization program. However, her range of motion improved only 50%. With her consent, we added Rosen Method Bodywork 6 weeks into her rehabilitation and she would then leave sessions pain-free and with full range of motion. Prior to this addition, she held herself stiffly during most of every session, although she would sometimes relax her more superficial musculature while deeper muscles stayed tense. With Rosen Method she could allow her armor to soften. After a year she began, quite unconsciously, to allow her body to relax more fully, and during one session, her breath changed—it deepened and more of her belly and pelvis moved with her breath. This differed greatly from her usual shallow chest breathing. Physically, the practitioner could feel her diaphragm move more easily and the deeper muscles of her spine soften. Movement was observable from her neck to her knees. It was not for another 2 months that she revealed the constant message she got at home in Germany as a child: to keep quiet and not talk or make a sound. If she made a sound, the Nazis might find her and her family. While she knew all of this intellectually, she had never been able to integrate this knowledge with any emotional qualities or somatic understanding. Although her original cervical symptoms had eased a year earlier, she could not enjoy the freedom of moving and expressing herself, the inhibition of which made her neck vulnerable to injury. She also had a deeper understanding of how the narrative facts of her life impacted her somatically.

VERBAL WORK

"You talk to the body and watch for a response."[2] The verbal part of Rosen Method Bodywork is one way of helping clients bring to consciousness what is unconscious. A practitioner, as always, pays close attention to what is happening in a client's body and may reflect this verbally to the client in a nonjudgmental way.

There are different ways in which the verbal part of the work occurs. Information obtained about the body through touch and vision may be presented to the client. If what is said by the practitioner has emotional truth for the client, she will respond physically, usually by unconsciously relaxing and allowing breath, or movement from the breath, to come into the held area. What is said by the practitioner is said to the body, not to the intellectual, rational mind of the client. What is said is based on the function of the held area of the body. More on this will be described later in a section on Body Maps.

For example, a nun who was in an automobile accident and being treated in physical therapy for a whiplash injury and thoracic dysfunction was lying prone on a treatment table. While treating her mid-thoracic region, integrating Rosen Method with soft tissue mobilization, the therapist said, "This area (rhomboids, middle trapezius region, bilaterally) seems to have forgotten how to receive." The client's breathing broadened to include this previously very tense area, and became deeper and more relaxed. After several minutes she responded, "Just before you said that about forgetting how to receive I thought to myself, 'I've been taken advantage of a lot.'" She sighed deeply and her entire upper body flowed with movement as she breathed. She had inhibited reaching out to receive (protraction of her scapulae) in order to not feel the pain of being taken advantage of.

Another client, a 42-year-old woman whose 2-year anniversary of her breast cancer diagnosis was on the day of treatment, had a great deal of tension and holding on the left side of her thoracic spine, just behind the heart. The practitioner's words, "This is where we sometimes hold when we feel betrayed," led to the patient crying and saying, "I've had a lot of that." However, her body did not respond to this; there was no relaxation or change in her breathing. The practitioner, thinking that the betrayal had to do with her body developing cancer, did not respond verbally. He maintained contact with her through touch. A few minutes later, as she stopped crying, she said, "My boyfriend broke up with me just after I was diagnosed." With this her diaphragm quivered with several breaths, then relaxed, and her back began to move and her breathing deepened. Her true feelings of betrayal had to do with her loss of relationship, not with her cancer. She had been referred to physical therapy for burning pain in her upper right thoracic region and decreased range of motion of her right shoulder as a result of a complete mastectomy. Her burning pain ceased and her range of motion increased to normal after this, her fourth treatment. She had been protecting herself from the emotional pain of feeling abandoned by splinting with her musculature. During subsequent physical therapy treatment, she was able to do the therapeutic exercises to strengthen and stabilize her upper body, which she had not been able to do previously because they reinforced her tension pattern and increased her pain.

Other times, clients will talk during a physical therapy treatment. As always, a practitioner pays close attention to the client's body to follow the emotional truth of the client. When the body responds, a practitioner may reflect back to the client what is happening in her body. There will be times when no verbal response is given but the contact with the client, through touch and awareness, is always maintained.

As a practitioner was mobilizing the thoracic spine of a client with a severely stiffened spine and strong spasms of her paraspinals due to neuromuscular changes resulting from aper-nicious anemia, the client was talking about her difficulties doing things around the house. She talked about her frustration at having to quit her job and shame about having to apply for MediCal (Medicaid) after losing her health care insurance. Although she was talking about very difficult events and the emotions she felt because of them, her breath did not change, nor did her held areas move any differently. She complained, too, about how her son just does things for himself, never wanting to help her. Her body tensed, particularly the back of her neck. She then started talking about how hard it had been for her 12-year-old son "having a mom who he has to help up and down the stairs because my balance is so bad." Her back started to relax a little and her breathing deepened. The practitioner reflected this back to her, "You have a lot of feelings about what your son must be going through." One tear rolled down her cheek; she breathed deeply and said, "That is the hardest part." Her body continued to relax as she lay on the table quietly. When she walked out of the clinic, her gait was more fluid in its rhythm, she could allow her legs to move at all of their joints without the scissoring hip pattern and locked knees, and her balance was better than it had been for 2 months.

Sometimes, a practitioner will have an image or thought independent from what a client says or, apparently, from what is happening in a client's body. This intuition might be verbalized to the client. If it rings true for the client, her body will respond. If not, the practitioner disregards it and realizes it is his own image and not one of the client's. This mode of gathering information can be effective but is also somewhat less reliable and must be used very cautiously.

For example, toward the end of a quiet, uneventful session, the practitioner kept seeing the color blue even though there was no new blue object in the room. After several minutes, the image of blue reappeared and the practitioner said to the client, "Does the color blue have any meaning to you?" With a deep sigh, the client described how the room she had as a little girl was blue. It was the only safe room in her house because her older brothers were not allowed in. This meant they could not "torment and hit me like they did outside. I would spend a lot of time in there. I have very fond memories of that room." As she was putting her clothes back on, she described how she was feeling more at ease in her body, "like the feeling I would get when I hid in my room."

BODY READING

A Rosen Practitioner will begin assessing a client's body as soon as she walks in the door of the office. The practitioner observes how a client moves and how and where she is holding tension and does not allow movement, distribution of body weight and density, breathing pattern, symmetry from top to bottom and side to side, and pace and aliveness of movement. Voice tone and quality as well as skin color also are noted. The practitioner is looking for areas that the client holds back, down, in, etc., and does not allow fullness and expression in her life, and areas where she allows herself movement and fullness without holding.

A client may have a compressed or inflated chest, elevated and pulled back shoulders and tense neck, held-in abdomen, erect or collapsed spine, pinched buttocks, legs held tightly together or spread apart, knees locked or collapsed, feet held toes up or dragging, or a client may exhibit other postures. The way a client holds herself reflects her internal unconscious processes and affects her ability to move. A practitioner will observe this while a client walks, undresses, and gets on the treatment table.

He will not interpret why a person holds tension in a particular way. This is allowed to unfold during the healing process. Even if a practitioner has some idea or thought about a client's stance or attitude in life, he will not burden the client with his own interpretation because the client's own somatic experience is the most important.

Part of the body reading will be performed tactiley as well. A practitioner may have a client stand while he palpates areas of her body that appear to be held or tense. A tactile body reading is the first thing done during each session while a client is lying on the treatment table. A practitioner gently runs his hands along the client's body, feeling for areas that are held and not moving with the breath.

This visual and tactile information, in addition to the client's verbal description of why she came for treatment, is used to help guide a practitioner to areas of treatment.

BODY MAP: FUNCTIONAL ANATOMY

Marion Rosen uses the body as a guide to understanding a client's emotional barriers. She maps the body based upon the functions of each area of the body. While these are generalizations, she has discovered a relationship of body segments to emotional holding by treating and listening to thousands of clients. To describe her map she uses common, heartfelt language a client will easily understand. Her map is as follows (see Figure 3-1).[2,3]

NECK AND TOP OF TORSO

Emotions of anger and sadness are held here. The scaleni and omohyoid are involved with holding in tears and yelling because these are the muscles used for expressing these emotions. The back of the neck bulges and hardens as a person holds back anger.

Responsibility may be reflected as tensely elevated shoulders, such as when a person "carries the world on his shoulders." Other emotional expressions include hiding, cringing, surprise, being wide-eyed, vigilance, etc.

HEART AND MID-TRUNK

Feelings towards others are held back by this area. This is the area of love on a personal level. When held back through the scapula, it is difficult to reach out to give and receive, and challenging to be creative. It is holding or pushing others away. A caved-in chest may reflect feelings about being loved, and tension behind the heart, as though one has been "stabbed in the back," is a way to protect the heart. An upright citizen might hold her spine erect and not allow flexibility in her life.

DIAPHRAGM

This is the most important muscle in the body because it is the primary muscle of respiration, and therefore, the link between the conscious and the unconscious. Fear and anxiety are held here. When relaxed and swinging freely, massaging the internal organs, a person will experience and feel self-acceptance and surrender—surrender to love.

PELVIS, DEEP IN THE BELLY

The pelvis is the body's support, and holding here may reflect a person's experience of feeling too much or too little support in life. Digestive problems and sexuality issues may be stored in this area as well. Held in this area are fear and repression of the deepest love. When this area lets go, true, deep love is experienced. "The emotion most held back is love."[3]

These are general guidelines; each client is unique and different and may experience barriers or tensions with different emotional roots. Many aphorisms describe body function but originate in emotional processes, including: keep a stiff upper lip, put a lid on it, hold your tongue, a gut feeling, kick up your heels, stand your ground, dig in your feet, hold your position, caved in under pressure, keep at arm's distance, hold it together. These and many more are physical descriptors of internal emotional processes that require muscular effort to maintain. Prolonged effort or tension can lead to vulnerable areas of the body which, paradoxically, was used as a protective mechanism by the client.

EXERCISES

Rosen Method is taught largely by apprenticeship. The 2-year classroom training includes many, many hours of practicing the work and is followed by a 350-hour internship with a supervisor. To give the reader a taste of the type of touch used by a Rosen Practitioner, the following two exercises are provided.

Some thoughts to keep in mind while you practice are:

- Your hands can listen and feel as well as touch.
- You are just meeting the client's tension, not trying to make it change.
- Be curious about who the person is who is doing the holding—who is under the barrier. This is the essence you are meeting.
- What do you feel (including tense areas, areas that move, the breathing pattern and location, temperature, etc.)?
- Does the client's body change as you touch?

Your partner can give you feedback about your touch by answering the following:

- Do you feel met?
- Is the pressure too much or too little?
- How engaged in the process do you feel?

HEAD, NECK, SHOULDERS

A client/partner can sit in a chair in front of the practitioner, who can stand or sit behind the client. The client can, if she is comfortable, remove her shirt or lower her collar enough so the practitioner can see and feel her neck and shoulders. Practitioner, rest your hands on your client's shoulders, just feeling her body in this area. After several minutes of feeling the tension, temperature, and breath, begin to adjust your pressure to match the client's tension. You may move your hands around or leave them in one place for now. Again, observe, through your hands. When you feel ready, begin to explore other areas of her shoulders, neck, and head. Always just meet the tension; be curious about it and do not try to make anything happen. Continue for 10 to 15 minutes in these areas. After you are done, you and your client/partner can discuss your experiences and then trade places.

BACK WHILE PRONE ON THE TABLE

The client/partner will lie prone on a treatment table with her back exposed and her lower legs on a pillow. The practitioner will stand alongside the table and place his hands on the client's back. Again, you are just feeling her holding or tension and not making anything happen to it. As in the first exercise, observe all the same autonomic nervous system functions. After several minutes, begin to curiously explore your client's back, meeting her tension as you empathically and respectfully move your hands. When you find areas that are held, remain with them for several minutes and note what happens. Continue for 10 to 15 minutes. After you are done, you and your client/partner can discuss your experiences and then trade places.

ROSEN METHOD MOVEMENT: "PHYSICAL THERAPY IN REVERSE"[7]

In 1956, Marion Rosen was asked how to prevent aches and pains between physical therapy treatments. Her answer to this question was to develop a movement class combining the exercises she had given to many of her private patients with her love of dance. She called it "physical therapy in reverse" because it focused on prevention of musculoskeletal problems.

The movement exercises in a Rosen Movement class use music and rhythm as adjuncts to movement because they help facilitate participants to move. Classes are about 45 minutes long and focus on releasing held areas so expansion and mobility are permitted. Marion Rosen designed the exercises around range of motion exercises so all joints in the body are moved in all directions, softening and toning muscles, increasing joint range and overall flexibility. Because the breath is a vital part of Rosen Method, movements encourage release of the diaphragm so the chest cavity has more space for breathing.

Some of the primary objectives of the movement classes include lubricating all body joints, expansion of the rib cage, lengthening of held muscles so habitual movement patterns can be modified and the body can reshape itself without pain, increased body awareness, prevention of injury, movement with joy, increased choice of movement, and social interaction.

The class provides a fun, social environment during which relaxation of the body is followed by simple, slow, single joint and double joint movements. Then, faster and more complex movements are added. Movements are always pleasurable and should not cause pain or discomfort. A significant part of the class consists of pausing for breath. This allows time for slowing down and conscious body awareness before starting more complex movements. The classes often end with large dance-like movements and movements with partners.

The movement classes can support the bodywork as a way for a client to feel movement with ease and relaxation. As an adjunct to physical therapy treatment, the movement classes provide an excellent source of exercise that is not painful but does require strength, endurance, and agility. Particularly for clients who cannot participate in rigorous exercise, the Rosen Movement classes provide a form of exercise as well as a way to limit the possibility of exacerbation.

SUMMARY

In Rosen Method Bodywork, healing does not necessarily mean fixing, as in contemporary physical therapy. While this does happen, and a client may no longer experience symptoms she had been having, it is not always the goal. Instead, a deeper healing process which includes mind, body, and spirit is engaged so a client will grow into her wholeness.

Unlike physical therapy, Rosen Method is about doing very little beyond being fully present with a client. It is a work that expands a practitioner's scientific, rational left brain approach into his intuitive, creative right brain. As Oliver Sacks wrote, "[I had to give to the] active, ordering masculine self which I had equated with my science, my self-respect," in order to heal.[8] It requires trust in the client's ability to heal without specific goals and guidelines set forth by the practitioner. When integrated with contemporary physical therapy, such as manual approaches, exercise, body mechanics, neuromuscular re-education, etc., a client can participate fully in her own healing process while also relying on the therapist for his knowledge and expertise.

Is all pain emotional? Marion Rosen is often asked this question.

> No, but all pain has an emotional background. How you deal with a structural problem must include this. What a person brings into healing, what her life experiences are when her pain started affects how she will heal. Pain results from the feelings that are held back, not expressed. They are the feelings left in the body when the event occurred that matters. What happened doesn't matter; how you hold is what matters.[2]

Rosen Method is concerned with facilitating a client's ability to express herself and her body's healing capacities for a fuller, richer, and healthier life.

REFERENCES

1. Hanna T. *Somatics: Reawakening the Mind's Control of Movement, Flexibility, and Health.* Boston, Mass: Addison-Wesley Publishing Company, Inc; 1988.
2. Rosen M. All quotations from Rosen were taken between 1985 and 1987 during the author's training in Rosen Method Bodywork and in 1994 during personal interviews.

3. Mayland E. *Rosen Method: An Approach to Wholeness and Well-Being Through the Body*. Elaine Mayland; 1991.

4. Berger D. A mind-body approach: psychophysical dimensions of treatment. *PT, A Magazine of Physical Therapy*. September 1994;2(9):66-75.

5. Reich W, Carfagno V, trans. *Character Analysis*. 3rd ed. New York, NY: Noonday Press; 1991.

6. Barrie L. Quote taken in 1986 during training with Barrie, a senior Rosen Method teacher.

7. Rosen M, Brenner S. *The Rosen Method of Movement*. Berkeley, Calif: North Atlantic Books; 1991.

8. Sacks O. *A Leg to Stand On*. New York, NY: Summit Books; 1984:170.

SUGGESTED READINGS

Duff K. *Alchemy of Illness*. New York, NY: Bell Tower; 1993.

Hanna T. What is somatics? *Somatics Magazine*. Spring/Summer 1986:1-4.

Johnson D. *Body*. Boston, Mass: Beacon Press; 1983.

Johnson D. *Body, Spirit and Democracy*. Berkeley, Calif: North Atlantic Books; 1994.

Keleman S. *Emotional Anatomy*. Berkeley, Calif: Center Press; 1985.

Lowen A. *The Language of the Body*. New York, NY: McMillan Publishing Company; 1958.

Mindell A. *Working With the Dreaming Body*. London, England: Arkan Publishers; 1985.

Shepard K, Jensen G, Schmoll B, et al. Alternative approaches to research in physical therapy: positivism and phenomenology. *Physical Therapy*. 1993;73(2):88-101.

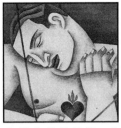

CHAPTER 4

ROLFING, HELLERWORK, AND SOMA

Jim Tavrazich, PT

INTRODUCTION

Structural Integration, or Rolfing as it is more popularly known, was developed by Dr. Ida P. Rolf (1896-1979). Born in New York City, she earned her PhD in biochemistry and was an associate at Rockefeller Institute. Her interests ranged beyond organic chemistry and she made intensive studies of osteopathy, yoga, homeopathy, and other body-centered therapies in the 1920s and 1930s. These interests were in part due to a motivation to improve her own health, and later, that of one of her sons. Through her studies, unique insights, and the application of the empirical methods of a research scientist, Dr. Rolf developed the theory and techniques of Structural Integration by the late 1950s. In 1973, she established the Rolf Institute. Today the Institute is a primary organization for training Rolfers and promoting public awareness of and supporting research related to Rolfing.

Rolfing is concerned with improving well-being and overall health. One of Dr. Rolf's central premises is the osteopathic concept that structure determines function.[1] The phys-

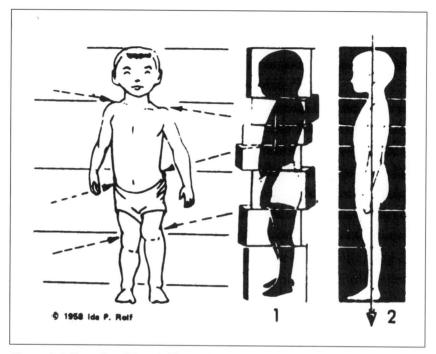

Figure 4-1. *Reproduced from Rolf IP. Rolfing the Integration of Human Structures. New York, NY: Harper and Row; 1978.*

ical relationships of the body's tissues (its structure) determine how the body functions, from gross movement to cellular activity.

Dr. Rolf realized that the optimal structure (and hence function) is one in which the body has a vertical relationship to gravity. Bodies cannot escape the influence of gravity. When the body is not in balance with gravity, as is evidenced when its segments are not balanced around a vertical line, the body segments are subjected to unrelenting unequal pull by gravity. The result is constant and progressive deterioration of structure and function. However, vertical alignment and balance can be improved. When this occurs, "the force of gravity can flow through. Then spontaneously, the body heals itself."[1]

Figure 4-1, taken from tracings of before and after photographs of a young child who was Rolfed, illustrates these ideas. The body segments of head, thorax lumbar spine, pelvis, thigh, and leg in the "before" tracing show the common structural relationships Dr. Rolf called random. The body is balanced, but not relative to a vertical line. Rather the anterior tilted pelvis causes the exaggerated lumbar lordosis which causes the thorax to compensate with excess kyphosis which results in forward head and shoulders. Similar leg imbalances exist which undermine pelvic support. The body segments are tilted and rotated, and their centers of gravity are displaced in a zigzag pattern of compensations. The body is subject to compressions and strains as it battles gravity to remain upright—a battle gravity eventually will win.

The "after" tracing shows the body balanced around the vertical line. Most significantly, the centers of gravity of the body segments are now located along the vertical line. Although not shown, the body is also symmetrical right to left. Gravity is not pulling down unequally on the segments, as there is now equal mass on each side of the line. The legs support a horizontal pelvis, which in turn reduces the excessive lumbar lordosis. As a result, the thoracic kyphosis is improved, the ribcage lifts, and the thorax forms a stable, level platform, allowing head and shoulder to come on line. With the centers of gravity of the segments supporting each other, the need for the zigzag of the compensations is removed. The body is able to attain its ideal length.

As physical therapists we might say, "Oh, Rolfing is just improving posture." We recognize the vertical line as the plumb line used to assess posture. But Dr. Rolf pointed out that structure is not posture.[2] Posture refers to how the body is positioned and held in position, often using muscular effort. Structure deals with how the tissues determine body alignment and support. Balanced structure is maintained without physical or conscious effort.

All this so far deals with static balance. Dynamic balance also improves with Rolfing because balanced structure allows balanced movement. Legs, for example, will track straight during ambulation and not in a toed in or toed out fashion. Also, in balanced movement, "when flexors flex, extensors extend."[2] In random bodies, the agonist-antagonist balance is often disturbed, causing distorted movement patterns and joint stresses.

CORE-SLEEVE RELATIONSHIP

Another aspect of balance is the core-sleeve relationship. The body's core can be envisioned as the spine and its supportive myofascia and the sleeve as the pelvic and shoulder girdles and limbs and the outer myofascia. Generally, the core is the axial skeleton and myofascia, and the sleeve is the appendages. The core ideally provides stable and resilient support. The working sleeve performs locomotion and manipulation. In a balanced body, the core supports the sleeve but is not disturbed by the activity of the sleeve. Also, the sleeve should not be engaged in the core functions of supporting the body. This is seldom the case in imbalanced body structure.

An additional important facet of balance recognized in Rolfing is mind-body balance. Dr. Rolf held that mind and body are different aspects of the same reality. Negative emotional response is often reflected in a physical response including a myofascial reaction. If

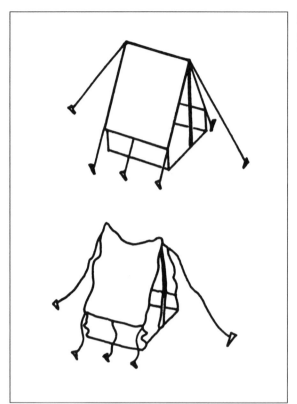

Figure 4-2. *Reproduced from Rolf IP. Rolfing the Integration of Human Structures. New York, NY: Harper and Row; 1978.*

the myofascial pattern persists, it can help perpetrate the emotional response. Similarly, structural imbalance may reinforce a sense of psychological insecurity—not feeling centered in the body may contribute to lessened emotional centeredness.

FASCIA

Dr. Rolf realized that the primary tissue of support and shape in the body is fascia.[2] Fascia is the most extensive body tissue; it wraps every muscle, vessel, organ, and nerve down to the level of the extracellular matrix. Additionally, fascia is a continuous structure throughout the body, from its superficial layers to its deepest investing layers. Fascia is a continuous, intricate, three-dimensional web determining the body's form. Where fascia thickens to form tendons and ligaments it displays dense innervation. And of central importance, fascia is changeable and plastic. Just as fascia can maintain imbalance, it can be brought into improved "span and tone."[1]

Dr. Rolf used the analogy of the body being a tent to demonstrate how myofascia supports the upright body (Figure 4-2).[2] The rigid tent poles are analogous to bones and the tent fabric and ropes to myofascia. In a tent, it is not only the poles that support and give form to the tent. Rather the downward pull of the fabric and ropes determines pole orientation and the shape of the tent. The poles act as spacers for the ropes and fabric, giving them the proper length and tension. If even a single rope is too taut, the poles are pulled out of alignment and the fabric and other ropes are stressed unevenly so that the tent leans in some places and sags in others. The tent is pulled out of shape by gravity.

Similarly, in the upright body the function of the bones is not to hold up the body by taking compression. Rather, the function of the bones is to give balanced span and tone to the myofascia. When the body segments are aligned, the bones permit the optimal balance of the myofascia. This is a circular situation because myofascial tone and span determine bone position which in turn affects tone and span. Rolfers maintain that the myofascia is the primary determinant of the body's form and that balancing the myofascia allows the bones to assume their ideal arrangement.

The tent analogy is also useful because it shows how the effects of local imbalance do not remain localized. Only one overly taut rope results in aberrant tensions throughout the entire tent—poles, rope, and fabric. This happens in bodies, as the extensive nature of myofascia may result in compensations seemingly remote from the location of insult.

Structural imbalances develop in many ways. A sprained ankle, for instance, may cause local myofascial restrictions at the ankle resulting from inflammation and immobilization. While in acute pain, the person alters his or her gait to favor the ankle, disrupting myofascial balance and alignment elsewhere in the body. Also, due to myofascial continuity, the ankle restriction may change myofascial tone and span up the leg and, consequently, in the pelvis and spine. These changes may persist even after the acute ankle pain is gone and they are seen as slight changes in stance, posture, and gait. The effects of these "minor" traumas occurring throughout life may be subtle but they are cumulative, resulting in "random" bodies.

There are other sources of structural imbalance. Negative emotional trauma may elicit a myofascial response. We feel grief, depression, and fear in our bodies, in our myofascia. These myofascial reactions produce effects similar to those caused by the twisted ankle. Additionally, the structural response may form a reinforcing loop with the persisting emotional response. Habitual patterns of body use and posture also may cause imbalances (eg, the worker who spends hours slouched at his desk). Another source of imbalance is emulation of others. We may consciously or unconsciously adapt the posture of others, for example, the child who copies his father's posture or walk. This list is not exhaustive.

The effects of structural imbalance are numerous. Look at the "before" tracing in Figure 4-1 again. Such a structure would cause joint strains and compressions (low back, neck); myofascial strain and eventual fibrosis as muscles constantly try to hold up the body (thoracic paraspinals, hamstrings); excessive muscular energy use to hold body segments; poor respiration due to rib position; and inefficient gait with abnormal joint function. The core is giving insufficient support. Sleeve activity will continually distort the core, perpetrating its weakness. Cellular exchange may be compromised because of myofascial tension on vessels; the result is poor nutrition and metabolite removal. Abnormal tension on nerves can affect their function and, thus, the function of their end organs; for example, a tight psoas can put pressure on the lumbar plexus. Dr. Rolf would describe these last two examples not as pathology but "perversion of physiology."[1]

Dr. Rolf developed a systematic approach to assessing structure and improving balance and support. The technique involves applying manual force to the myofascial restriction and then having the client perform small movements. By placing the structure "nearest to the place it should be"[1] the elicited movement will be more balanced. Dr. Rolf described what she was doing as softening the fascia by using energy in the form of manual force, essentially taking it from a semisolid gel state to a more liquid sol state,[3] to allow improved movement and myofascial balance. Recently, Rolfers have been addressing the probable neurological component of the technique. They note that deep pressure also may inhibit abnormal myofascial tension via the Golgi tendon reflex and muscle spindles.[3,4] This creates an opportunity for more balanced movement as well. Schleip's explanation that the immediate short-term effect of a Rolfing manipulation is mainly a neuromuscular tonus change that feeds into long-term changes in fascial density and arrangement seems reasonable.[5]

THE ROLFING SERIES

The basic Rolfing series involves 10 1-hour sessions of myofascial mobilization and movement re-education aimed at establishing the vertical line in the body. Sessions 1-3 are the superficial sessions. The focus is the outer fascial layers and sleeve. Session 1 goals are to free the rib cage from the spine; free the pelvic and shoulder girdles from the spine; improve rib mobility and breathing; and lengthen the front of the trunk. Session 2 aims to improve the foot, ankle, and knee myofascial balance and, complementing Session 1, to lengthen the back of the trunk. Session 3 lengthens an imaginary "lateral line" extending from ear to lateral knee. The lateral line is where the front and back (addressed in Sessions 1 and 2) intersect. Session 3 concludes with lengthening the quadratus lumborum to begin getting the pelvis horizontal—that is, out of its anterior tilt.

Sessions 4-7 are the deep sessions. They are deep because the structures worked are those of the deep, supportive tissues of the body, not because deeper pressure is applied.

As Session 3 lengthened the lateral line, Session 4 lengthens the "medial line" running from the pubic ramus to the medial malleolus. The goal is to balance the hip-knee-ankle tissues and to free the pelvis (which is the lower end of the body's "core") from below. Session 5 works the front of the pelvis. Goals include establishing balance between the psoas (core) and rectus abdominus (sleeve); lengthening the body's front; and further horizontalizing the pelvis. Additional tissues worked include diaphragm, pectorals, and quadriceps. Session 6 works the back of the pelvis. Posterior leg, gluteal, and hip rotator balance are the focus. Session 7 balances head, neck, and shoulder relationships. Dr. Rolf observed that the head could be effectively righted only after support and balance from below has been achieved.

Sessions 8, 9, and 10 focus on integrating the balances established in the superficial and deep sessions. Sessions 8 and 9 work the upper and lower halves of the body. Long myofascial connections are the focus. Integrating core and sleeve is the goal. The core should lengthen to initiate movement and support the sleeve while not being distorted by sleeve activity. Session 10 works the entire body to even out remaining snags and send the client out balanced and on his or her line.

Note that Rolfing is not only about releasing myofascial restrictions, but is also about building in support. For example, a horizontal pelvis is key to ideal spinal alignment; it supports this alignment. To be horizontal, the pelvis requires balanced support from the legs as well.

Notice the progressive nature of the 10 sessions. Superficial work precedes deep work and both are integrated in the late sessions. The client's structure is improved a little in each session. This improves the way the client functions between sessions and prepares the way for the next session. "There's a steadiness, a gradual straightening that organizes the body."[1]

Also note the balance inherent in the sessions. A session focusing on the front of the body is followed by one balancing the back. Lateral line work is followed by medial line. The sessions balance each other. This allows the body to accept and integrate the work in an organized progression that feels "right." Throughout, the critical measure is how the body segments relate to the vertical line, that is, how they relate to gravity. Much of Dr. Rolf's genius lies in her insights into human structure and function and her development of an objectively based, teachable approach to assess and improve structure.

This bare bones description of Rolfing has emphasized the anatomical aspects familiar to physical therapists. Dr. Rolf's text, *Rolfing: The Integration of Human Structures*,[2] gives a sense of her larger vision of Rolfing. Examples of topics include: the physiological basis of psychology; the energy body; monism and dualism; and Structural Integration as an aid to personal evolution.

ROLFING MOVEMENT INTEGRATION

Complementing Rolfing is Rolfing Movement Integration. This approach focuses on the way people hold tension and how they experience and use their bodies. Awareness exercises and movements are used to release tension and integrate body movement. A client may benefit from Rolfing Movement Integration after the basic series, or Movement work may be done independently.

People who have been Rolfed typically report positive results. Energy levels may increase, because the body is expending less muscular effort maintaining inefficient posture. Ease of movement improves. The client may gain height, because length is not being lost to body segment displacements. There is a sense of "lift" to the body, which is the subjective experience of alignment to the client's vertical line. There may be emotional changes; for example, less negativity, more openness in social contact, and a greater sense of security (possibly due to increased physical security in gravity).[2] Chronic aches and pains may improve, although Rolfing is not about relieving pain and Rolfers tell clients that any improvement in symptoms is coincidental and not the object of the sessions.

RESEARCH CONDUCTED ON THE EFFECTS OF ROLFING

There have been numerous studies on the effects of Rolfing. Hunt et al[6] administered electromyelograms during common activities of daily living, electroencephalograms of right and left hemispheres, and the State-Trait Anxiety Inventory, and took Kirlian photographs of experimental (Rolfed) subjects and controls. Results indicated that Rolfing decreased anxiety states; had a positive effect on hemispheric dominance; increased emanations of auric fields; and produced a major improvement in the efficacy of motor performance. The authors suggest this last effect could reduce muscular pain and strain and conserve energy.

Perry, Jones, and Thomas[7] measured lower extremity passive range of motion, muscle strength and balance, and gait in subjects with cerebral palsy. They found that locomotor gains were measurable in young, mildly involved patients, while patients with severe impairment displayed no gains. The authors suggest Rolfing may be useful as an adjunct to conventional treatments with appropriately selected patients.

Cottingham, Porges, and Richmond[8] studied the effects of a 45-minute Rolfing pelvic mobilization on subjects and found the session significantly decreased standing pelvic tilt angle and significantly increased vagal tone. In another study, Cottingham, Porges, and Lyon[9] assessed the effect of a Rolfing technique, the pelvic lift, on parasympathetic tone, and found the technique significantly increased parasympathetic tone.

Silverman et al[10] measured electroencephalogram averaged evoked responses of stimulus intensity and perceptual differentiation, eye saccadic movements, urinary levels of 17-Hydroxycorticosteroid, and blood levels of creatine phosphokinase in Rolfed subjects. Results indicated that Rolfing increased openness and improved sensitivity to environmental stimulation. Weinberg and Hunt[11] found that Rolfing reduced levels of state anxiety compared to a control group.

Rolfing lends itself to research on its observed effects. More research studies are needed and hopefully will be forthcoming.

DISTINCTION BETWEEN ROLFING AND TRADITIONAL PHYSICAL THERAPY

Despite some obvious commonalities between Rolfing and physical therapy, for example, the use of physical intervention and movement re-education to improve structure/posture, there are important differences. Dr. Rolf felt the Rolfer should not deal with acute injury; rather, Rolfers are concerned with chronic conditions.[1] This is not the case with physical therapy. Also, while physical therapy treats specific local dysfunctions and problems in the related region, Dr. Rolf taught that local treatment only shifts the area of strain elsewhere in the body; hence, Rolfing's holistic approach. Most importantly, Dr. Rolf emphasized that Rolfing is not a form of therapy, but an educational process assisting the client in establishing a vertical relationship to gravity.[1] This relationship is the "structural pattern of health."[1] As such, Rolfing is nonmedical and does not "treat" symptoms or disease. Additionally, unlike physical therapy, Rolfing does not employ techniques such as joint mobilization, stretching, and strengthening.

Despite their differences, Rolfing and physical therapy can complement each other very well. For example, Rolfing can enhance stretching because Rolfing affects not only muscle groups but also whole body patterns of muscle and fascial relationships. Rolfing can augment joint mobilization by balancing the myofascia around the joint. Also, by improving the client's body awareness and physical balance, Rolfing can enhance body mechanics instruction and movement re-education by the physical therapist. These are only a few of the possibilities.

The physical therapist might refer a client with a musculoskeletal condition for Rolfing once the acute condition has stabilized or after physical therapy is concluded. Most of the musculoskeletal conditions seen by the physical therapist would benefit further from Rolfing. Rolfing may help to correct the whole body patterns and compensations which may have resulted from the injury or may have contributed to causing the patient's condition in the first place. Rolfing is especially useful if the client has a good understanding of Rolfing goals. The myofascial imbalances related to neurological conditions such as mild cerebral palsy and cerebral vascular accident may benefit from Rolfing concurrent with physical therapy and occupational therapy. Improving myofascial balance may allow neuromuscular re-education to be more effective. Of course, the greater the severity of neurological damage, the less likely Rolfing would help. Physical therapists whose clients engage in physical performance, such as athletics and dance, may find Rolfing helpful in restoring and enhancing performance.

The physical therapist should not view Rolfing as a "fix-it" approach. More correctly, the physical therapist may view Rolfing as a process that supports and enhances therapy. More ideally, the physical therapist will view Rolfing as a unique process that can optimize health and well-being at many levels.

HELLERWORK AND SOMA

Joseph Heller was trained as a Rolfer and a Structural Patterner (ie, a practitioner of the Aston-Patterning movement system). In the late 1970s he developed Hellerwork, a technique that has much in common with Rolfing, while adding several unique elements. Organized around a series of 11 sessions, the hands-on bodywork portions of the first 10 sessions essentially are identical to the basic 10-session Rolfing series. Additionally, Hellerwork incorporates movement lessons into the sessions, while Rolfing tends to address these separately using Rolfing Movement Integration. Hellerwork also employs verbal dialogue during the sessions to help the client explore relevant mind-body connections. Emotions, attitudes, and patterns of body tensions and use are associated with each session and the dialogue helps the client discover and utilize these relationships to facilitate change. There is a strong psychological emphasis.

Session 11 is concerned with completion of the work. There may or may not be any body manipulation done. Client and Hellerworker review issues and responses raised during the sessions and feedback is encouraged. A personalized movement session may be created. Support is given for the client to own the results of the work.

Bill M. Williams, PhD studied under Dr. Rolf, and he developed SOMA Bodywork in

1978. SOMA is even more similar to Rolfing than Hellerwork. Like Rolfing, SOMA Bodywork involves 10 sessions of myofascial manipulation directed at aligning the body with gravity. The SOMA sessions closely parallel the basic Rolfing series. SOMA Bodywork also aims to facilitate access to the functioning of each of the brain's hemispheres. SOMA training addresses psychological facilitation, right/left hemisphere integration, and mind/body integration.

CASE EXAMPLE

NB is a 46-year-old male referred for Rolfing by his physician. NB complains of sharp costochondral pains of insidious onset 6 months ago. Pain is worse with full thoracic flexion, carrying heavy loads, and occasionally, with deep inspiration. Rest, cervical and thoracic manipulations, and medications have not helped.

NB's structure is one of an anteriorly inclined pelvis, exaggerated spinal physiological curves, depressed rib cage, hyperextended knees, and genu valgum bilaterally. Rib excursion is limited and there is considerable muscular tension and tenderness of thoracic paraspinals, shoulder girdles, diaphragm, hip flexors, and adductors.

NB is educated about Rolfing and its goals. He understands that the aim is to improve his entire structure and that the rib pain will probably be the *last* thing to resolve.

Structural alignment shows good improvement during the sessions. As leg and pelvis balance improve, the spinal curvatures are able to normalize considerably and the rib cage does not collapse down. Pain complaints decrease throughout the sessions, but by Session 10 NB still has some irritation. Verbal follow-up 8 weeks after Session 10 reveals the pain complaints have resolved.

By improving NB's overall structure (posture), Rolfing created the support and balance to relieve the over-stressed joints. This allowed the body to heal in a way the previous physical therapy treatments did not facilitate.

CONCLUSION

In many ways, the Rolfing approach to health and well being embraces both the traditional and alternative perspectives. The importance Rolfing places on anatomical relationships and their objective assessment, myofascial and neurological contributions to body balance, and research reflect traditional features. The emphasis placed on holism, the unity of mind and body, energy relationships, and the promotion of growth and knowledge of self through personal evolution gives a sense of Rolfing's unconventional aspects. Therapists who refer their clients for Rolfing will find it an alternative therapy that is effective and meaningful on many levels for a wide variety of clients and conditions.

REFERENCES

1. Rolf IP. *Rolfing and Physical Reality*. Rochester, Vt: Healing Arts Press; 1990.

2. Rolf IP. *The Integration of Human Structures*. New York, NY: Harper & Row Publishers; 1978.

3. Cottingham JT. *Healing Through Touch: A History and a Review of the Physiological Evidence*. Champaign, Ill: Broadside Press; 1985.

4. Schleip R. The golgi tendon reflex arc as a new explanation of the effect of Rolfing. *Rolf Lines*. 1989;17(1):18-20.

5. Schleip R. Rolfing and the neuro-myofascial net. *Rolf Lines*. 1993;21(1):22-30.

6. Hunt VV, Massey W, Weinberg RS, Bruyere R, Hahn P. *A study of structural integration from neuromuscular, energy field, and emotional approaches*. Project Report: Rolf Institute of Structural Integration, Boulder, Colo; 1977.

7. Perry J, Jones MH, Thomas L. Functional evaluation of Rolfing in cerebral palsy. *Dev Med Child Neurol*. 1981;23:717-729.

8. Cottingham JT, Porges SW, Richmond K. Shifts in pelvic inclination angle and parasympathetic tone produced by Rolfing soft tissue manipulation. *J Amer Phys Ther Assn*. 1988;68(9):1364-1370.

9. Cottingham JT, Porges SW, Lyon T. Effects of soft tissue mobilization (Rolfing pelvic lift) on parasympathetic tone in two age groups. *J Amer Phys Ther Assn*. 1988;68(3):352-356.

10. Silverman J, Rappaport M, Hopkins HK, et al. Stress stimulus intensity control, and the structural integration technique. *Confinia Psychiatrica*. 1973;16:201-219.

11. Weinberg RS, Hunt VV. Effects of structural integration on state-trait anxiety. *J Clin Psych*. 1979;35(2):319-322.

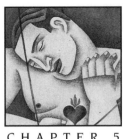

CHAPTER 5

NON-CONTACT THERAPEUTIC TOUCH

Guy L. McCormack, MS, OTR
Mary Lou Galantino, MS, PT

INTRODUCTION

Throughout history, various forms of touch have been used to comfort, console, reassure, show acceptance, and facilitate the healing process. Non-Contact Therapeutic Touch (NCTT) may be described as a modern derivative of the "laying on of hands," but this treatment does not require that it be performed in a religious context nor does it require a professed faith or belief by either the practitioner or the patient.[1] Granted, the intent of the practitioner is essential to the successful administration of therapeutic touch, but the mechanism seems to have a "lawfulness" about it that is grounded in the principles of physics. In recent years, Dolores Krieger[2-4] and Dora Kunz[5] have been credited as being the first to introduce health professionals to the ancient art of therapeutic touch.

QUANTUM THEORY AS EXPLANATORY OF OBSERVATIONS

By definition, NCTT is a learned process by which the practitioner centers his or her mind or induces a state of consciousness similar to a meditative state, becomes clear about the intent to help or heal, and moves the palms of the hands slowly as if to form a silhouette around the body of the recipient in an effort to assess or influence an individual's energy system. In this context, energy is perceived in terms of quantum physics, that is, all matter is simply composed of various forms of vibrations and energy waves. Drawing from quantum physics and field theory, there is an assumption that matter is energy and all living things generate vibratory fields which are interconnected by mathematical laws.

For example, Bell's Theorem[6] states that two particles, originally united but eventually separated, continue to affect one another regardless of whether they are in close proximity or at a distance. Said another way, if a molecule is broken up so that the electrons fly apart, and the spin is changed on one electron, the spin on other electrons originally joined to it will immediately correspond, regardless of the distance between them. In theory, NCTT follows the belief that universal energy connects all living things within the immediate environment, throughout the planet and the universe as well.[7] According to Gerber[8] and Becker,[9] the human body produces a bioelectric field that is composed of low frequency electromagnetic energy. This field may be the sum total of several subtle energies which are produced by the movement of positive and negative molecules as they pass through cell membranes. Considering that the skin is the largest organ of the body and every movement involving muscles, bones, and nerves creates measurable currents by piezoelectricity,[10-12] it is not too hard to believe that a field exists around the human body the same way an electrical current exists around an insulated copper wire.

Although the therapeutic value of touch is rarely refuted, many health professionals remain skeptical about the validity of NCTT. Skeptics were quick to critique early attempts in the 1970s to quantify the benefits of NCTT using experimental research designs which were fraught with methodological inconsistencies. In a critical view of the research literature, Clark and Clark[13,14] argued that there were too few double-blind studies of statistical significance and not enough independent replication to support the claim that NCTT was anything more than a placebo. Other skeptics have focused their criticisms on the language or terminology used to explain the process of an energy exchange, which often is interpreted from an intuitive perspective. Such terms as "universal energy," "depletion," or "blocked" energy defy good operational definitions that satisfy an empirical mind set. Yet many researchers[4,15-17] have argued convincingly that it is not plausible to restrict biological or psychological phenomena to operationalism. For instance, if quantum physics were restricted to narrow operational definitions, how would one identify the qualities or meanings of the Theory of Relativity, the Black Hole, or theories on Consciousness?

However, in the last two decades there has been a growing interest in non-experimental design and qualitative studies employing phenomenology, grounded theory, single system design, and ethnographic investigations, which has generated a richer body of knowledge that speaks to other ways of knowing.[18] A review of the literature will reveal that much of the support for the practice of NCTT, which is holistic in nature and thus does not comply with reductionistic analytical methods, is anecdotal; however, reductionist research methods have steadily improved in the last 20 years and many of the current studies possess acceptable scientific rigor.[13,15,19,20]

Efforts to isolate possible mechanisms responsible for the relaxation outcomes experienced by the recipient of NCTT can be located in four main categories:

1. electromagnetic field studies
2. pain studies
3. stress and anxiety studies
4. wound healing.

ELECTROMAGNETIC FIELD STUDIES

A critical factor in understanding the mechanisms which underlie the effects of NCTT stems from the field studies in quantum physics. Humans and other living organisms are composed of subatomic particles that form matter and energy. This is supported by Einstein's famous equation $E = mc^2$, which postulates that energy and matter are interchangeable and related to the speed of light.[6] Thus, solid matter, such as the human body, can be subdivided into smaller and smaller molecules and particles with the end result being a field of energy. For example, water makes up 99% of the molecules composing the human body.[8] Magnetic resonance imaging (MRI) scanners employ the magnetic properties of protons (hydrogen atom in water, H_2O) as an emitting source for computed imagery. In essence, MRI uses hydrogen atoms' resonant frequencies which penetrate through the radio waves to produce a clear image of soft tissues on a computer monitor. If the body were not potentially energetic, this would not be possible.

Several researchers have explored the properties of the skin in respect to direct current (DC) and electromagnetic energy.[8,12,21-24] The results of these studies concluded that the human body generates subtle yet measurable alternating current (AC) and DC at all times. For example, electrocardiograms, electromyographic biofeedback units, and electroencephalograms are all evidence of alternating currents that are both measurable and generated by specific tissues of the body.[25] DC has been shown to be produced by the movement of ions in the stratum cornium of the skin, and by cell to cell communications called gap junctions.[12,25] In physics, it is well understood that any time a current moves through a linear pathway, such as electrons through a wire, a field is produced around the structure through which the energy passes. Since the human body is a heat-producing organism, it seems likely that resonant wave forms are produced within the electromagnetic spectrum. To date, the most compelling studies have been conducted by Green[26] at the Menninger Foundation. Green's "copper wall studies" have examined the anomalous electrical potentials and voltage surges in so-called healers while performing NCTT. Green's (1992) data has been analyzed by Tiller (1992) and the voltage charges were reported to be electromagnetic in nature. Although the results are preliminary, Green has reported voltage surges of as much as 80 volts in healers during the time they perform NCTT. These voltages were dipoles or localized spots seen in the chest region.

In a related study, Fahrain[27] has analyzed brain wave patterns of both practitioners and recipients during the NCTT procedure. Fahrain concluded that during the NCTT process, the brainwaves of both individuals (receiving and giving) come into synchrony through some unidentifiable process of consciousness. Could this unidentifiable process be intentionality?

The process of intentionality is the conscious intent to help or heal another person while holding to the emotion of unconditional love. This is a mind set which the therapist engenders that is nonjudgmental and completely focused on the interaction between the two people.

PAIN STUDIES

Connell and Meehan[28] explored the effects of therapeutic touch on the experience of acute pain in postoperative patients by testing the hypothesis that there will be a greater decrease in post-test acute pain experience scores in subjects treated by NCTT than in subjects treated by sham therapeutic touch. The sham therapeutic touch was applied with the same hand gestures but the main difference was the practitioner counted to him or herself backwards from two hundred to one. This process focused the practitioner's consciousness or intent on the act of counting rather than the intent to help or heal. Their experimental design used multiple regression analysis with post-hoc comparison which indicated no significant differences between the two test groups. They suggested that a less conservative measure might be appropriate; that the 5-minute treatment time may not have been long enough for an analgesic effect. Additionally, the pain medication standard medical treatment might have been a confounding factor in measuring the effects of NCTT.[29]

In another study by Meehan[7] on postoperative pain, some interesting questions were raised about the use of experimental research design for investigating therapeutic touch. In this study, 108 hospitalized patients who had undergone abdominal or pelvic surgery were randomly assigned to one of the following groups: a therapeutic touch group, a placebo control group, or a standard intervention group receiving intramuscular narcotic analgesic.

At first glance, the hypothesis that therapeutic touch would decrease postoperative pain when compared to the placebo control and intervention group was not supported by statistical significance. However, this finding might represent a Type I error because the null hypothesis was rejected when it should not have been.[18] The real significance of the study was found on a secondary finding of the data. After reviewing the data, the researchers discovered that it should be analyzed from a different perspective. Although the 13% pain reduction may not be significant in and of itself, the combination of NCTT and the narcotic intervention shows that it is effective when used in combination with other analgesics. Although the group receiving narcotic intervention reported 42% pain relief, the group receiving NCTT reported 13% pain relief, and the placebo group reported no pain relief as measured by the Pain Visual Analogue Scale. Simply said, 13% pain reduction does not support the use of NCTT alone as a postoperative analgesic, but it does suggest that it validates its use as an adjunct to analgesic. What is more, NCTT seems to beat the odds of pain relief by placebo. This observation has been recently reported by Jonasen,[30] who performed NCTT in a perioperative nursing unit. In Jonasen's words, "…by holding one's hands 10 to 15 cm away from the skin's surface and slowly moving the hands over the client's field…a sense of well-being is imparted."

Keller and Bzdek[31] examined the effects of NCTT on tension headache pain, building on previous work by Heidt (1989) and Quinn (1989), which indicated that NCTT decreased anxiety. Because anxiety is known to influence the etiology of tension headaches, Keller hypothesized that subjects receiving NCTT would not only experience pain relief, but the duration of relief would exceed that of the placebo group. Data analysis revealed a highly significant decrease in pain scores of subjects treated with therapeutic touch. Pain scores dropped an average of 70% in the NCTT group and 37% in the placebo group. There have been other quantitative reports of pain relief from therapeutic touch, studies which have not employed double-blind methodology to rule out the placebo effect.[29,32-35]

A recent investigation by Wirth and Cram[36] supported the premise that NCTT produces observable physical changes which essentially constituted a relaxation response.[37] The authors used a double-blind experimental design where NCTT was assessed by multi-site surface EMG recording located at the frontalis, cervical, thoracic, and lumbosacral segments. The results of this study showed that, in addition to a reduction of muscle tone, other physiologic indicators, such as skin temperature, heart rate, and end tidal CO_2 levels showed a reduction in sympathetic tone or the manifestations of a shift to the parasympathetic end of the continuum.

These findings contribute to the observation that NCTT not only alleviates pain, but produces a relaxation response which is known to ameliorate levels of state anxiety or the situational occurences of anxiety. For instance, Heidt[32] has conducted extensive research on decreased state anxiety following NCTT intervention. In 1991, Heidt reported that among hospitalized cardiovascular patients, a therapeutic touch group had more significantly decreased levels of psychologic anxiety post-treatment than did either of two other groups—one of which received casual touch, which is a light pat on the shoulder or some other contact that indicated support; the other received no touch. The patients' anxiety levels were measured on a standardized self-evaluation questionnaire before and after treatment. The results showed that the therapeutic touch groups' anxiety levels were significantly lower than those of the control groups.

Gagne and Toye[38] investigated the effects of NCTT in a psychiatric facility. Their study compared reported measures of anxiety in a relaxation training group, an NCTT group, and a control group. A statistically significant reduction in reported anxiety was present in those treated with NCTT.

Fedoruk[39] studied the effects of therapeutic touch on infants in Neonatal, Intermediate, and Intensive Care Units. The analysis indicated that there was a significant difference between infants treated with therapeutic touch and those who were treated with sham therapeutic touch, where the intent to help or heal was omitted from thought processes, or no therapeutic touch in decreasing arousal states to a more relaxed state during observation time. However, the study was criticized because the data presented did not make it possible to determine if the reported differences in infant scores among the three treatment types were a function of the effectiveness of therapeutic touch in reducing arousal or the fact that the sham therapeutic touch appears to have increased arousal.

Parkes[40] studied the effects of therapeutic touch on the state anxiety of elderly hospitalized patients. Parkes used NCTT and a sham therapeutic touch treatment. Comparison of post-test means using analysis of covariance (ANOVA) revealed no statistically significant difference between groups. Findings of this study were consistent with the findings of

Quinn,[15] who reported that a low but significant negative correlation was noted in both the giver and the recipient during therapeutic touch. A negative correlation suggests that the two groups, the sham group and the group that received NCTT, were inversely related. In other words, there was no relationship between the fake group and the real group. Samarel[1] examined the experience of receiving therapeutic touch in a phenomenological study. The narrative findings showed that for the 20 participants receiving treatment who were analyzed and coded for word patterns, the consensus of the group stated that it was a "fulfilling multidimensional experience that facilitated personal growth."

More recently, Mackey[41] provides testimony to the value of NCTT for terminally ill patients. In addition to helping the patient cope with death, NCTT has been shown to alleviate dyspnea (especially acites-induced dyspnea) which is not relieved by repositioning or medication. Mackey reports that after NCTT is administered for a few minutes, the patient relaxes and his or her "breathing becomes slow and even, allowing the patient to let go and die in peace."[41]

WOUND HEALING STUDIES

Smith[42] examined the potential effects of a healer and a magnetic field on the enzyme trypsin in vitro, that is, in separate beakers. The investigator had NCTT applied to four solutions of the enzyme trypsin:

1. control
2. a solution exposed to ultraviolet light and treated by the healer
3. a solution held by the healer
4. a solution exposed to a magnetic field.

While no statistical tests of significance were reported, standard deviation of the activity levels of the various solutions were shown on graphs. After two replications of this study, Smith concluded that the healer produced similar effects on the enzyme trypsin as did the magnet field produced by electromagnets. These results have been reported by other investigators as well.[43]

In a classic study, Krieger[4] reported a significant increase in hemoglobin values in response to therapeutic touch (treatment group) versus routine hospital care (control group). However, this study was criticized for the absence of operational definitions, lack of random assignments to groups, and no control for the placebo effect. In a follow-up study, Krieger[2] reported significant increases in hemoglobin values in response to NCTT.

Grad[16] conducted a pilot study on wound healing in mice. A surgical incision was per-

formed on the backs of 300 mice and each wound was measured. The mice were randomly assigned to an experimental group treated by a folk healer named Esterbantz who was
well known throughout Canada, a control group treated by medical students who were
volunteers and randomly assigned, or to a non-treatment group. On the 15th and 16th
days of the study, the investigator found significantly smaller wound sizes for the mice
treated by the healer. The mice in the no-treatment group showed better signs of healing
than the ones treated by the skeptical medical students. Because the medical students did
not claim to have any paranormal healing abilities, it is curious that the group of mice
treated by them were the slowest to heal. It appears that the attitude or intentionality projected by the medical students was counterproductive to the healing process in the mice.

Wirth[17] conducted a study demonstrating the potential for therapeutic touch in the
healing of full thickness human dermal wounds. Full thickness dermal wounds were incised
on the lateral deltoid muscle using a skin biopsy instrument by a physician. Incisions were
dressed and wound surfaces were measured on Days 0, 8, and 16 using a direct tracing
method. Active control and treatments were comprised of daily sessions of 5-minute expo-
sures to a hidden therapeutic touch practitioner or to sham exposure. Results showed that
subjects treated with therapeutic touch experienced a significant acceleration in the rate of
wound healing as compared to nontreated subjects. Subjects were not informed of group
assignment or the true nature of the active treatment modality in order to control placebo
and expectation effects. The findings of this study produced significant results under experimental conditions which indicate that non-contact therapeutic touch may be a effective
healing modality on full thickness human dermal wounds in human subjects.[6]

INTEGRATION OF THERAPEUTIC TOUCH WITH PHYSICAL THERAPY—METHOD

NCTT can be an integral part of the plan of care. Indications for performing NCTT
include pain, anxiety, tension, stress, and facilitation of wound healing. This section will
present various case studies through the use of exclusive NCTT along with the integration
of physical therapy modalities. A brief summary outline of general information, procedures, and written documentation will be presented.

GENERAL INFORMATION

1. NCTT takes only 15 to 20 minutes to administer.
2. Two conditions must exist in order to do the process:

    a. Intentionality—a form of meditation and a way of calming the mind so the practitioner is nonjudgmental and intending to help or heal.

    b. Assessment—performed by scanning over the person's body about 3 to 6 inches away from the skin to detect differences in temperature, electrical potential, or other perceivable sensations.

3. Treatment—the transfer of energy can occur from a healthy person who intends to help or heal a client.

4. Human beings are open systems in constant flux, and they experience input and output of energy. Humans are energy fields who are continually, simultaneously exchanging energy with the environment. There appears to be a universal order or properties that conform to the principles of physics.

PROCEDURE

NCTT can be provided through the following series of steps:

1. *Centering oneself, physically and psychologically*: this is a process by which the caregiver finds a calm, focused state of being. This is done by conscious direction of his or her attention inward. It can be achieved by various methods, such as deep breathing, visualization, and focusing.

2. *Assessment of the client*: this is a process by which the caregiver notes areas of balance and imbalance in the patient's energy field by scanning the client's energy field from head to toe with the caregiver's hands. Perception of heat, cold, tingling, congestion, or pressure indicate imbalances or obstructions in the field.

3. *Unruffling the field*: this is a process by which the client's energy field congestion, sluggishness, or static is removed or lessened. This is performed by making slow brushing sweeps with the caregiver's hand over the client's body without touching the body itself, sweeping from head to toe. This allows the energy to move more freely.

4. *Direction and modulation of energy*: once the field has been cleared, treat areas that have been blocked or congested. The therapist lets the hands rest on or near the body where the block or congestion was detected or in other areas of energy imbalance. Energy is directed to the area in order to balance or correct the "blockage" or modulate energy by changing the outflow to meet the client's needs. This is performed as an act of consciousness as the caregiver images a flow or movement of particles, color, fluid, or whatever visualization is clearly formulated in the mind.

5. *Recognize when it is time to stop*: stop when there are no longer any cues, when the body is symmetrical and there are no perceivable differences bilaterally, such as

magnetic-like repulsions, heat, cold, static electricity, emptiness, or fullness.

DOCUMENTATION

1. Complete a therapeutic assessment sheet.
2. Identify the presenting problem on picture and describe in patient words.
3. Identify from assessment process the area of blockage, congestion, and imbalance.
4. List methods of intervention used and describe.
5. Evaluate the procedure.
6. Plan for the next intervention.[44] Make a chart or mark anatomical drawings where the field felt different, compare history and physical findings. Use initial chart as a baseline measure.

SUBJECTIVE OBSERVATIONS

1. Generalized feelings of warmth expressed.
2. Spontaneous verbal response, a sigh or comment ("I feel relaxed").
3. Description of change in pain levels.

OBJECTIVE OBSERVATIONS

1. Lowering of the client's voice.
2. Slowing and deepening of the client's respiration.
3. Peripheral flush of the skin, especially in areas treated.
4. Physiological changes in the relaxation response, such as decreased pulse, lowered blood pressure.

CASE EXAMPLE 1

A 7-year-old pianist was preparing to participate in his Tae Kwon Do class when the door to the studio closed abruptly and amputated the distal interphalangeal joint of his right fifth finger. Since his mother, a nurse also trained in NCTT, was immediately present to assist him, she implemented NCTT to maintain the energy field of the amputated finger until they were able to seek medical attention.

Unfortunately, the physician who assessed the finger stated that it was not viable for surgical repair. The patient's mother requested that the procedure take place despite the grim outlook for the ability to optimize her child's piano career. Throughout the discussion and subsequent procedure, she continued to perform NCTT. The physician surgically repaired the finger without need for anesthetizing the right hand (that is, no radial nerve blocks were required since pain management was evident from the mother's treatment with NCTT). The microsurgery was successful due to the increased blood supply and hemoglobin values facilitated by the NCTT.

The patient was then referred to a plastic surgeon who also presented a poor prognosis for the function of this finger. He anticipated that the patient would reject the surgically reconnected finger within a few months. During this entire period, however, the patient continued to receive daily NCTT and range of motion by his mother. The former prognosis was, in time, reversed. NCTT was performed for 8 weeks, with the end result of no loss of sensation or function of his right hand. Today, he is a classical pianist performing professionally.

CASE EXAMPLE 2

Pat is a 34-year-old female who was thrown from her horse and fractured her left ankle, which was placed in a cast for 6 weeks. After the cast was removed, she developed reflex sympathetic dystrophy syndrome (RSDS). Physical therapy was ordered and the patient complained of severe pain despite the use of modalities for pain control and manual therapy techniques to restore range of motion and strength of the left lower extremity. She sought the intervention of a nurse trained in NCTT to complement her PT sessions. The course of events were as follows:

SESSION 1 OF NCTT (1 YEAR POST INJURY)

Pat arrived in a wheelchair. NCTT was initiated for 20 minutes. The five-step process described above was performed by a trained practitioner. The patient reported a feeling of warmth in her cold left extremity. She ranked her pain initially at a level 10, but with the initiation of NCTT it was reduced to 5 in the first session. PT continued for two additional sessions between the NCTT. Treatments consisted of joint mobilization, stretching, strengthening, and the initiation of gait training at the parallel bars.

SESSION 2 OF NCTT

Pat received NCTT one time during the second week and reported that the pain was decreased to a level 4. She was advanced to a straight cane and therapists noted a greater normalization of gait. Increased range of motion and strength continued and were measured in PT sessions.

SESSION 3 OF NCTT

The third therapeutic touch session resulted in a normalization of the entire body in addition to the left lower extremity. Pat was able to ambulate without any assistive device and her pain decreased to a very tolerable level of 2. PT continued with aggressive joint mobilization, gait, and endurance retraining.

Given the seemingly progressive nature of RSDS, it can be said that this patient made a remarkable recovery with the addition of NCTT. In the studies on NCTT, the relaxation response and pain amelioration have high reliability.[1] NCTT seems to accelerate the healing process, and in the case of this patient, post injury, remarkable progress was made with NCTT in addition to PT. We also can state that the benefits of PT and NCTT are related to a shift in the parasympathetic nervous system continuum. The research demonstrates growing evidence to support this physiologic alteration.

SUMMARY

Selected research on NCTT has been presented in this chapter. Clearly, more recent studies continue to elucidate the physiological benefits of NCTT. Since Dolores Krieger[2] introduced NCTT in 1974, it has become, for many, a standard nursing intervention.[2] Many nursing curricula teach the skills of NCTT, and nursing research has been the forerunner of the studies which report the positive benefits of this technique. Physical and occupational therapists continue to perform manual contact skills through massage and soft tissue mobilization with good results. The additional aspect of NCTT may be added to the PT and OT treatments to maximize the available options, especially in chronic conditions. However, it is important to receive proper training in NCTT in order to maximize the beneficial effects of this intervention.

To the skeptic, assessing and then smoothing out the invisible energy field around the patient seems like "magic" or pure placebo. However, research confirms that: a) all people have energy fields surrounding their bodies,[9] b) the quality of these energy fields can be perceived by practitioners trained in the use of therapeutic touch,[2,3] and c) knowledgeable practitioners can affect the energy fields by hand movements that result in accelerated healing of the entire body, not just the skin.[17]

CONCLUSION

The NCTT process may be perceived with skepticism and suspicion, for it appears rather mystical as it is being performed. However, endogenous bioelectrical circuits have been measured in both superficial layers of the skin and in the deep connective tissues. The field which projects outward from the surface of the visible body is not visible to the eye but is perceivable to the tactile and touch senses. Although it seems like a magical act or apparent placebo, there is enough good research evidence to support the claim that physiological benefits result from those who have experienced the techniques.

Research confirms that:

1. All biological life plants, animals, and humans produce a subtle field of energy that appears to operate within the electromagnetic spectrum. This field appears to be influenced by the integrity of the soft tissues of the body.[8,9]

2. The qualities or characteristics of these fields are perceivable as the hands move slowly through the field. In areas where there is pathology or pain the field feels different. Caregivers describe the differences metaphysically or by temperature changes, electrical, magnetic or empty/full, pins and needles, etc.[7,11,30]

3. Skilled practitioners use both the slow, sweeping motions of their hands and their consciousness to affect the energy fields. The motion elicited by the movement of the hands seems to affect the accumulation of positively and negatively charged molecules or ions which readily pass through the cell membranes, causing minute changes in electrical potentials. The human body is not solid, but is composed of molecules which are constantly being exchanged and influenced by factors in the environment.[2,6,12,24]

REFERENCES

1. Samarel N. The experience of receiving therapeutic touch. *J Adv Nurs.* 1992;17:651-657.

2. Krieger D. Therapeutic touch: two decades of research, teaching and clinical practice. *NSNA/Imprint.* 1990;37(3):83,86-88.

3. Krieger D. *The Therapeutic Touch: How To Use Your Hands to Help or to Heal.* Englewood Cliffs, NJ: Prentice-Hall, Inc; 1979.

4. Krieger D. Healing by the "laying on" of hands as a facilitator of bioenergetic change: the response on in-vivo human hemoglobin. *Psychoenergetic Systems.* 1979,1:121-129.

5. Kunz D (compiler). *Spiritual Aspects of the Healing Arts.* Wheaton, Ill: The Theosophical Publishing House; 1985.

6. Dossey L. *Meaning and Medicine.* New York, NY: Bantam Books; 1991.

7. Meehan TC. Therapeutic touch and postoperative pain: a Rogerian research study. *Nursing Science Quarterly*. 1993;6(2):69-78.

8. Gerber R. *Vibrational Medicine*. Santa Fe, NM: Bear & Company; 1988.

9. Becker RO. An application of direct current neural systems to psychic phenomena. *Psychogenetic Systems*. 1977;2:189-196.

10. McCormack G. *Therapeutic Use of Touch for the Health Professional*. Tucson, Ariz: Therapy Skill Builders;1991.

11. McCormack G. The therapeutic benefit of the relaxation response. *Occup Ther Pract*. 1992;4(1):51-60.

12. Tiller WA. Explanation of electrodermal diagnostic and treatment instruments: part 1. Electrical behavior of human skin. *J Hol Med*. 1982;4(2):105-127.

13. Clark MJ. Therapeutic touch: Is there a scientific basis for practice? Reply. *Nurs Res*. 1984,33(5):296-297.

14. Clark PE, Clark MJ. Therapeutic touch: is there a scientific basis for practice? Reply. *Nurs Res*. 1984;33:37-41.

15. Quinn JF. *An Investigation of the Effects of Therapeutic Touch on Anxiety of Open Heart Surgery Patients*. Washington, DC: National Institutes of Health, Center for Nursing Research, Grant number R23 NU 01067; 1984.

16. Grad B. Some biological effects of the "laying on of hands": a review of experiments with animals and plans. *J the Amer Soc for Psychical Research*. 1965;59(2):95-129.

17. Wirth D. The effects of non-contact therapeutic touch on the healing rate of full thickness dermal wounds. *Subtle Energies*. 1990;1(1):1-20.

18. Depoy E, Gitlin LN. *Introduction to Research Multiple Strategies for Health & Human Services*. St Louis, Mo: Mosby; 1994.

19. Gagne P, Toye RCA. The effects of therapeutic touch and relaxation therapy in reducing anxiety. *Arch Psychiatr Nurs*. 1994;8:184-189.

20. Mackey RB. Discover the healing power of therapeutic touch. *Am J Nurs*. 1995;95:26-32.

21. Baker A, Jaffe L, Vanable J. The glabrous epidermis of cavies contains a powerful battery. *Amer Physiol Soc*. 1982;242:360-365.

22. Becker RO. An application of direct current neural systems to psychic phenomena. *Psychogenetic Systems*. 1977;2:189-196.

23. Becker RO, Selden A. *The Body Electric: Electromagnetism and the Foundation of Life*. New York, NY: William Morrow; 1985.

24. Edelberg C. Relation of electrical properties of skin to structure and physiologic state. *J Invest Dermatol*. 1977;69:324-327.

25. Guyton MA. *Textbook of Medical Physiology*. 8th ed. Philadelphia, Pa: W.B. Saunders; 1986.

26. Green E. Anomalous human potential data: parallels between biofeedback and subtle energies in the science, consciousness and practice of healing traditions. Presented at the Third Annual Conference for the International Society for the Study of the Subtle Energies and Energy Medicine; June 1993; Monterey, Calif.

27. Fahrian SL. EEG, amplitude, brain mapping and synchrony in and between a bioenergy prac-

titioner and client during healing. *Subtle Energies.* 1992;3:19-51.

28. Connell M, Meehan M. The effect of therapeutic touch on the experience of acute pain in post-operative patients. Dissertation Abstracts International. 1985;46:795B. (University Microfilm No. DA8510765.)

29. Quinn JF. Therapeutic touch as energy exchange: republication and extension. *Nursing Science Quarterly.* 1989,2(2):79-87.

30. Jonasen AM. Therapeutic touch: a holistic approach to perioperative nursing. *Today's OR Nurse.* 1994;16:7-12.

31. Keller E, Bzdek VM. Effects of therapeutic touch on tension headache pain. *Nurs Res.* 1986;35(2):101-106.

32. Heidt P. Effect of therapeutic touch on the anxiety level of hospital patients. *Nurs Res.* 1991;30(1):32-37.

33. Heidt P. Helping patients to rest: clinical studies in therapeutic touch. *Holistic Nurs Prac.* 1991;5(4):57-66.

34. Quinn JF. Building a body of knowledge: research on therapeutic touch 1974-1986. *J Holistic Nurs.* 1988;6(1):37-45.

35. Thayer MB. Touching with intent: using therapeutic touch. *Ped Nurs.* 1990;16(1):70-72.

36. Wirth DP, Cram JR. Multi-site electromyographic analysis of non-contact therapeutic touch. *Int J Psychsom.* 1993;40:47-55.

37. Benson H. *The Relaxation Response.* New York, NY: William Morrow; 1975.

38. Gagne P, Toye RCA. The effects of therapeutic touch and relaxation therapy in reducing anxiety. *Arch Psychiatr Nurs.* 1994;8:184-189.

39. Fedoruk RB. Transfer of the relaxation response: therapeutic touch B as a method for reduction of stress in premature neonates. Dissertation Abstracts International. 1984;46:978B.

40. Parkes B. Therapeutic touch as an intervention to reduce anxiety in elderly, hospitalized patients. Dissertation Abstracts International. 1985;47:573B.

41. Mackey RB. Discover the healing power of therapeutic touch. *Am J Nurs.* 1995;95:26-32.

42. Smith MJ. Paranormal effects on enzyme activity. *Human Dimension.* 1972;1:15-19.

43. Tiller WA. Towards explaining the anomalously large body boltage surges on "Healers" in the Menninger Cooper Wall Experiments. Presented at the Third Annual Conference for the International Society for the Study of Subtle Energies and Energy Medicine; June 1993; Monterey, Calif.

44. Krieger D. *Living the Therapeutic Touch: Healing as a Lifestyle.* Wheaton, Ill: Quest Books; 1989.

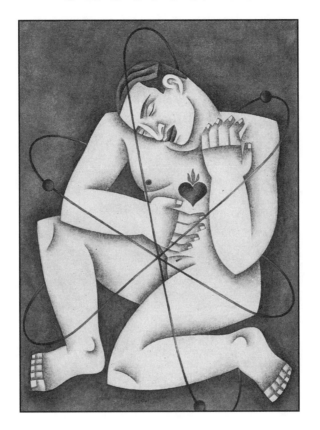

MIND-BODY
INTERVENTIONS

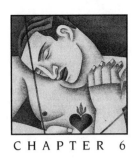

CHAPTER 6

BIOFEEDBACK
CONNECTING THE BODY & MIND

Jennifer M. Bottomley, PhD, MS, PT

INTRODUCTION

The suggestion that hemiplegia, migraine and tension headaches, asthma, hypertension, cardiac arrhythmias, toricollis spasms, pain, hyperkinesis, and functional disorders of any of the body's systems all may be relieved by a single form of treatment sounds more like a 19th-century pitch for snake oil than a true reflection of research. Yet biofeedback has been investigated extensively and has promising clinical applications in an astounding number of conditions.[1-76]

The last two decades have seen an increasing convergence of body and mind therapies. These new therapies are often labeled *psychosomatic* or *psychophysical* medicine.[1] As both names imply, these approaches to healing deal with the effect of the mind on the body. With them tremendous strides have been made in understanding mental influences on body systems ranging from the muscular to the immune system. This has led to treatment procedures that exploit this connection between mind and body. Biofeedback techniques for stress-related disorders and dysfunction and mental imaging using autogenic feedback (a method of mind-over-body control based on a specific discipline for relaxing parts of the body by means of auto-suggestion) to enhance the responsiveness of the autonomic nervous system and/or the immune system response are two good examples of this process. Biofeedback is one of the earliest and most accepted ways that rehabilitation professions have employed that integrates rather than separates the mind and body.[2]

Biofeedback, meaning "life-feedback," is a process of electronically utilizing information from the body to teach an individual to recognize what is going on inside of his or her own brain, nervous system, and muscles. Biofeedback refers to any technique that uses instrumentation to give a person immediate and continuing signals on changes in a bodily function that he or she is not usually conscious of, such as fluctuations in blood pressure, brain-wave activity, or muscle tension. Theoretically and very often in practice, information input enables the individual to learn to control the "involuntary" function.

Biofeedback acts as an output-input system whereby output is based in the motor unit and the input is via sensory pathways comprising proprioceptors, exteroceptors, and interoceptors.[2] Biofeedback provides a means of measurement of a physiological response using an electronic device. It aids the sensory side of a feedback mechanism assisting a compensated sensation, such as with a cerebral vascular accident or other brain injury, in responding appropriately (ie, motor unit training) by increasing conscious awareness of intact but usually unfelt sensation. Basically, biofeedback acts as a sixth sense by providing an artificial proprioception feedback. Via operant conditioning, a new association between a stimuli and a response is developed. The action the learner takes is voluntary and under his or her own control. The response is instrumental in producing a reward or removing a negative stimulus, and this reinforcement shapes behavior and function with successive stages.

Biofeedback transfers the responsibility for final success to the patient. Often, individuals seek medical help, hoping to place the responsibility of "curing" their problems on the clinician, while the patient takes an almost passive role in the treatment process. This is commonly known as an external locus of control. Patients should understand that they have the ability, with assistance from the appropriate medical professionals, to help themselves. Biofeedback provides a modality to accomplish this.

PRINCIPLES OF BIOFEEDBACK

The prefix "myo" is derived from the Greek word for muscle. In combination with the Greek word "graphos," meaning to write, and the additional prefix "electro," the word becomes electromyograph, an instrument for recording the electrical activity of the muscles. Electromyographic (EMG) biofeedback is a modality for measuring and display-ing muscle activity, and is used primarily where any modification of muscular behavior is indicated. With its use, an individual can learn to become more aware of his or her own muscle activity, and thus gain more complete control of functional activity. It also pro-vides an ideal method for rehabilitation practitioners to record a patient's day-to-day progress.

The biofeedback device imparts objective information about the degree of activity occurring in a muscle through surface electrodes, in audio and/or visual form, in much the same way that an EKG provides information about cardiac activity or an EEG displays brain wave activity. In an EMG biofeedback system, the electrical signal originating in the muscle under study is amplified and then translated into sound and visual readings which correspond to increased and decreased muscle activity. Electromyography is the process of recording and interpreting the electrical activity of muscle. When a muscle contracts, it produces a characteristic spike (pulse) waveform that can be detected easily by placing an electrode on the skin over the muscle belly. For example, if you tightly grasp an object in your hand, the muscles in your arm will generate a specific electrical voltage, usually mea-sured in millivolts (.001 volt) or microvolts (.000001 volt). As you squeeze the object tighter, the electrical voltage will increase as more motor units are recruited. As you relax your hand, the electrical voltage will decrease dramatically. EMG is, therefore, a direct physiological index of muscular activity and the state of relaxation.

The interior of a nerve cell is electrically negative with respect to the exterior during its resting phase. This negative potential, typically 50 to 100 millivolts, exists because of the "selective permeability" of the cell wall. On the outside of the cell membrane, $Na+$ ions are more concentrated, and on the inside, $K+$ ions are more concentrated, along with $Cl-$ and other large, negative ions. The semipermeable membrane acts as a barrier to the free interchange of these ions, bringing about a condition like that of a charged battery. The membrane is, therefore, polarized, giving rise to a potential gradient across the cell membrane. This phenomenon is known as the resting potential of the cell.[43]

When a nerve cell is stimulated, its normal resting potential disappears. The perme-ability of the cell wall changes, permitting $K+$, $Na+$, and $Cl-$ ion migration through the wall. $Na+$ ions move from the interstitial tissue fluid surrounding the nerve cell into the nerve fiber. Eventually the sodium ion concentration inside the nerve fiber exceeds that in the interstitial fluid. Potassium ions move from within the nerve fiber to the interstitial fluid. The $Na+$ and $K+$ ion movements cause a reverse potential to build up (ie, the inte-rior of the cell becomes more positive then the exterior) because the inside of the cell has been flooded with sodium ions. This reverse potential may reach a value of 30 to 50 millivolts. After a short time, the membrane regains its original permeability characteristics, and the normal ion distribution is reestablished via the sodium-potassium pump. This changing potential produced when the nerve cell "fires" and then regains its resting voltage is known as the *action potential*.[2,3]

When a nerve cell fires, it influences adjacent cells and causes them to fire. These cells, in turn, cause firing of the nerve cells adjacent to them. In this manner, the action potential spreads rapidly from cell to cell. This traveling action potential is known as an impulse. Impulses move along nerve fibers to stimulate the associated muscle fibers, and along the muscle fibers to cause contraction. An impulse can travel in both directions away from the point of stimulation, but cannot reverse direction toward the starting point. Such reversal of direction is prevented because each nerve cell along the path of the impulse becomes momentarily refractory, that is, insensitive to stimulation for a short time after it has fired.[2,3]

The motor unit is a basic configuration of neuromuscular activity. It consists of a collection of muscle fibers controlled by a singe nerve fiber. When the nerve provides the "triggering" electrical impulse, the muscle fibers contract practically simultaneously. A motor unit may have only a few muscle fibers or thousands, and many motor units are needed to provide the mechanical force required to impart movement to the body.

The motor point is normally the most excitable point of a muscle and represents the area of the greatest concentration of nerve endings. It generally corresponds to the level at which the nerve enters the belly of the muscle.

The frequency spectrum is the range of frequencies present in a given electrical event, as measured in hertz. An example of such a frequency is the 60 cycle (hertz) waves given off from wall outlet voltage. The frequency spectrum of EMG signals covers the range from 20 to 5000 hertz.[3]

The raw, unprocessed EMG signal when amplified can be heard in a set of earphones or a speaker. These "muscle sounds" have been variously described as popping, crackling, hissing, freight train, airplane, and chugging sounds.[2] The raw EMG sound, however, is of little use as a feedback signal since the ear's ability to discern changes in signal amplitude is very limited. For this reason, the EMG signal is usually processed and converted to a variable frequency signal because the ear is much more sensitive to changes in tone.[2,3]

Both surface and needle electrodes have been used in electromyography. Although the voltage from a single muscle fiber can be monitored by the use of a fine-tipped needle electrode, surface electrodes are commonly used for biofeedback in the rehabilitation setting. The voltage picked up by the surface electrodes is actually an average for the many muscle fibers below and near the electrodes. Although muscle action potentials as picked up by the electrodes could possibly be as high as 1000 microvolts, values between 100 and 500 microvolts are more representative.[3]

The principal advantage of needle electrodes is their high sensitivity to individual motor unit potentials, usually without interference from nearby muscles.[2] Therefore, they usually are used for diagnostic purposes. However, since physical therapists normally use EMG biofeedback for muscle re-education and relaxation purposes, surface electrodes have a number of advantages. For example, they eliminate the necessity of keeping all materials sterile and can be used easily on a home basis by the patient.

EMG biofeedback has been reported as being a successful procedure for assisting the rehabilitation of patients with a wide variety of neuro-muscular problems,[2-76] providing muscle re-education and/or muscle relaxation in conditions which may include:

1. Relaxation in spasmodic torticollis[2]
2. Migraine headache pain[6-12]
3. Tension headache pain[6-12]
4. Improvement of functional deficits in paraplegia and quadriplegia[13,14]
5. Improvement of postural instability, proprioception, and reduction of falls[14-16]
6. Treatment of cerebral palsied children for muscle re-education and relaxation[17,18]
7. Cerebral vascular accident rehabilitation[19-25] for:
   a. Foot drop and other gait problems
   b. Posture and muscle tone improvement
   c. Improved voluntary control of involved muscles
   d. Muscle relaxation in associated reactions
   e. Speech problems
8. Muscular training after nerve, muscle, ligament, or tendon injury, repair, or transfers:[26-29]
   a. Carpal tunnel syndrome
   b. Rotator cuff and other shoulder pathologies
   c. Lateral epicondylitis
   d. Thoracic outlet syndrome
   e. Patellofemoral pain
   f. Achilles tendon repairs
9. Early joint mobilization after surgery:[26-29]
   a. Total joint replacements and other orthopedic surgeries
   b. Re-education of affected muscle following radical mastectomy
10. Measurement of endurance with sustained activity[30,31]
11. Functional training and reduction of myoclonus following brain injury[32,33]

12. Control of urinary incontinence and other pelvic floor disorders[34-43]
13. Relaxation for intractable constipation symptoms[44,45]
14. Respiratory control in asthma, emphysema, and chronic obstructive lung disease[46-48]
15. Modification of hypertension[49,50]
16. Autogenic training of temperature control in diabetes, vascular disease, and symptoms of intermittent claudication[51,52]
17. Parasympathetic control of cardiac arrhythmias[53]
18. Stress management[54-59]
19. Intervention for dysphagia and other swallowing disorders[60,61]
20. Muscle re-education following Bell's palsy[62,63]
21. Pain management and reduction in chemotherapy-related symptoms in cancer patients[64-74]

TYPES OF BIOFEEDBACK INTERVENTIONS

Primarily, in the field of rehabilitation medicine, biofeedback techniques are used that focus on muscle re-education, or voluntary inhibition (relaxation) of the muscle. In these approaches, electrodes are placed directly over the belly of the target muscle.

Success is measured by appropriate muscle activation or relaxation. Techniques that are aimed at autonomic nervous system control include: placement of surface electrodes on the frontalis muscle and measurement of physiologic variables such as heart rate, blood pressure, breathing pattern and rate, and galvanic skin response. Another approach for biofeedback intervention is the use of a digital temperature monitor for measurement of physiologic response though body temperature.[23]

In addition to instrumentation for feedback purposes, treatment techniques often include guided imagery training or progressive muscle relaxation, which are forms of autogenic relaxation techniques.[3] Deep breathing techniques have been shown to effectively regulate mental states,[55-57] and often are employed in combination with the above mentioned biofeedback techniques to enhance a state of relaxation. Guided imagery frequently is used as an adjunct to biofeedback to facilitate a state of excitation for athletic training. Blumenstein et al[55] found that significant tachypnea was observed during imagery of sprint running, and in most cases studied, EMG biofeedback substantially augmented the physiological responses.

MUSCLE RE-EDUCATION

When using biofeedback for muscle re-education, it is important to place the muscle to be examined in the easiest position for the patient to elicit movement. For example, in testing the strength of the vastus medialis of the quadriceps muscle group, the patient might be positioned on his or her side, attempting to straighten the lower leg. Another useful position might be with the patient supine and the lower leg hanging off the edge of the table. For other patients, this movement might best be accomplished from a sitting position. It is generally easier to elicit motor unit firing when a muscle is in a fully stretched condition and the patient is asked to move through a full range of motion. Visual observation by the patient of the motion to be performed often can be of great benefit.

At the initial treatment session, it is important for the therapist to familiarize the patient with the operation of the biofeedback unit. Placing electrodes on a normal muscle or on the corresponding muscle of the uninvolved extremity when possible, and going through the full range of motion or tensing and relaxing the muscle, will help prepare the patient to work with the affected muscle or muscle group. This approach will also give the patient practice in reading the meter and hearing the "muscle sounds."

To aid the patient in eliciting motor responses, all forms of exercise, proprioceptive neuromuscular facilitation (PNF) techniques, and body positioning may be employed. The objective is to discover any functional motor units in the muscle. If no active motor units are discovered at a particular therapy session, it does not necessarily mean that none are present. In a weakened muscle, there may be only a few active motor units, as compared to the thousands in a normal muscle. What we are searching for is "potential activity" of motor units in what appears to be a "paralyzed" muscle.

When active motor unit responses are found, the next step is to bring the responses under voluntary control. It should not be expected that when responses in an involved muscle are detected they will remain at the same high level of activity at future therapy sessions. A great degree of variability can be expected initially, especially in the neurologically compromised muscle. Over an extended period of treatment, a muscle given regular, continued exercise is likely to show a continuing increase in strength and less tendency toward wide fluctuations in readings.

Motivation of the patient is the key. If the therapist approaches the patient optimistically with the attitude that EMG biofeedback can be of significant benefit in the rehabilitation process, and continually emphasizes reachable goals with good exercise programs, then real progress can be achieved and objectively measured. As the return of functional components for a desired task occurs, and the speed and accuracy of performance improves, biofeedback instrumentation may be gradually withdrawn.

It is important to remember that it is extremely easy for a person who has obtained some functional use of a muscle group to later let those muscles regress to a decreased level of function. This generally happens when muscles are not exercised for a period of time. It must be stressed to the patient that the natural sensory feedback mechanism of the muscles he or she is attempting to strengthen has been diminished, and that constant attention on a daily basis is required to increase muscle strength and function to an optimum level.

EMG biofeedback can also be used as a monitor for evaluation of progress with home exercise programs in subsequent follow-up sessions. A home unit is often helpful, and most EMG biofeedback units manufactured today have memory capabilities of 30+ treatment sessions, so that progress can be downloaded, and compliance with the exercise program monitored. Since it is a natural tendency to decrease exercise as strength increases, patients should be re-evaluated on a periodic basis, and the therapist should reinforce the necessity of continuing their exercise programs. It is important to remember that if a total program of objective measurement of muscle activity is undertaken, clear, concise records must be kept to facilitate reimbursement by third party payers.[76]

MUSCLE RELAXATION

The procedure for training a patient in muscle relaxation techniques is much the same as for muscle re-education. The difference lies in the fact that instead of teaching the patient to increase motor unit firing, we are trying to inhibit or decrease the level of firing created by the tension or tone in the muscle. Again, electrodes should be attached over an unaffected muscle for demonstration of how muscle tension can be lowered after an initial muscle contraction. Only when the patient has thoroughly understood the relationship between muscle contraction and relaxation and the corresponding changes in auditory and visual displays should the electrodes be placed on the affected muscle.

The patient must understand that relaxing a muscle that has abnormal tone will not be as easy as relaxing a normal muscle, but that it can be done with practice and perseverance. Repeated orientation is necessary. Patients must understand that they control the feedback and that the equipment does not control them. Among the best tools to assist a patient in decreasing muscle tension are deep breathing techniques focusing in on the abdominal region, music, relaxation tapes, and progressive relaxation exercises, such as those designed by Jacobsen.[3]

To assist patients who have difficulty in decreasing muscle activity, the therapist should point out any strained posture, labored breathing, or noted lack of focus, etc., interfering with the ability to relax. Ideally, for training practice sessions, the patient should be in a quiet, dimly-lit room, free from outside distractions, and positioned for maximum comfort. It is sometimes helpful to begin training or practice sessions by having the individual imagine pleasant scenes or experiences. This allows the patient to clear his or her mind of any of the "built-in" tensions of everyday life. Clinical training sessions generally last 30 minutes on a two- to three-time per week basis. As the patient makes progress in decreasing the microvolts level in a structured situation, he or she should be encouraged to practice these relaxation techniques in the environment where the tension arises.

When working with patients who have muscle contraction or tension headaches, the electrodes are often placed on the skin over the frontalis muscle, about two inches apart and approximately one inch above the eyebrows. It should be explained to patients that the electrodes are measuring the amount of muscle tension they are producing, and that this tension is a reflection of the tension throughout their whole body.

Some clinicians feel that the frontalis is not necessarily the best reflector of body tension for every patient, and this author would agree. Another effective lead placement is suggested using a global technique. With this technique, the electrodes are attached to the flexor surface of each forearm. This electrode placement allows monitoring tension of all the muscles of the upper body, which comprise approximately 60% of the controlled muscles of the body.

In order to develop a complete program of muscle re-education or relaxation, it is important that the patient be instructed in the use of the EMG biofeedback unit at home. This approach allows patients to monitor and maintain the optimum level that they have achieved in the clinical environment.

CLINICAL RESEARCH IN THE USE OF BIOFEEDBACK TECHNIQUES

IMMUNOLOGY

The role of the mind in healing the body is a fascinating subject which is steadily gaining in importance even within traditional medical practice. Mentally influencing the immune system, for example, is an exciting new field given the name *psychoneuroimmunology* (literally, the effect of the mind through the nervous system on the immune system). This topic has been extensively covered in Chapter 1 of this book and is only mentioned here as it relates to the utilization of biofeedback techniques.

The effect of biofeedback-assisted relaxation on cell-mediated immunity, cortisol, and white blood cell count was investigated by McGrady et al[4] under low-stress conditions. Interestingly, the group of subjects trained in biofeedback-assisted relaxation techniques showed increased blastogenesis and a decreased white blood cell count, indicating a clear effect on the immune system.

The results of immunological responses of breast cancer patients to behavioral interventions is remarkable and promising.[5] Gruber et al[5] reports the results of an 18-month study of immune system and psychological changes in Stage 1 breast cancer patients provided with relaxation, guided imagery, and biofeedback training. Significant effects were found in natural killer cell activity, lymphocyte responsiveness, and the number of peripheral blood lymphocytes. This study clearly indicates that relaxation, guided imagery, and related biofeedback techniques have the potential for modifying the immune system's response in a positive manner.

MIGRAINE AND TENSION HEADACHE PAIN

Behavioral therapies such as biofeedback are commonly used to treat migraine and tension headaches.[9,12] Controlling sympathetic activity is effective for controlling the pain in both disturbances.[9] Grazzi and Bussone[9] confirmed the clinical efficacy of EMG biofeedback treatment for tension and common migraine headaches. In this study, the basal stress indices (plasma catacholamines and cortisol) were significantly different in the experimental group, compared to no change in the controls, and the study group experienced a substantial decrease in frequency of headaches reported.

Functional activities of daily living are often restricted in the presence of tension headaches.[6-8] In a study by King,[6] EMG biofeedback was used to decrease upper trapezius activity related to tension headaches. It was this study's finding that headaches are caused by general tension and anxiety and affected the individual's ability to attend to activities of daily living adequately, including child care, homemaking, and vocational activities. The program combined deep-breathing exercises, progressive muscular relaxation exercises, resisted shoulder elevation exercises, and EMG monitoring during upper extremity tasks and a home exercise/relaxation program. EMG biofeedback was successful in helping to eliminate tension headaches, and the patients reported an increased ability to attend to activities of daily living.[6]

Other studies[10,11] also strongly support the use of biofeedback-assisted relaxation techniques in the treatment of tension[10] and migraine[11] headaches.

IMPROVEMENT OF FUNCTIONAL DEFICITS IN PARAPLEGIA AND QUADRIPLEGIA

The efficacy of enhancing muscle function in spinal cord patients when administered in conjunction with physical rehabilitation therapy has been substantiated.[13] Evidence from the study by Klose et al[13] indicated that spinal cord injury patients in the study group using biofeedback and a conventional exercise program increased the amount of improvement seen, compared to the control group who used a conventional exercise program alone to regain muscle strength and function.

POSTURAL INSTABILITY, PROPRIOCEPTION, AND FALLS

Postural instability, deficits in proprioception, and kinesthesia are associated with many neuromuscular pathologies and increase the potential of falling. Postural instability may be developmental, as in the case of the severely motorically impaired child with cerebral palsy, or acquired later in life secondary to neural disease or trauma.[14] Beyond the pathological conditions creating postural instability, aging is also associated with trunk weakness, alterations in neuromuscular and musculoskeletal efficiency, and an increased incidence of falling.[15,16] In contrast to the use of biofeedback for neuromuscular re-education of muscles that are over-active or under-active, biofeedback for postural instability has been used to augment achievement of functional skills, such as head or trunk control, or symmetry of standing balance.[14] EMG biofeedback instrumentation is effective in detecting muscle activity and giving the patient objective information about the physiological functioning and movements not ordinarily perceived by the individual. In the case of postural instability, auditory and visual biofeedback signals provide the patient with information regarding head and trunk orientation, and about symmetry of weight bearing through the lower extremities.[17-20]

CEREBRAL PALSY

In addition to the physical problems inherent in cerebral palsy, speech problems can often create a frustrating communication deficit in these individuals. In a study by Howard and Varley,[22] the use of electopalatography biofeedback was used to treat patients with severe speech production problems affecting articulation, phonation, and resonance. It was found that this form of instrumented biofeedback provided a valuable form of visual feedback for patients and revealed and clarified aspects of oral movements for speech and nonspeech activity which had been difficult to capture via auditory perception.[22]

CEREBRAL VASCULAR ACCIDENT

Rehabilitation for individuals sustaining a CVA has been shown to be enhanced by employing EMG biofeedback for neuromuscular re-education.[23] These authors found that problems such as foot drop and other gait problems, posture and muscle tone, voluntary control of involved muscles, and muscle relaxation in associated reactions were all improved with the use of biofeedback as an adjunct to physical and occupational therapy.

Sunderland et al[24] did a detailed study to determine the recovery of upper extremity function following an acute stroke, comparing orthodox physical therapy interventions with therapy regimes enhanced by the use of EMG biofeedback to encourage motor learning with behavioral methods. Six months following strokes, it was found that study subjects had a statistically significant advantage in recovery of strength, range, and speed of movement. Moreland and Thomson[25] showed that a small but significant effect on muscle function was realized utilizing EMG biofeedback compared to conventional physical therapy for improving upper extremity function in patients following a stroke.

MUSCULAR RE-EDUCATION/RELAXATION FOLLOWING INJURY

The effects of biofeedback on carpal tunnel syndrome shows promise in preventing this problem from recurring. In a study by Thomas et al,[26] behavioral modification based on audible electromyographic biofeedback signals was used to discourage awkward hand postures and the exertion of excessive force with the fingers, which are suspected of causing carpal tunnel syndrome. They found a reduction in symptomatology and a learning affect related to proper ergonomic posturing.

Reynolds[27] describes a rehabilitation approach for keyboard operators following radial tunnel compression and release of the extensor origin of the right elbow.[27] An EMG biofeedback device was employed in this study to determine which work activities individuals should avoid or alter to reduce strain in the wrist musculature. It was found that recurrence of carpal tunnel symptoms was significantly reduced by re-educating workers through the use of biofeedback.[27]

Rotator cuff and other shoulder pathologies often are accompanied by protective muscle guarding in the supraspinatus, infraspinatus, anterior, and middle portions of the deltoid, and the descending part of the trapezius. By using biofeedback surface electrodes, it has been found that subjects could reduce the EMG activity voluntarily in the trapezius.[28] This was not true for the other muscles investigated. When the trapezius activity was reduced, there was a tendency toward an increase in EMG activity in the other shoulder muscles, particularly the infraspinatus. Palmerud et al[28] suggests that the findings may be related to relaxation from an initial overstabilization of the shoulder, or redistribution of load among synergists. It is suggested that the possibility of reducing trapezius activity may be of ergonomic significance.[28]

Voluntary posterior dislocation of the shoulder is a difficult condition to treat successfully. It has been shown that EMG biofeedback is a nonoperative treatment that has been successfully used to prevent recurrent dislocation.[29]

MEASUREMENT OF ENDURANCE

The effect of psychological strategies upon cardiorespiratory and muscular activity during aerobic exercise has been widely employed in sports therapy. Hatfield et al[30] demonstrated that all cardiovascular parameters (for example, heart rate, respiratory rate, depth of ventilation, blood pressure) could be consciously altered using biofeedback monitoring.[30] Leisman et al[31] investigated the effects of fatigue and task repetition on the relationship between integrated electromyogram and force output of working muscles.[31] This study showed that with fatigue, integrated EMG activity increased strongly and functional force output of the muscle remained stable or decreased. Fatigue results in a less efficient muscle process. Through training using biofeedback, the efficiency of muscle contraction could be improved with volitional control, and the level of fatigue reduced.[31]

BRAIN INJURY

Biofeedback has traditionally been used in the context of relaxation therapy along with stress management. Some recent studies have looked to extend the applicability of biofeedback by using it as a didactic tool for neuromotor rehabilitation. Duckett and Kramer[32] applied biofeedback with anoxic head-injury patients unable to participate in transfers owing to severe myoclonicity. They trained the patients using autogenic relaxation along with EMG biofeedback to reduce the myoclonus and therefore participate actively with stand pivot transfers.

The mechanisms of feedback not controlled by our consciousness play an essential role in the functions of the central nervous system in the process of programming of activities and behavior, and control of these functions. In cases of deviations or errors of activities imposed by brain injury and stroke, the possibility of their immediate correction exists.[33] Brain damage after trauma or caused by tumor disturbs normal feedback mechanisms, producing varying symptom complexes. Kwolek and Pop[33] found that EMG biofeedback was advantageous in providing afferent information to the brain-damaged patient and enhanced the return of motor function more substantially than conventional physical therapy interventions.

URINARY INCONTINENCE AND OTHER PELVIC FLOOR DISORDERS

Stress incontinence is a debilitating condition affecting a large proportion of the female population. Pelvic floor exercising with the aid of EMG biofeedback is well established as an effective treatment regime.[34-43] Current EMG monitoring devices are effective, as they also may be employed in community-based home therapy.[34,35] Many of the units are compact, accurate, and suitable for ambulatory monitoring of vaginal pressure. McIntosh et al[36] found that both urinary and fecal incontinence was improved through the use of EMG biofeedback-assisted pelvic floor exercise. These authors clearly demonstrated that a pelvic floor rehabilitation program is an effective alternative to surgical intervention in reducing the frequency of urinary and fecal leakage. Brubaker and Kotarinos[37] also demonstrated that pelvic floor muscle training utilizing EMG biofeedback was beneficial in the treatment of urinary incontinence. Numerous studies confirm that urinary incontinence can be managed conservatively through physical therapy interventions utilizing biofeedback-assisted pelvic floor muscle training.[36-42]

Postoperative complications following radical prostatectomy usually include urinary incontinence.[41] Milam and Franke[41] found that beyond surgical interventions, such as modified apical dissection and construction of a tubularized neourethra, EMG biofeedback provided a reliable alternative to management of urinary incontinence after prostatectomy.

The effective use of biofeedback for gynecological problems such as vulvar vestibulitis syndrome, marked by moderate to severe chronic introital dyspareunia and tenderness of the vulvar vestibule, also has been clearly demonstrated.[43] Women instructed in a home program employing biofeedback-assisted pelvic floor muscle rehabilitation exercises experienced an increase in pelvic floor muscle contraction strength, a decrease in resting tension levels of the pelvic floor muscle, a decrease in the muscle instability associated with this syndrome, and a remarkable decrease in pain.[43]

INTRACTABLE CONSTIPATION

Some individuals have difficulty relaxing the striated muscles of the anal sphincters, sometimes referred to as animus. In a study by Turnbull and Ritvo,[44] a biofeedback-based relaxation program was developed to teach patients with intractable constipation to relax the "voluntary" anal sphincter muscle. This research evaluated the efficacy of this treatment approach in reducing symptomatology. The study group consisted of patients who were unresponsive to a high-fiber diet and required persistent laxative dosing to achieve regular bowel frequency. A dual-therapy approach was employed in which patients were taught to relax the anal sphincter muscles via biofeedback from a manometric anal sphincter probe. Concurrently, patients were instructed in general biofeedback-relaxation techniques (autogenic relaxation). In all subjects studied, stool frequency increased, pain and bloating decreased, and follow-up of 2 to 4.5 years post-therapy showed continued improvement in bowel function.[44,45]

ASTHMA, EMPHYSEMA, AND CHRONIC OBSTRUCTIVE LUNG DISEASE

The use of biofeedback techniques also has been shown to have an impact on respiratory resistance in conditions of asthma and other resistive lung problems.[46-48] Hypothesis for the positive impact of both visual and auditory biofeedback effectiveness in these respiratory conditions is the activation of the parasympathetic nervous system providing more available oxygen, and the influence of relaxation and deep breathing techniques in calming the system, thereby reducing respiratory resistance.[46,48] Blanc-Gras et al[47] provided substantial evidence for support of the learning effect facilitated by the use of visual feedback in control of respiratory pattern. This information indicates that EMG biofeedback could have a great deal of merit in the treatment of asthma and other stress-related breathing problems.

Laryngeal dyskinesis is a functional asthma-like disorder refractory to bronchodilator regimes.[48] Nahmias, Tansey, and Karetzky[48] showed that patients treated with EMG biofeedback demonstrated clinical improvement with reversal of their variable extrathoracic upper airway obstruction.

MODIFICATION OF HYPERTENSION

The central mechanisms and possibilities of biofeedback on systemic arterial pressure have been investigated extensively.[30,49,50] McGrady[49] studied a group of patients with essential hypertension for the effects of group relaxation training and thermal biofeedback on blood pressure and other psychophysiologic measures—heart rate, frontalis muscle tension, finger temperature, depression, anxiety, plasma aldosterone, plasma renin activity, and plasma and urinary cortisol. A significant decline in blood pressure was observed in 49% of the experimental group. Of that group, 51% maintained a lower blood pressure at a 10-month follow-up examination, suggesting that relaxation training has beneficial effects for short-term and long-term adjunctive therapy of essential hypertension in selected individuals.

DIABETES, VASCULAR DISEASE, AND INTERMITTENT CLAUDICATION

Saunders et al[51] examined the therapeutic effects of thermal biofeedback-assisted autogenic training in a group of diabetic and vascular disease patients with symptoms of intermittent claudication. The individuals received thermal feedback from the hand for five sessions, then from the foot for 16 sessions, while hand and foot temperatures were monitored simultaneously. Within the session, foot temperatures rose specifically in response to foot temperature biofeedback, and starting foot temperatures rose between sessions. Post-treatment blood pressure was reduced to a normal level. Attacks of intermittent claudication were reduced to zero after 12 sessions, and walking distance increased by about a mile per day over the course of the treatment. It would appear that thermal biofeedback and autogenic training are potentially promising therapies for persons with diabetes and peripheral vascular disease.

Of interest is a study by Freedman et al[58] comparing the sympathetic activation using temperature feedback compared to autogenic training alone. Thirty-nine normal volunteers of both sexes were randomly assigned to receive 8 sessions of temperature biofeedback or autogenic training to increase finger temperature. Temperature feedback subjects produced significant elevations in finger temperature during training, whereas those who received autogenic training did not. This study indicates that autogenic training alone may not produce vasodilatation.

Rice and Schindler[52] investigated the effect of relaxation training/thermal biofeedback on blood circulation in the lower extremities of diabetic subjects. A within-subject experimental design was used. During phase 1, all subjects used a self-selected relaxation method and recorded toe temperatures daily. During phase 2, subjects were taught a biofeedback-assisted relaxation technique designed to elicit sensations of warmth in the lower extremities and increase circulation and temperature. Subjects relaxed at home with the use of a designated relaxation tape. Each phase of the study lasted 4 weeks. Mean temperature change scores between phases 1 and 2 were 8.73% (phase 1) and 31.88% (phase 2). The greater increase in phase 2 was attributed to the biofeedback-assisted relaxation technique. These authors concluded that diabetic patients show significant increases in peripheral blood circulation with this technique. This noninvasive method could serve as an adjunct treatment for limited blood flow in some complications of diabetes, such as ulceration.

CARDIAC ARRHYTHMIAS

Respiratory sinus arrhythmia, the peak-to-peak variations in heart rate caused by respiration, can be used as a noninvasive measure of parasympathetic cardiac control. In a study by Reyes del Paso et al,[53] they showed that subjects could actually alter their respiratory sinus arrhythmia, that is, decrease or increase the rate, by monitoring respiratory biofeedback apparatus in conjunction with consciously concentrating on their depth and rate of respiration. Shahidi and Salmon[54] also demonstrated that individuals classified as Type A adults were able to modify their heart rates volitionally when instructed in relaxation techniques using EKG biofeedback monitoring.

STRESS MANAGEMENT

When we are truly relaxed, very definite and measurable changes take place in the body.[49,55-57] These changes distinguish relaxation from the opposite states of tension or arousal. Some of the most significant changes are triggered by the two branches of the autonomic nervous system. The sympathetic branch of the nervous system controls body temperature, digestion, heart rate, respiratory rate, blood flow and pressure, and muscular tension. The parasympathetic nervous system lowers oxygen consumption and reduces the following bodily functions: carbon dioxide elimination, heart and respiratory rates, blood pressure, blood lactate, and blood cortisol levels.[49,55-59] These bodily changes are collectively referred to as the "relaxation response."

Recent research also suggests that among the biochemical changes triggered by relaxation there is an increase in the body's manufacture of certain mood-altering neurotransmitters.[57,58] In particular, production of serotonin (the biochemical equivalent to Prozac) is increased. Serotonin is associated with feelings of calmness and contentment.

Lehrer et al[57] isolated the types of biofeedback techniques that worked most effectively in various conditions. Their study showed that instrumentation using biofeedback electrodes placed over the involved muscles was most effective in treating disorders with a predominant muscular component, eg, muscle strength and/or tone changes, tension headaches, carpal tunnel, etc. Disorders in which autonomic dysfunction predominates, for example, hypertension and migraine headaches, are more effectively treated by techniques with a strong autonomic component, such as lead placement on the frontalis muscle, or digital temperature monitoring, and progressive relaxation techniques.

DYSPHAGIA

Electromyography and biofeedback techniques are well established in the disciplines of physical medicine for the retraining of muscle groups to approximate functional performance in swallowing.[60,61] The management of dysphagia presents a major problem in the comprehensive rehabilitation of stroke and head injury patients. Dysphagia is a disorder of the swallowing process. Oral dysphagia refers to abnormalities in the oral phase of the swallowing mechanism.[60] As this disorder is primarily based in muscle over- or under-activity, biofeedback devices rendering feedback of biomechanical parameters characterizing the oral phase of swallowing have been shown to be extremely effective in re-establishing swallowing patterns in neuromuscularly impaired individuals.[60] Leplow, Schluter, and Ferstl[21] demonstrated that the use of biofeedback was instrumental in assessment of muscle activity in facial and oral musculature. These authors demonstrated that proprioception of neuromuscularly involved patients was enhanced, especially in muscles richly supplied with muscle spindles and afferent fibers, that is, the masseter muscle and zygomatus major muscle.

BELL'S PALSY

Neuromuscular rehabilitation can reduce the severity of chronic facial paralysis, but complete recovery is frequently impeded by synkinesis.[62,63] It has been determined that synkinesis could be minimized by preventing its possible reinforcement during rehabilitation by employing EMG biofeedback with the goal of eliciting smaller movements. Muscular re-education in Bell's palsy patients who have intact facial-motor innervation has clearly been found to be enhanced by the use of EMG biofeedback. Facial function typically improves with a more rapid recovery of symmetry and a decrease in synkinesis.[62,63]

PAIN MANAGEMENT IN CANCER PATIENTS

Pain is one of the most feared consequences of cancer. Control of pain from cancer has been shown to decrease discomfort and diminish the need for drugs that may induce other negative side effects.[64-66] Relaxation and related biofeedback techniques have been shown to be effective in the management of cancer pain.[66-68] Utilizing such interventions as progressive muscle relaxation, relaxation and systemic desensitization, hypnosis, and biofeedback and relaxation, researchers have determined that nonpharmaceutical interventions for pain management have a great deal of potential.[66-69] Filshie[68] compared many specific methods in the management of pain, including electrical nerve stimulation, acupuncture, sympathetic blockade, epidural and intrathecal blocks, and neurosurgical and psychological biofeedback techniques. This comparison showed that the noninvasive procedure of relaxation and biofeedback had the greatest overall effect on pain.

Chemotherapy protocols that induce severe protracted nausea and vomiting are stressful for cancer patients, and the fear that may be associated with chemotherapy often outweighs other negative aspects of the cancer experience. Stoudemire, Cotanch, and

Laszlo[65] showed that many of the associated side effects of chemotherapy could be managed through pharmacologic approaches and maintenance of hydration, in addition to reducing stress levels through emotional support and the use of behavioral relaxation techniques supported by EMG biofeedback. Recent research provides evidence that sensory-behavioral pretreatments can ameliorate radiation therapy-induced nausea and vomiting[69-72] and significantly diminish and in some cases eliminate pain in the cancer patient.[64,71,73]

SUMMARY

As a literate civilization, we are now more than 5000 years old. Physical needs have always kept the mind well occupied. Technologies have granted us a comfortable control over our environment. Yet, these technologies are costly. It is clear that medical problems can be caused by or aggravated by the mental status of the individual. Understanding this, it is an intriguing paradox that western medicine has created in its concentrated efforts on developing extensive drugs and elaborate surgical techniques to deal with physical and mental compensations. With the evolution of managed care, the trend needs now to seek less costly alternatives of care. This involves reaching inward and developing technologies which will allow us some insight into our inner world. It's time to equal the balance and attempt to solve some of the physical manifestations of pathologies from within.

Biofeedback has shown a remarkably positive benefit on the functional and treatment outcomes of numerous conditions.[75] Biofeedback instrumentation has been a growing part of physical therapy practice for over 20 years,[76] and physical therapists have contributed to researching its efficacy in treating varying conditions. Sophisticated contemporary equipment does much more in quantifying the worth of biofeedback techniques than was originally envisioned. The importance of relating quantified movement-based data to functional measures has influenced the level of appropriate reimbursement for physical therapy services utilizing biofeedback.

Physical therapy, as an integral member of the health care community, needs to continue to investigate self-awareness and self-control as a probable rehabilitative tool in the treatment of a multitude of conditions.

REFERENCES

1. Ford CW. *Where Healing Waters Meet.* Barrytown, NY: Station Hill Press, Inc; 1989.

2. Peper E, ed. *Mind/Body Integration: Essential Readings in Biofeedback.* New York, NY: Plenum, Inc; 1979.

3. Wirth DP, Barrett MJ. Complementary healing therapies. *International Journal of Psychosomatics.* 1994;41(1-4):61-67.

4. McGrady A, Conran P, Dickey D, Garman D, Farris E, Schumann-Brzezinski C. The effects of biofeedback-assisted relaxation on cell-mediated immunity, cortisol, and white blood cell count in healthy adult subjects. *J Behav Med.* 1992;15:343-354.

5. Gruber BL, Hersh SP, Hall NR, et al. Immunological responses of breast cancer patients to behavioral interventions. *Biofeedback & Self Regulation.* 1993;18(1):1-22.

6. King TI. The use of electomyographic biofeedback in treating patients with tension headaches. *Am J Occup Ther.* 1992;46:839-842.

7. Sheffied MM. Psychosocial interventions in the management of recurrent headache disorders: policy considerations for implementation. *Behav Med.* 1994;20(2):73-77.

8. Penzien DB, Holroyd KA. Psychosocial interventions in the management of recurrent headache disorders: description of treatment techniques. *Behav Med.* 1994;20(2):64-73.

9. Grazzi L, Bussone G. Effect of biofeedback treatment on sympathetic function in common migraine and tension-type headache. *Cepahalgia.* 1993;13(3):197-200.

10. Arena JG, Bruno GM, Hannah SL, Meador KJ. A comparison of frontal electromyographic biofeedback training, trapezius electromyographic biofeedback, and progressive muscle relaxation therapy in the treatment of tension headache. *Headache.* 1995;35:411-419.

11. Grazzi L, Bussone G. Italian experience of electromyographic-biofeedback treatment of episodic common migraine: preliminary results. *Headache.* 1993;33:439-441.

12. Blanchard EB. Psychological treatment of benign headache disorders. *J Consult Clin Psychol.* 1992;60:537-551.

13. Klose KJ, Needham BM, Schmidt D, Broton JG, Green BA. An assessment of the contribution of electromyographic biofeedback as an adjunct in the physical training of spinal cord injured persons. *Arch Phys Med Rehabil.* 1993;74:453-456.

14. Moore S, Woollacott MH. The use of biofeedback devices to improve postural stability. *Phys Ther Pract.* 1993;2(20):1-19.

15. Leonhardt C. Posture biofeedback for improved sitting [in German]. *Fortschritte der Medizin.* 1992;110(1-2):33-34.

16. Hawken MB, Jantti P, Waterston JA. The effect of sway feedback and loss of sensory cues in older women with a history of falls. In: Woollacott MH, Horak F, eds. *Posture and Gait-Control Mechanisms.* Vol II. Eugene, Ore: University of Oregon Books; 1992:263-266.

17. Nashner LM, Shumway-Cook A, Marin O. Stance posture control in select groups of children with cerebral palsy: deficits in sensory organization and muscular coordination. *Exp Brain Res.* 1983;49:393-409.

18. Woolridge CP, Russell G. Head position training with the cerebral palsied child: an application of

biofeedback techniques. *Arch Phys Med Rehabil.* 1976;57:407-414.

19. Shumway-Cook A, Anson D, Haller S. Postural sway biofeedback: its effect on reestablishing stance stability in hemiplegic patients. *Arch Phys Med Rehabil.* 1988;69:395-400.

20. Wolf SL, Binder-MacLeod SA. Electromyographic biofeedback applications to the hemiplegic patient. *Phys Ther.* 1983;63:1404-1413.

21. Leplow B, Schluter V, Ferstl R. A new procedure for assessment of proprioception. *Perceptual & Motor Skills.* 1992;74(1):91-98.

22. Howard S, Varley R. Using electropalatography to treat severe apraxia of speech. *Eur J Disord Commun.* 1995;30(2):246-255.

23. Schleenbaker RE, Mainous AG III. Electromyographic biofeedback for neuromuscular re-education in the hemiplegic stroke patient: a meta-analysis. *Arch Phys Med Rehabil.* 1993;74:1301-1304.

24. Sunderland A, Tinson DJ, Bradley EL, Fletcher D, Langton Hewer R, Wade DT. Enhanced physical therapy improved recovery of arm function after stroke: a randomized controlled trial. *J Neurol Neurosurg Psychiatry.* 1992;55:530-535.

25. Moreland J, Thomson MA. Efficacy of electromyographic biofeedback compared with conventional physical therapy for upper-extremity function in patients following stroke: a research overview and meta-analysis. *Phys Ther.* 1994;74:534-547.

26. Thomas RE, Vaidya SC, Herrick RT, Congleton JJ. The effects of biofeedback on carpal tunnel syndrome. *Ergonomics.* 1993;36:353-361.

27. Reynolds C. Electromyographic biofeedback evaluation of a computer keyboard operator with cumulative trauma disorder. *J Hand Ther.* 1994;7:25-27.

28. Palmerund G, Kadefors R, Sporrong H, et al. Voluntary redistribution of muscle activity in human shoulder muscles. *Ergonomics.* 1995;38:806-815.

29. Young MS. Electromyographic biofeedback use in the treatment of voluntary posterior dislocation of the shoulder: a case study. *J Ortho Sports Phys Ther.* 1994;20:171-175.

30. Hatfield BD, Spalding TW, Mahon AD, Slater BA, Brody EB, Vaccaro P. The effect of psychological strategies upon cardiorespiratory and muscular activity during treadmill running. *Med Sci Sports Exer.* 1992;24:218-225.

31. Leisman G, Zenhausern R, Ferentz A, Tefera T, Zemcov A. Electromyographic effects of fatigue and task repetition on the validity of estimates of strong and weak muscles in applied kinesiological muscle-testing procedures. *Percept Mot Skills.* 1995;80:963-977.

32. Duckett S, Kramer T. Managing myoclonus secondary to anoxic encephalopathy through EMG biofeedback. *Brain Injury.* 1994;8:185-188.

33. Kwolek A, Pop T. Use of biological vicarious biofeedback in the rehabilitation of patients with brain damage [in Polish]. *Neurologia I Neurochirurgia Polska.* 1992;(suppl 1):321-327.

34. Jones KR. Ambulatory biofeedback for stress incontinence exercise regimes: a novel development of the perineometer. *J Adv Nurs.* 1994;19:509-512.

35. Phillips HC, Fenster HN, Samsom D. An effective treatment for functional urinary incoordination. *J Behav Med.* 1992;15:45-63.

36. McIntosh LJ, Frahm JD, Mallett VT, Richardson DA. Pelvic floor rehabilitation in the treatment of incontinence. *J Reprod Med.* 1993;38:662-666.

37. Brubaker L, Kotarinos R. Kegel or cut? Variations on his theme. *J Reprod Med.* 1993;38:672-678.

38. McCandless S, Mason G. Physical therapy as an effective change agent in the treatment of patients with urinary incontinence. *J Miss State Med Assoc.* 1995;36:271-274.

39. Stein M, Discippio W, Davia M, Taub H. Biofeedback for the treatment of stress and urge incontinence. *J Urol.* 1995;153:641-643.

40. Rayome RG, Johnson V, Gray M. Stress urinary incontinence after radical prostatectomy. *J Wound, Ostomy, & Continence Nurs.* 1994;21:264-269.

41. Milam DF, Franke JJ. Prevention and treatment of incontinence after radical prostatectomy. *Seminars in Urol Oncol.* 1995;13:224-237.

42. Smith DA, Newman DK. Basic elements of biofeedback therapy for pelvic muscle rehabilitation. *Urol Nursing.* 1994;14:130-135.

43. Glazer HI, Rodke G, Sencionis C. Hertz R, Young AW. Treatment of vulvar vestibulitis syndrome with electromyographic biofeedback of pelvic floor musculature. *J Reprod Med.* 1995;40:283-290.

44. Turnbull GK, Ritvo PG. Anal sphincter biofeedback relaxation treatment for women with intractable constipation symptoms. *Diseases of the Colon & Rectum.* 1992;35:530-536.

45. Anonymous. Anismus and biofeedback. *Lancet.* 1992;339(8787):217-218. Editorial.

46. Mass R, Dahme B, Richter R. Clinical evaluation of respiratory resistance biofeedback training. *Biofeedback & Self Regulation.* 1993;18:211-223.

47. Blanc-Gras N, Esteve F, Benchetrit G, Gallego J. Performance and learning during voluntary control of breath patterns. *Bio Psych.* 1994;37:147-159.

48. Nahmias J, Tansey M, Karetzky MS. Asthmatic extrathoracic upper airway obstruction: laryngeal dyskinesis. *New Jersey Medicine.* 1994;91:616-620.

49. McGrady A. Effects of group relaxation training and thermal biofeedback on blood pressure and related physiological and psychological variables in essential hypertension. *Biofeedback & Self Regulation.* 1994;19:51-66.

50. Vasilevskii NN, Sidorov YA, Kiselev IM. Biofeedback control of systemic arterial pressure. *Neurosci Behav Physiol.* 1992;22:219-223.

51. Saunders JT, Cox DJ, Teastes CD, Pohl SL. Thermal biofeedback in the treatment of intermittent claudication in diabetes: a case study. *Biofeedback & Self Regulation.* 1994;19:337-345.

52. Rice BI, Schindler JV. Effect of thermal biofeedback-assisted relaxation training on blood circulation in the lower extremities of a population with diabetes. *Diabetes Care.* 1992;15:853-858.

53. Reyes del Paso GA, Godoy J, Vila J. Self-regulation of respiratory sinus arrhythmia. *Biofeedback & Self Regulation.* 1992;17:261-275.

54. Shahidi S, Salmon P. Contingent and non-contingent biofeedback training for Type A and B healthy adults: can Type A's relax by competing? *J Psychosom Res.* 1992;36:477-483.

55. Blumenstein B, Breslav I, Bar-Eli M, Tenenbaum G, Weinstein Y. Regulation of mental states and biofeedback techniques: effects on breathing pattern. *Biofeedback & Self Regulation.* 1995;20:169-183.

56. Montgomery GT. Slowed respiration training. *Biofeedback & Self Regulation.* 1994;19:211-225.

57. Lehrer PM, Carr P, Sargunaraj D, Woolfolk RL. Stress management techniques: are they all equivalent, or do they have specific effects? *Biofeedback & Self Regulation.* 1994;19:353-401.

58. Freedman RR, Keegan D, Rodriguez J, Galloway MP. Plasma catecholamine levels during temperature biofeedback training in normal subjects. *Biofeedback & Self Regulation*. 1993;18(2):107-114.

59. Van Zak DB. Biofeedback treatments for premenstrual and premenstrual affective syndromes. *Inter J Psychosom*. 1994;41:53-60.

60. Sukthankar SM, Reddy NP, Canilang EP, Stephenson L, Thomas R. Design and development of protable biofeedback systems for use in oral dysphagia rehabilitation. *Med Eng Physic*. 1994;16:430-435.

61. Bryant M. Biofeedback in the treatment of a selected dysphagic patient. *Dysphagia*. 1991;6:140-144.

62. Segal B, Hunter T, Danys I, Freedman C, Black M. Minimizing synkinesis during rehabilitation of the paralyzed face: preliminary assessment of a new small-movement therapy. *J Otolaryngol*. 1995;24:149-153.

63. Segal B, Zompa I, Danys I, et al. Symmetry and synkinesis during rehabilitation of unilateral facial paralysis. *J Otolaryngol*. 1995;24:143-148.

64. Ferrell BR, Ferrell BA. Easing the pain. *Geriatric Nursing*. 1990;11:175-178.

65. Stoudemire A, Cotanch P, Laszlo J. Recent advances in the pharmacologic and behavioral management of chemotherapy-induced emesis. *Arch Intern Med*. 1984;144:1029-1033.

66. Foley KM. The treatment of pain in the patient with cancer. *CA: A Cancer Journal for Clinicians*. 1986;36:194-215.

67. Contanch PH. Relaxation techniques as an independent nursing intervention for onocology patients. *Cancer Nursing*. 1987;10(suppl 1):58-64.

68. Filshie J. The non-drug treatment of neuralgic and neuropathic pain of malignancy. *Cancer Surveys*. 1988;7:161-193.

69. Blum RH. Hypothesis: a new basis for sensory-behavioral pretreatments to ameliorate radiation therapy-induced nausea and vomiting. *Cancer Treatment Reviews*. 1988;15:211-227.

70. Moher D, Arthur AZ, Pater JL. Anticipatory nausea and/or vomiting. *Cancer Treatment Reviews*.1984;11:257-264.

71. Schafer DW. The management of pain in the cancer patient. *Comprehensive Therapy*. 1984;10:41-45.

72. Burish TG, Jenkins RA. Effectiveness of biofeedback and relaxation training in reducing the side effects of cancer chemotherapy. *Health Psychology*. 1992;11:17-23.

73. Steggles S, Fehr R, Aucoin P, Stam HJ. Relaxation, biofeedback training and cancer: an annotated bibliography, 1960-1985. *Hospice Journal*. 1987;3:1-10.

74. Ahles TA. Psychological approaches to the management of cancer-related pain. *Sem Onocol Nurs*. 1985;1:141-146.

75. Cassetta RA. Biofeedback can improve patient outcomes. *American Nurse*. 1993;25:25-27.

76. Wolf SL. The relationship of technology assessment and utilization: electromyographic feedback instrumentation as a model. *Int J Technol Assess in Health Care*. 1992;8:102-108.

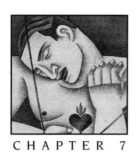

CHAPTER 7

UNTYING THE KNOT
YOGA AS PHYSICAL THERAPY

Judith Lasater, PhD, PT

INTRODUCTION

Physical therapy is much more than physical. All physical therapists know this, consciously or unconsciously, and most are acutely aware of how much the patient's mind influences the progress of treatment. Awareness of this existent mind-body connection is becoming increasingly more obvious to Western science.[1] However, the mind-body connection has been acknowledged and understood by the classic and ancient philosophers of yoga for thousands of years, and is in fact the basis for the practice of yoga.

The teachings of yoga are believed to have been spread from Egypt to India more than five thousand years ago. There are Egyptian carvings showing figures sitting in the lotus pose, the cross-legged sitting posture so often associated with yoga and other forms of meditation. These physical postures are perhaps the most familiar part of yoga for Westerners.

The postures of yoga, called *asanas*, have been created to liberate the natural flow of energy (called *prana*) throughout the body. But critical to the success of the postures is the proper breathing and slow, meditative assumption of the poses. In other words, the benefits of yoga are not simply achieving the postures, but rather integrating the attitude of wholeness that their proper practice engenders. These principles are seated in the Hindu tradition in India.

Actually, the postures are part of a wider system that includes ethical precepts, breathing, and meditation. While concerned in part with higher states of meditation, traditional yoga also is concerned with the way one stands, sits, breathes, and interacts with others. Because of the universality of all aspects of yoga philosophy, it is quite a useful practice for modern society.

The most important reason that yoga is relevant for us today is that while culture and technology have certainly changed, the body and mind which interact in that society and with ever-changing technology have not. I may be writing this chapter on a portable computer sitting out in nature (actually I am literally writing while out of doors) but the spine I use to sit upright and the mind I use to think of my next sentence have changed very little in thousands of years. We have "primitive" bodies which are attempting to cope with "civilized" environments. (I put "civilized" in quotes because I am reminded of a statement made by Mahatma Gandhi, the modern-day saint and political activist of India. When asked what he thought of Western civilization, Gandhi is reported to have replied, "Sounds like a good idea.")

It is becoming increasingly obvious that our nervous systems are geared to a very different life than the one we are living, and the result is the phenomena we term "stress."[2] Occasional stress in and of itself is not harmful; for example, we must stress a muscle in order to strengthen it. Stressing the heart muscle within safe guidelines is what cardiovascular training is all about. What is harmful to the body, to the emotions, and eventually to the psyche, is the unrelenting and unresolved stress of modern life. And this is common for a large number of Western, and increasingly, Eastern and third world people. Stress affects virtually everyone, even children.

Stress can affect every organ system and every physiological process in the body.[3] It plays a part in every disease, especially in immune deficiency diseases, migraines, cardiovascular diseases, and sexual and gastrointestinal dysfunction.

Because of the stressful environment in which we live, there are two important aspects from the philosophy of yoga that would be beneficial to all of our patients, regardless of their diagnoses: deep relaxation and a practice which I will term *awareness*. Both of these are at the heart of the philosophy of yoga, and are powerful tools for improving the quality of life, and hopefully, specific dysfunctions or disease processes.

The point is to share these techniques to help patients enhance the quality of their lives. Sometimes patients will get better, sometimes not, but deep relaxation and awareness practice will always improve the quality of life experienced. In the words of physician Bernie Siegel, a well-known cancer treatment specialist, "Some people get well, but are not healed, and some get healed and die anyway. Since we all eventually die, the point of life is to be healed."[4]

In order to teach these life-affirming tools well, we must practice them ourselves; otherwise, we are teaching from the "outside" and our words will not have the power they could if those words were deeply rooted in our own experience. Think of the music of J.S. Bach. Some of it is the most joyous and transcendental music ever written. He could not have composed this type of music unless he had experienced joy and transcendence himself. His music is not something that can be faked or intellectualized.

Likewise, if we are to "teach" physical therapy we are most effective when we practice what we teach, or, in other words, *become* what we are teaching. Remember the story attributed to King Solomon and occasionally to other great leaders and teachers. Solomon was approached by a mother asking him to tell her child to stop eating so much sugar. The mother was told to come back in 3 days. In 3 days she reappeared and Solomon promptly told the child to stop eating so much sugar. When the mother asked why it took so long for him to be able to tell the child to stop eating sugar, Solomon replied, "Three days ago I was still eating sugar myself."

The first of these two important practices is deep relaxation. Physical therapists can no longer ignore the results of recent research which has shown the incredible benefits of 20 minutes of deep relaxation.[5-7] When we consciously relax, all physiological parameters are affected: blood pressure drops, as does heart rate and respiratory rate. Norepinephrine levels drop dramatically in the blood stream; blood becomes more alkaline, thus decreasing the leaching of calcium from the bones. Blood moves away from the extremities and toward the abdomen, facilitating digestion and elimination. Immune function measurably improves. The experience of pain may be lessened while a general feeling of anxiety is decreased. Deep relaxation is definitely a habit that the modern American needs to learn and practice to improve quality of life and help prevent stress-related illnesses.

Besides the physical benefits of deep relaxation, there may be psychological ones as well. When we were worried about an occasional problem as a child, we were usually told that things would no doubt be better in the morning. It was usually true. The problem had remained the same but we had changed. Not only were we more rested but also we had a little perspective on the problem and on ourselves. It was easier to find the courage or creativity necessary to solve the problem.

Deep relaxation is like that. When one deeply lets go of muscular tension, when breathing slows and the mind quiets a bit, we are given a respite from the onslaught of physical or mental dysfunction. It as if for those 20 minutes we are on a mini-vacation. It is a familiar phenomenon to have a new perspective on our life after returning from a trip or vacation. Deep relaxation is in effect that little vacation; it can help us to have some perspective and therefore we are better able to handle whatever needs handling. This shift in focus not only has mental benefits but can spill over into beneficial physical effects as well.

The other important thing we as physical therapists can teach our patients and practice ourselves is what I call awareness. While this is a simple practice, it is not easy. Similar to what is taught in Gestalt therapy, awareness practice is simply paying attention to what we are feeling at any given moment, in fact, paying attention to the exact sensations we are feeling at any given moment.

How does this help? Consider the patient with back pain. If each person were aware of the sensations associated with sitting, standing, or lifting poorly, a great deal of back pain could be avoided. Each person would feel the tightness beginning to build up in the lower back, for example, and take immediate and necessary steps to correct the situation.

With awareness of what we are feeling and when we are feeling it, we know exactly when that knot begins to tighten in the belly with anger. With that observation one has a choice about that anger. We may want to express it verbally; we may want to express it by running laps at the track. As with many of the mind-body intervention and movement awareness techniques described in this text, because self-awareness has afforded a choice, we are able to release that reflex anger as it forms instead of ignoring it, denying it, or avoiding it until it manifests as a bad back or some other dysfunction. If we can be aware of how we create our problems, then there is a great chance that we can short-circuit the process and change from trying to undo damage to preventing it.

In summary, yoga is not only an ancient practice consisting of the assumption of various postures (asanas), but it is an entire philosophy or approach to living which improves the flow of energy (prana) throughout the body. Physical therapists are ideally suited to teach yoga in that we can diagnose musculoskeletal imbalances and assist clients in assuming postures that will work to diminish these imbalances. But it is important that even before learning postures themselves, physical therapists practice (and help their patients learn) the processes of deep relaxation and awareness. The remainder of this article is devoted to introducing these two practices.

PRACTICE

DEEP RELAXATION

Begin by finding a quiet room away from the telephone where interruptions can be avoided. Bring with you three blankets and one face towel. If you are practicing on a bare floor you will need an extra blanket.

Spread out your first blanket or sit down on a comfortable rug. Loosen your belt and remove your shoes, socks, and watch. If time is an issue, you may want to set your watch, alarm, or timer for 20 minutes so that you can forget the time and enjoy the relaxation.

Fold a blanket into a shape of 2 feet by 3 feet. Make a small fold at one of the long ends, then roll the entire blanket into a tight roll and place it under the knees to reduce lumbar strain. If a round bolster is available, that will work well.

Fold one blanket into a shape approximately 18 by 12 inches and place it behind you where your shoulders will rest on the floor. When you lie down, about 3 inches or so of the end of the blanket will support your upper thoracic spine down to the spine of the scapula.

Lie down on this blanket. The lateral proximal humerus should be supported as well as the proximal scapula. Reach up and curl the loose end of the blanket to support the cervical curve. Make sure that this support feels comfortable; the amount of curl necessary varies from person to person. Make sure that the forehead and chin are parallel and the neck is not in extension. The head and neck should feel comfortable and supported.

Fold the face towel in half lengthwise and place it over your eyes and forehead, being careful not to cover the nose or obstruct the breathing in any way. Pull the third blanket over you now if you think that you might get too cool. Spend a moment making sure that your arms and legs are equidistant from the midline and that thighs are slightly and easily externally rotating and your palms are supinated.

Spend the first few minutes of your relaxation letting the body grow quiet and soft. Imagine that your body is getting longer, looser, and warmer. When you start to feel relaxed, begin to pay attention to your breathing.

Notice that as soon as you notice your breathing you begin to change it. Notice yourself noticing this change. After a few minutes begin to take several long, slow breaths through your nose. Take a long inhalation and follow it with a long exhalation of the same length. Then take a short, normal breath in and out. It may take you several breaths in order for you to feel that you are using your full lung capacity. Take your time. Again take a long, slow breath and follow it with a short, normal breath.

Make sure that you are not straining or forcing the breath. One of the signs that you may be forcing the breath is that you will feel breathless at the end of the exhalation. If this happens, stop the breathing practice and breathe normally again for a few breaths; then resume the breathing practice. But this time make the long breaths shorter; the inhalation and exhalation should still be equal in length to each other, but shorter.

After 5 minutes or so of this breathing practice, finish with a long exhalation, and let your breath become natural while continuing to keep your attention on it. Notice any changes that may have occurred in your breath. Allow yourself to relax for another 10 minutes or so. Most people spontaneously come out of the relaxation in about 20 minutes.

To come out of the relaxation, once again take a deep inhalation and let it out slowly. Bending one knee and then the other, roll onto your side, open your eyes, and use your arms to help you come to a sitting position. Sit quietly on the floor for a few minutes before getting up and resuming your normal activities. You may want to be careful about driving immediately after practicing the deep relaxation.

To maximize the benefits of deep relaxation, it should be practiced on a daily basis. It may be practiced at any time of day that fits into your busy schedule. This practice is not an "extra," but rather an essential to a healthy life today.

AWARENESS

To practice awareness, sit in a comfortable chair with your feet flat on the floor, taking care to establish all the normal curves of the spine. Place your hands easily in your lap. Breathe normally and spend a few minutes relaxing in this position. You can either keep your eyes open or close them.

Use the breathing pattern suggested in the deep relaxation practice for a few minutes and then let the breath resume its normal rhythm. The next thing to do is nothing. Simply remain present with your sensations. Immediately the mind will try to escape by planning future activities or bringing up memories. Return to your bodily sensations.

The mind will continue to try other tricks, like going to sleep. Whatever happens, for 20 minutes keep coming back to your bodily sensations. Do not try to shut out any sounds; remain motionless and breathe normally. Sometimes during practice you will realize that you are thinking about your sensations rather than merely experiencing them directly. Whenever you realize that you are doing this, do not judge yourself, simply return to noting your bodily sensations. After 20 minutes or so, slowly and carefully get up and go about your normal activities.

Ultimately you will find that you have periods during your day when you are noting your bodily sensations. This practice will serve the dual purpose of allowing you to be more fully present in the moment as well as relaxing and refreshing you. This is a practice that you can do anywhere and anytime.

Whatever your life situation, learning to consciously relax life's inevitable tensions in deep relaxation is an imperative skill for patients of all ages. Even more importantly, learning the awareness technique can help prevent a myriad of health problems. Practiced every day, these two practices can help us to untie the knot we may have made of our bodies and minds, and even of our own lives. Only then will we be truly ready to assist our patients with improving the quality of their lives and preventing further illness and injury.

REFERENCES

1. Chopra D. *Quantum Healing.* New York, NY: Bantam Books; 1989.

2. Jacobson E. *You Must Relax.* New York, NY: McGraw-Hill; 1934.

3. Sapolsky RM. *Why Zebras Don't Get Ulcers.* New York, NY: W.H. Freeman and Company; 1993.

4. Siegel B. *Love, Medicine and Miracles.* New York, NY: HarperCollins Publisher, Inc: 1986.

5. Benson H, Stuart EM. Staff of the Mind/Body Institute of New England Deaconess Hospital and Harvard Medical School. *The Wellness Book.* New York, NY: Carol Publishing Group; 1992.

6. Cole R. Personal communication, August 1994.

7. Ornish D. *Dr. Dean Ornish's Program for Reversing Heart Disease.* New York, NY: Random House; 1990.

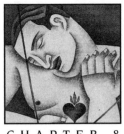

CHAPTER 8

T'AI CHI
CHOREOGRAPHY OF BODY & MIND

Jennifer M. Bottomley, PhD, MS, PT

INTRODUCTION

The use of T'ai Chi is an alternative therapeutic approach that can greatly enhance the practice of physical therapy. It is a form of exercise that recognizes the mind/body connection.[1] The movements are graceful, the tempo is slow, the benefits are great. It can positively augment physical therapy programs aimed at improving balance and posture, coordination and integration of movement, endurance, strength, flexibility, and relaxation.[2-11] T'ai Chi exercise has cardiovascular,[3,5,8] neuromuscular,[2,4,6,7,9] and psychological[1,10,11] benefits that are clinically observed. It is a form of exercise that allows the individual to assume an active role in obtaining maximal health and focusing on the prevention of disease, rather than the passive acceptance of illness as a consequence of life, aging, fate, or genetics. It is an exercise form that is particularly helpful in an elderly population because of its slow, controlled, non-impact-type movement which displaces, thereby "exercising," the center of gravity. This exercise form incorporates all of the motions that often become restricted with inactivity and aging. It improves respiratory status, stresses trunk control, expands the base of support, improves rotation of the trunk and coordination of isolated extremity motions, and helps to facilitate awareness of movement and position.[2,4,6,7,9] An additional benefit is the interaction on a social basis, as most T'ai Chi is done in group settings.

WHAT IS T'AI CHI?

T'ai Chi is an ancient physical art form, originally a martial art, where the defendant actually uses his attacker's own energy against him or her by drawing the attack, sidestepping the attacker, and throwing the opponent off balance. There are numerous forms of T'ai Chi[12] involving as many as 108 posturings and transitions of controlled movement, each style with slightly different philosophical foundations. Family surnames came to be associated with the different styles of T'ai Chi that have been passed on from generation to generation, for example, Wu style, Yang style, Ch'en style, Chuan style, etc. Each style is distinctive, but all follow the classic T'ai Chi principles.

T'ai Chi is a way of life that has been practiced by the Chinese for thousands of years. It is a Taoist philosophical perspective which forms the foundation of an exercise regime developed to balance mind and body. Unlike Western civilization, which separates body from mind and allows spiritual development only in terms of religious and mystical beliefs, T'ai Chi integrates the connections between mind, body, and spirit in a quest for the highest form of harmony in life through the combination of exercise and meditation.[13-15] The Chinese conceived the human mind to be an unlimited dimension and focused on simplification of beliefs. They also viewed the human body as limitless in its physical capabilities. These beliefs were the keystones for the evolution of what we know as T'ai Chi Ch'uan today.[12]

Since ancient times, Taoist philosophy has been concerned with the question of how to reproduce and maintain the essential kind of energy required to prolong life and enhance creativity of the individual. The answer can be found in the T'ai Chi methods of Taoist meditation, in which a combination of movement, breathing, and mental concentration is used to purify the essential life energies, distill out its pure Yang aspect, the vital energy (ch'i), and transmit it through the eight body/mind channels to every cell in the body. The regular practice of these methods has been shown to result in longevity, good health, vigor, mental alertness, and creativity far beyond what is experienced by most people.[16]

In order to obtain the full benefit from the practice of T'ai Chi, it is essential to understand the principles underlying the methods. Hence, it is the aim of this chapter to not only describe the methods of meditation and exercise, but also to explain how they are based on the philosophy of Taoism.

The "spiritual" component of T'ai Chi is what makes many Westerners uncomfortable with this and other Eastern practices.[13-15] However, the concentration required to accomplish the rhythmic and coordinated movement patterns and integrate these motions with respiration in T'ai Chi induces a level of concentration that edges on meditation.[1,10] Movement is vital to preventing disability and maintaining health and well-being. The capability of cognitively understanding the movements is an essential element in the successful practice of the T'ai Chi exercise form. T'ai Chi requires practice (preferably throughout the life cycle) and commitment.[10,11] There would be a total lack of consistency and benefit from this exercise form if the mind/body connection was not made.

PHILOSOPHICAL BACKGROUND OF T'AI CHI

Behind every T'ai Chi movement is the philosophy of Yin and Yang. As described in the chapters in Section IV, *Traditional Chinese Medicine*, the Yin-Yang principle has been the basis of the Chinese understanding of health and sickness since ancient times. Good health requires a balance between opposing forces within the body. If one or the other is too predominant, sickness results. It is the aim of Eastern medical practices, including acupuncture, qi gong, and herbal medicine, to discover the source of the imbalance and restore the forces to their proper proportions. In the Western world, exercise concentrates on outer movements and the development of the physical body. T'ai Chi develops both the mind and body.[1] It embodies a philosophy that not only promotes health but can be applied to every aspect of life. T'ai Chi emphasizes the development of the whole person, promoting personal growth in all areas.[16]

T'ai Chi means "the ultimate" energy. This ultimate power is ch'i. According to the legendary theory of Yin and Yang, ch'i exercises its power creating a balance between the positive and negative energies of nature.[12] T'ai Chi's philosophical basis is directed towards improving and progressing toward the unlimited and immense inter-relationship between the self and all other things in existence. T'ai Chi is guided by the theory of opposites: the *Yin* and the *Yang*, the negative and the positive. This is the *original principle* of Taoist thought.[17] According to the T'ai Chi theory, the abilities of the human body are capable of being developed beyond their commonly conceived potential. Creativity has no boundaries, and the human mind should have no restrictions or barriers placed upon its capabilities.

The fundamental principle of Taoist philosophy, the joining together of opposites, is the basis for the practice of T'ai Chi. The Taoist philosophy that underlies T'ai Chi exercise and meditation is somewhat more complex in its application of the relationship between Yin and Yang within the body. It is not denied that a general balance is necessary to avoid illness; however, it is the aim of *meditation* to greatly *increase* the *Yang* and to reduce and *diminish* the *Yin*. One of the fundamental beliefs of Taoist philosophy is that the reason people become old and weak and eventually die is that they lack essential energy (ch'i) that sustains life.[12,16,18] Thus the goal of *exercise* is to greatly *reduce Yang* and to *increase* and enhance *Yin*.[16,18] Thus, the combined practice of meditation and exercise balances these opposing energies.

One reaches the ultimate level of health and physical and mental well-being through exercise and meditative means of balancing the opposing powers and their natural motions: Yin, the negative (yielding) power, and Yang, the positive (action) power. The theory is that the interplay and balance between opposite yet complementary forces of equal strength promotes health. These two opposing manifestations have universal significance and apply to the phenomena of the cosmos as well as the operations of the human body. On the largest scale, heaven is Yang, while earth is Yin. Day is Yang; night is Yin. Bright and clear weather is Yang; dark and stormy weather is Yin. On the scale of living things, the male is Yang, the female Yin. Spirit is Yang; body is Yin. This opposition applies to the parts of the body and their functions as well. In the circulatory system, the arteries are Yang; the veins are Yin. Muscle contraction is Yang; relaxation is Yin. In breathing, exhalation is Yang; inhalation is Yin. In human activities, movement is Yang; rest is Yin.[19]

Hundreds of years ago, those who searched for a way to elevate the human body and spirit to their ultimate level developed the ingenious system known as T'ai Chi Exercise. It has since proven to be the most advanced system of body exercise and mind conditioning ever created.[12,19] It makes intuitive sense from a clinical perspective to apply the idea of a natural harmony and a balancing of life forces to the integration of body and mind.

HISTORICAL BACKGROUND OF T'AI CHI

A systematic description of the relationships of Yin and Yang is found in the hexagrams of I Ching, the oldest and most important book of Chinese philosophy.[17]

One of the pioneers of the philosophy of Taoism was Lao Tzu.[12] He emphasized that "the soft overcomes the hard." Later, this idea permeated the practice of T'ai Chi Ch'uan. After Lao Tzu, the second great master of Taoism was Chuang Tzu.[20] To the philosophy of soft over hard he added the component of "breathing", not only as the process of the movement of air in and out of the lungs, but the process involving the whole body, including the circulation of oxygen to the extremities through the blood. In other words, the flow of Ch'i, or vital energy. T'ai Chi Ch'uan was not actually developed until centuries after Chuang Tzu, though there is clear evidence that he was practicing methods of exercise coordinated with breathing[21] which is the basis of T'ai Chi exercise.

Approximately 1700 years ago (third century a.d.), a famous Chinese medical doctor, Hua-Tuo, emphasized physical and mental exercise as a means of improving health.[19] He believed that human beings should exercise and imitate the movements of animals to recover physical/cognitive abilities that had been lost to "civilization." Hua-Tuo organized a martial arts form called the Five Animal Games.[12] Since then, these exercises have become popular with the Chinese, who wish to maximize their health through exercise.

Huang Ti, the so-called Yellow Emperor of 2700 B.C., practiced a form of exercise called Tao Yin with the aim of increasing his life span.[12] Tao means "guide" and Yin is translated here as "leading." These terms give a hint of how the exercise works: the movement of the limbs guide the circulation of the blood so that the tissues throughout the body can be repaired and cleansed more efficiently. The movement also leads the breath in and out of the lungs to nourish and energize the body through inhalation and rid the body of poisons through exhalation. Thus, movement is the foundation of a discipline that guides and leads the automatic bodily processes so that they will function efficiently.[16] The essential element of Tao Yin was the way in which the movements of the limbs were combined with breathing. Huang Ti's exercises were also known as T'u Na (t'u = exhale; na = inhale) exercises.[19] There is little doubt that Huang Ti's health practices, consisting of an alternation of movement and rest, and his form of exercise involving breathing in and out were direct applications of the Yin-Yang principle.

Ko Hung (325 A.D.), an alchemist, developed a series of eighteen forms of "health exercise" to complete the evolution. Ko's system is only for health, not for self-defense.[18] He also combined exercise, breathing, and meditation.

These exercise forms were precursors of the methods of Taoist meditation and of the form of exercise known as T'ai Chi Ch'uan. Unlike movements of martial arts, which are generally strenuous and sometimes very quick, the movements developed in what we know as T'ai Chi Ch'uan today are done slowly, gently, and evenly from beginning to end, each posture unfolding with the same continuous rhythm. In this evolutionary way, the modified form of T'ai Chi became today's T'ai Chi Ch'uan, or the so-called T'ai Chi Exercise. This is the T'ai Chi practiced publicly in China today.[12] It is the "T'ai Chi Dance," also called the Chinese Ballet by some Westerners.[5]

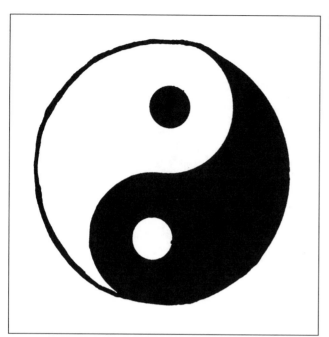

Figure 8-1. Yin and Yang: *Diagram of the Supreme Ultimate: T'ai Chi T'u.*

PRINCIPLES OF T'AI CHI CH'UAN

An important insight to be attained through an understanding of Taoist philosophy concerns the way in which the practice of exercise, such as T'ai Chi Ch'uan, and meditation should complement one another. The relationship between them manifests as a subtle interweaving of opposite tendencies. This relationship can be seen in the famous diagram known as the T'ai Chi T'u (Diagram of the Supreme Ultimate) (Figure 8-1).

This diagram represents rest in the black portion which is called the "greater Yin", and the white portion, representing movement, is called "greater Yang." Within each figure there is a smaller circle of the opposite color. The black circle within the white figure is called the "lesser Yin" and the white circle within the black portion is called the "lesser Yang." This inner component represent the way in which each of the opposing forces, Yin and Yang, contains its opposite and continuously originates from its opposite. T'ai Chi, essentially a form of movement, is Yang—the white portion. Meditation, which involves quiet and rest, is Yin—the black segment of the T'ai Chi T'u. This distinction takes into account only the external aspects of these activities. To perform T'ai Chi Ch'uan exercise effectively requires inner peacefulness and quiet while executing outwardly visible movements. Conversely, the meditator uses breath and mental concentration to move the vital energy through the psychic channels while remaining externally at rest. Thus, the inner aspect of each of these practices is opposite to its outer aspect. In other words, just as the greater Yang contains the lesser Yin within it, the greater Yin embraces the lesser Yang. This diagram is a pictorial representation of how exercise and meditation grow out of one another as alternating practices. The movements of T'ai Chi Ch'uan tend to increase the Yang side of the Yin-Yang balance. When the Yang reaches a high point of energy and vitality, it generates the need to sit quietly in meditation, which procludes a more peaceful condition and increases the Yin side of balance. And this is cyclic. When Yin reaches its peak, it generates a need to increase the Yang once again. Thus, it is through the alternate practice of these two opposite methods that one can obtain the beneficial effects of this form of exercise/meditation: T'ai Chi Chaun.[16,18-21]

The traditional Chinese concept of the human body differs somewhat from the Western one. Physiological foundations are based in descriptions of ch'i, or vital energy. The body is hypothetically composed of eight energy (psychic) channels and has twelve meridians that run along the surface of the body. These channels and meridians form the basis of the highly sophisticated theories in acupuncture and acupressure.[14-16]

The eight channels systematically include all parts of the trunk and extremities. The *Tu Mo*, or Channel of Control, runs along the spinal column from the coccyx through the base of the skull and over the crown of the head to the roof of the mouth. The *Jen Mo*, or Channel of Functions, goes through the center and front of the body from the genital organs to the base of the mouth. The *Tai Mo*, or Belt Channel circles the waist from the navel to the small of the back. The *Ch'eug Mo*, or Thrusting Channel, passes through the center of the body between *Tu Mo* and *Jen Mo*, extending from the genitals to the base of the heart. The *Yang Yu Wei Mo* is the Positive Arm Channel, beginning at the navel, passing through the chest, and going down the posterior aspect of the arms to the middle fingers, while the *Yin Yu Wei Mo*, or Negative Arm Channel, extends along the inner aspect of the arms from the palms and ending in the chest. Likewise, there are Positive and Negative Channels for both lower extremities. The *Yang Chiao Mo* is the Positive channel that goes down the sides of the body, down the outer aspect of the lower extremity ending the soles. The Negative Channel is called the *Yin Chiao Mo*, and starts in the soles and extends upward on the inside of the legs through the center of the body to a point just below the eyebrows.[19] These energy channels are represented in Figure 8-2.

Twelve "psychic centers" of the human body are identified in Taoist thought.[12,17,19] They are represented in the I Ching[17] by twelve hexagrams which represent not only the twelve pathways in the body, but also the twelve months of the year and the twelve times of the day. According to Taoist thought, the circulation of energy through these twelve psychic centers reflects the cyclic pattern of the universe, which brings about the alteration of light and darkness as well as the changing of the seasons.[19] The following diagram

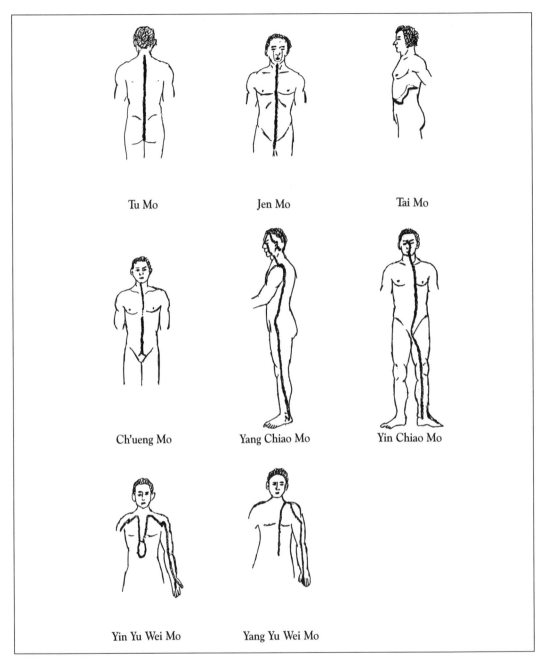

Tu Mo   Jen Mo   Tai Mo

Ch'ueng Mo   Yang Chiao Mo   Yin Chiao Mo

Yin Yu Wei Mo   Yang Yu Wei Mo

Figure 8-2. *The Eight Energy Channels.*

relates the twelve psychic centers to the twelve hexagrams that symbolize them, and indicates how the cycle reflects the times of the day and year and the center of the body that they represent (Figure 8-3).

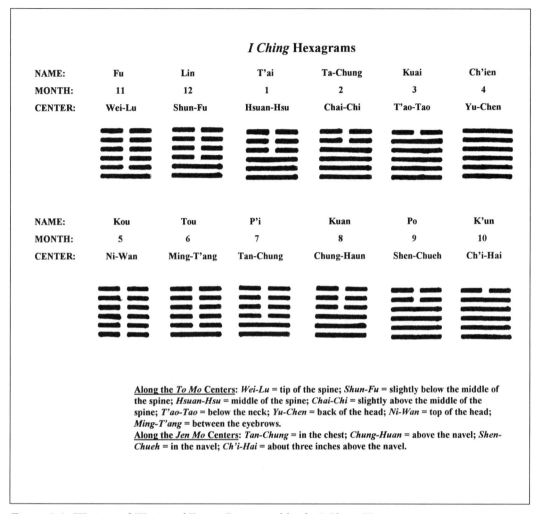

Figure 8-3. *Waxing and Waning of Energy Represented by the* I Ching *Hexagrams.*

According to Chinese astrologists, the *Yang* movement begins with the eleventh month, which is identified with *fu*. This *Yang* movement increases through the twelfth month up to the fourth month as represented by the increase in solid lines in the hexagrams. At the fifth month, the *Yang* movement begins to decrease until it reaches the tenth month when *Yin* reaches complete dominance. The *Yin* movement is the opposite of the *Yang*.[16,17,19]

In addition to the psychic centers there are twelve pathways of energy at the surface of the body called meridians (refer to Chapter 12, *Acupuncture in the Physical Therapy Clinic*). The twelve pathways take their names from the specific inner organs to which they correspond. The development of the T'ai Chi postures and movements are related to these meridians in the human body.[12,16,19] The transition from one posture to the next, combined with breathing, reflects the flow of energy through these meridians.

The importance of breathing techniques has long been stressed in Chinese medicine as a means of preventing illness, prolonging youth and achieving longevity.[22] The rationale behind this is that, besides oxygen, the air we breathe contains many other essential elements such as iron, copper, zinc, fluorite, quartz, zincite, and magnesium,[12,16,18,19,22,23] and that the combination of exercise and breathing provides an efficient and effective method of taking these precious elements in and getting rid of wastes and poisons. It is believed that the breathing techniques of abdominal or "inner" breathing facilitates the flow of energy throughout the body. Inhalation "stores" energy while exhalation "releases" energy.[23]

The classic methods of T'ai Chi combine movement with breathing. The movements are performed to assist and guide the circulation of vital energy, *ch'i*, through the eight channels and twelve meridians. The mind consciously "lifts" the energy during inward breathing from the solar plexus region, which is considered the central energy source of the body.[12,18,19,23] During exhalation, concentrated directing of the energy is from the solar plexus region towards the lower abdomen.[12,16,18,19,23] It is through this conscious directing of the energy that each of the eight channels is supplied with energy during the movement of T'ai Chi. It is hypothesized that in T'ai Chi exercise the circulation of ch'i through the channels does not occur automatically as a result of the arm and leg movements combined with breathing. Rather, it is the mind's power of concentration that combines with the breathing to move the *ch'i* through the channels. The outer movements aid and guide the inner concentration. T'ai Chi is regarded as a method of "moving meditation."[18,19]

Both the movements of the limbs and the way they are coordinated with the breathing cycle constitute the T'ai Chi form of exercise. The movements are relatively simple, involving only the bending and unbending of the knees while the hands are lowered or raised. The movements are an effective way of directing the flow of energy through the channels. Several kinds of movement of the body and limbs during T'ai Chi exercise involve movements such as shifting the weight from one leg to another, rotating the body to the right or left, taking a step, moving forward or backward, and fine hand and foot movements, all put together and coordinated in more or less complicated combinations and sequences.

A T'AI CHI ROUTINE

The mastering of the T'ai Chi exercise form requires the guidance of a knowledgeable teacher. However, the following is offered as a recommended routine for the elderly. This progression is an example of movement through a sequence of 45 classic T'ai Chi postures, diagrammed with their Chinese names. Each movement should be practiced several times until it can be performed fluidly. It is recommended that transition through each posture be built upon, so that the individual starts with the first fifteen postures and gradually adds additional postures in the sequence until all 45 postures are perfected. Any exercise can be omitted if it presents difficulty for the individual. It is important to take note of the positions of the hands and feet, and to keep the spine straight. For comfort, wearing loose-fitting clothing and slippers or aerobic sneakers is recommended. This author generally divides this exercise routine into three segments, starting with double stance exercises (exercises 1-19), progressing to single stance postures (exercises 20-30), and cooling down with mostly double stance, stetching-type postures (exercises 31-45).

Each T'ai Chi exercise session should be preceded by stretching. It is essential to stretch before a T'ai Chi workout in order to prevent injury and prepare for the best possible practice. Flexibility allows concentration on breathing, position, pace, etc. rather than on the limits of motion in poorly stretched muscles. General flexibility improves the effectiveness and benefits of T'ai Chi exercises. The following instructions teach a series of 45 movements. To practice them, have someone read the text to you, or make an audiotape of the text for yourself.

To start the exercise routine, assume an erect standing posture. Turn your right foot out 45 degrees and sink down slightly on your right leg. Shift all your weight onto the right leg and extend your left leg, flexing your foot and crossing your hands in front of your chest (1. Salutation to the Buddha). Step back onto your left foot, turning it out, and move your hands to waist level as you shift your weight to the left leg (2. Grasp Bird's Tail). Swing your arms to the right and press forward, shifting some of your weight to the right leg (3. Grasp Bird's Tail). Pivot left, shifting your weight to your right leg, bringing your left foot around and opening your arms (4. Single Whip). Step forward, leading with your right leg (5. White Crane Spreads Its Wings). Your right hand, elbow, knee, and toes should be in alignment. Slide your left foot forward and move your right arm parallel to the floor (6. White Crane Spreads Its Wings). Step back on your left foot as you raise your left hand and twist to the right (7. Brush, Knee, Twist, Step). Step back on your right foot (8. Parry, Punch); parry with your left arm and punch with your right. Rock back onto your right leg and bring your arms up (9. Closing). Pivot 90 degrees to the right, crossing your arms (10. Embracing Tiger). Slide forward, dropping your left hand to waist level and extending your right hand (11. Fist Under Elbow). Step back with your left foot and straighten your right leg and arm (12. Repulse Monkey). Pivot and step out, opening your arms (13. Diagonal Flying). Come forward, shifting your weight to your right leg, and extend your left arm (14.

DOUBLE STANCE EXERCISES

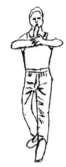

1. Salutation to the Buddha

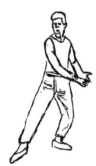

2. Grasp Bird's Tail

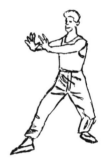

3. Grasp Bird's Tail

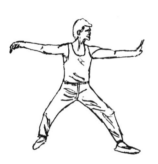

4. Single Whip

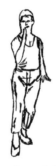

5. White Crane Spreads Its Wings

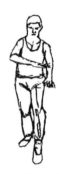

6. White Crane Spreads Its Wings

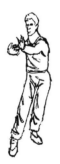

7. Brush, Knee, Twist, Step

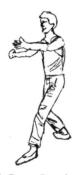

8. Parry, Punch

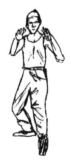

9. Closing

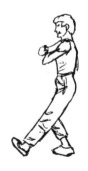

10. Embracing Tiger

DOUBLE STANCE EXERCISES

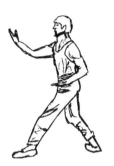
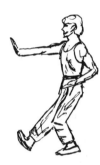
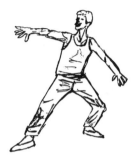

11. Fist Under Elbow   12. Repulse Monkey   13. Diagonal Flying

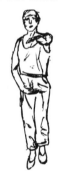
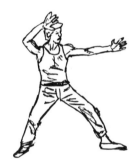
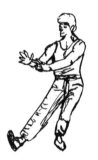

14. Raise Left Hand   15. Fan through the Arms   16. Green Dragon Dropping Water

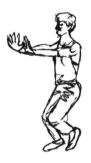
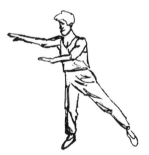
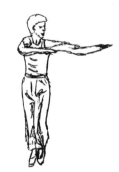

17. Step Up and Push _   18. Cloud Hands   19. Cloud Hands

SINGLE STANCE POSTURES

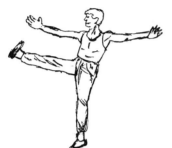

20. Separation of Legs

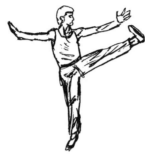

21. Separation of Legs

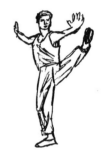

22. Separation of Legs

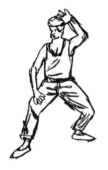

23. Wind Blowing Lotus

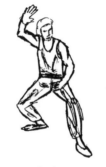

24. Wind Blowing Lotus

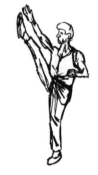

25. Double Jump Kick

SINGLE STANCE POSTURES

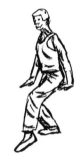
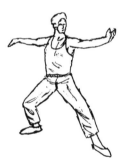

26. Step Back, Hands to the Side

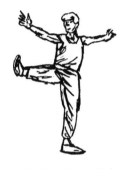
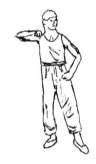

27. Kick with the Sole

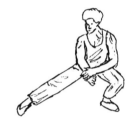

28. Clap Opponent with Fist

29. Diagonal Single Whip

30. Parting of Wild Horse's Mane

DOUBLE STANCE, STRETCHING-TYPE POSTURES

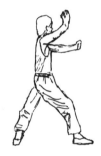

31. Fair Lady Works the Shuttles

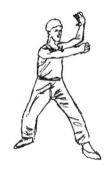

32. Fair Lady Works the Shuttles

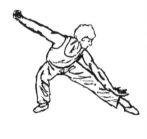

33. Single Whip Down

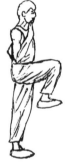

34. Golden Cock Stands on One Leg

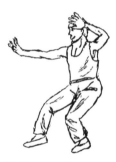

35. Cannon through the Sky

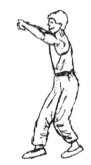

36. Cannon through the Sky

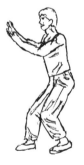

37. Cannon through the Sky

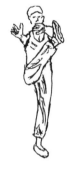

38. Lotus Kick

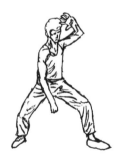

39. Downward Punch

DOUBLE STANCE, STRETCHING-TYPE POSTURES

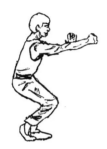

40. Step Up to Form Seven Stars

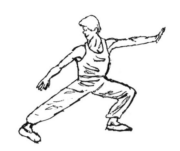

41. Retreat to Ride the Tiger

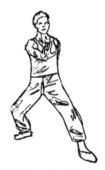

42. Turn the Moon

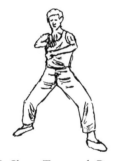

43. Shoot Tiger with Bow

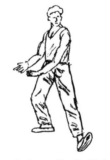

44. Grasp Bird's Tail

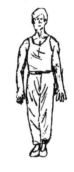

45. Conclusion

Raise Left Hand). Then pivot and step out with your left foot, moving your right hand up to your temple (15. Fan through the Arms). Pivot right (16. Green Dragon Dropping Water). Step up, with knees bent, and push out with hands flexed (17. Step Up and Push). Pivot right, so that you face straight ahead, and extend your left leg out as your arms and torso rotate right (18. Cloud Hands). Rotate to the left as you bring your feet together (19. Cloud Hands). Rotate right and then left four times, ending in a single whip position (4. Single Whip). This ends the portion of exercise postures in which both feet are in contact with the ground. As this is mastered, progress to the single leg stance postures.

From the single whip position (4. Single Whip), rotate your torso right and kick your right leg straight out as you open your arms (20. Separation of Legs). Shift your weight to your right leg and kick with your left (21. Separation of Legs). Lower your left leg almost to the floor, turn your right foot out, and kick again with your left leg (22. Separation of Legs). Drop your left leg back, shift your weight onto it, and parry high and low with your arms (23. Wind Blowing Lotus). Pivot on your left foot and switch hand positions (24. Wind Blowing Lotus). Then pivot on your right foot, jump onto your left foot and kick your right leg—without straining—toward your extended right arm (25. Double Jump Kick). Step back on your right leg, drop your arms, and shift backward onto your left foot (26. Step Back, Hands to the Side). Pivot in a full circle, coming around to stand on your left leg, and kick with your right (27. Kick with the Sole). Drop down on your left leg, keeping your right leg straight and your feet parallel; cover your right wrist with your left palm (28. Clap Opponent with Fist). Swing your right leg back and open your arms (29. Diagonal Single Whip). Step forward, moving your fists to your chest and hip (30. Parting of Wild Horse's Mane). This concludes the second segment of the exercise routine.

The third portion of this exercise routine starts with the Fair Lady Works the Shuttles (31 & 32. Fair Lady Works the Shuttles) by turning to one side. Parry with one hand and punch with the other. Then pivot 90 degrees to your left and punch and parry again. Repeat the 90-degree pivot, along with the punch and parry, two more times, bringing you full circle. Finish with a single whip position (4. Single Whip). Shift your weight to your right leg and extend your torso and left arm towards your left foot (33. Single Whip Down). Swing around to face left; shift your weight onto your left leg and raise your right leg (34. Golden Cock Stands on One Leg). Extend your right leg straight out and step forward. Turn and block your temple with your left hand as you move your right arm and leg forward (35. Cannon through the Sky). Step onto your right foot. Bring your arms out in loose fists, as though you were punching an opponent's ears (36. Cannon through the Sky). Then repeat the stepping movement and punch both fists in an uppercut (37. Cannon through the Sky). Step onto your left foot and kick your right leg high and slightly left, so that it moves across your extended palms (38. Lotus Kick). Step to bring your feet into a "T" position and block up with your left hand. Pivot to face left, sink down on your left leg, and punch and parry at chest level (40. Step Up to Form Seven Stars). Extend your right leg and arm back in a reverse lunge (41. Retreat to Ride the Tiger). Shift back onto your right leg and pivot to face forward, extending your right arm (42. Turn the Moon). Follow up with two short punches (43. Shoot Tiger with Bow). Form a mirror image of position 2, but with your forward foot flexed (44. Grasp Bird's Tail). Swing your hands up, crossing your palms at chest level, then lower your arms and turn so that you face forward in an erect posture (45. Conclusion).

Once this routine is mastered, it takes approximately 20 minutes to complete. Stretching exercises should be added to complete the T'ai Chi exercise routine.

PREVENTIVE QUALITIES OF T'AI CHI

Greater than 80% of all illness has been shown to have stress-related etiologies.[24] Medical and rehabilitation practices that seek only to "fix" the physical symptoms (body) without addressing the impact of emotional well-being on disease are missing the target. Although the origins of T'ai Chi exercise are based in ancient Eastern philosophy, it is a suitable form of exercise for tense Westerners. It has the advantage of regular exercise [1-11] combined with an emphasis on gracefulness and slowness of pace that Western society so conspicuously lacks. T'ai Chi can give those who live in a fast-paced environment a compensating factor in their lives.

From ancient Chinese medicine, it has long been recognized that there is mental as well as physical aspects of disease.[20-24] Traditionally, according to Eastern philosophies, the mental state of the individual was considered to be more important than the physical symptoms. Recently, a new basic science of Western medical research, called psychoneuroimmunology, has emerged.[1,10,11,24] This area of science is the study of the effect of emotions on disease. The new studies strongly indicate that virtually every illness, from a common cold to cancer and heart disease, can be influenced either positively or negatively by an individual's mental status. Today, Western health care professionals in both the physical and mental health professions are increasingly recognizing the role of the mind in the prevention and cure of illness. The health practitioner may encounter clients who do not seem to respond to traditional health care. Psychoneuroimmunology confronts these problems by employing the health traditions of other cultures and viewing the body and mind as a balanced whole.[1]

T'ai Chi is a specific technique for attaining peaceful mental states and therefore it can be extrapolated that it may help prevent or reverse disease processes. T'ai Chi integrates the body and mind through breathing and movement. The open and closed movements of T'ai Chi are coordinated with breathing. The benefits of this exercise form seem to be based in the fundamental combination of movements and breathing techniques in the basic T'ai Chi exercise routines. The entry level of the exercise has many similarities with medical treatments for respiratory illness, for example, Deep Breathing Exercises, Segmental Expansion Exercises, etc., and with walking exercise, the most recommended aerobic exercise for coronary artery disease.[3,5,8]

CURRENT RESEARCH OF EFFECTS OF T'AI CHI

In a study by Lai et al,[5] it was determined that the elderly T'ai Chi exercisers showed a significant improvement in VO2 uptake compared to an age-matched control group of sedentary elders. Lai and colleagues concluded that the data substantiated the practice of T'ai Chi as a means of delaying the decline in cardiorespiratory function commonly considered "normal" for aging individuals. In addition, T'ai Chi was shown to be a suitable aerobic exercise for older adults.[5] A subsequent study by Lai et al[8] further substantiated that T'ai Chi exercise is aerobic exercise of moderate intensity. In the past, it was believed, though never studied, that T'ai Chi exercise forms did not have a significant cardiorespiratory component and therefore were deemed non-aerobic. It has been clearly demonstrated in these studies that, despite the slow, steady, smooth pace of T'ai Chi exercise routines, there is a significant positive effect on the cardiorespiratory system.[3,5,8]

The potential value of T'ai Chi exercise in promoting postural control, improving balance, and preventing falls also has been substantiated by several researchers.[2,4,6,7,9] Tse and Bailey[2] found that T'ai Chi practitioners had significantly better postural control than the sedentary nonpractitioner. Province et al[4] found that treatments directed towards flexibility, balance, dynamic balance, and resistance, all components of T'ai Chi exercise, reduced the risk of falls for elderly adults. Wolfson et al[6] demonstrated that short-term exposure to "altered sensory input or destabilizing platform movement" during treatment sessions, in addition to home-based T'ai Chi exercises, elicited significant improvements in sway control and inhibited inappropriate motor responses. The outcome measure of functional balance improved more substantially in the exercise group that combined the treatment sessions with the home program of T'ai Chi. Wolf et al[7] compared a balance training group, in which balance was stressed on a static to moving platform using biofeedback, to a group of T'ai Chi Quan exercisers. A third group served as a control for exercise intervention. This article did not provide information on the results of the effects of the two different exercise approaches on balance and frailty measures, although it provides a superb set of assessment tools for measuring balance. In a subsequent interview with Steven L. Wolf, PhD, PT, FAPTA by Jan P. Reynolds of the *PT Magazine of Physical Therapy*,[25] Wolf spoke positively about the therapeutic value of exercise forms such as T'ai Chi in delaying or possibly preventing the onset of frailty. The benefits of T'ai Chi in fall prevention also has been supported by a study by Judge et al[9] in which these researchers demonstrated improvements in single-stance postural sway in older women with T'ai Chi exercises.

The stress reduction effects of T'ai Chi exercise, as measured by heart rate, blood pressure, urinary catecholamine, and salivary cortisol levels, were compared to groups of brisk walkers, meditators, and quiet readers.[10] In general, it was found that the stress-reduction effect of T'ai Chi characterized those physiological changes produced by moderate exercise. Heart rate, blood pressure, and urinary catecholamine changes for the T'ai Chi exercise group were similar to those changes occurring in the walking group. Additionally, it was reported that the T'ai Chi group expressed the enhancement of "vigor" and a reduction in anxiety states. In a study by Brown et al[11] unequivocal support is provided for the hypothesis that T'ai Chi exercise, which incorporates a cognitive strategy as part of the training program, is more effective than exercises lacking a structured cognitive component in promoting psychological benefits.

CASE EXAMPLE: MANAGED CARE AND T'AI CHI

Mr. K is an 84-year-old white male, admitted to the nursing home from home in a markedly deconditioned state, with diagnoses of coronary heart disease, tuberculosis, confusion, recent history of falls, depression, and malnutrition. He was referred to physical and occupational therapy for screening and recommendations. Screening by physical therapy resulted in an initial evaluation which revealed a significantly compromised cardiopulmonary response to any activity, flexed posturing in standing with occasional loss of balance during directional changes, ambulation with moderate assistance of one requiring verbal cueing, and a fluctuating cognitive status. He was quite congested and occasionally expectorated blood, especially with exertion. He had remarkable shortness of breath at rest and significant rubor of all extremities with 1+ pulses distally. He was withdrawn, minimally verbal, and obviously quite depressed. Based on our assessment, his prognosis was deemed poor for functional recovery to his premorbid state and discharge unlikely.

Mr. K was placed on a fall prevention program that included trunk extensor strengthening, extremity strengthening, and flexibility exercises. Deep breathing exercises were initiated and a reconditioning walking program using a 12-minute test protocol was started. Buerger-Allen exercises were initiated for his circulation and to promote postural changes and mobility. He also was referred to a nutritionist and nursing was consulted regarding his skin and circulatory status. Patient's gains were marginal in both physical and occupational therapy over a 3-week period. He continued to require minimal to moderate assist during ambulation, had a poor physiological response to activity of any sort, remained short of breath at rest, and was still withdrawn, now being virtually non-verbal and severely depressed.

Due to the restrictions placed on duration of intervention in a managed care delivery system driven by critical pathways, aggressive "skilled" intervention could no longer be justified. The insurer agreed to a 4-week trial of T'ai Chi exercises to be done 5 days per week in a group setting. The patient was initially instructed in breathing techniques and standing postures utilizing a set of T'ai Chi movements that did not significantly displace his center of gravity. Remarkable improvements were noted in respiratory status, that is, he was no longer short of breath at rest, and standing posture was distinctively improved by the end of the first week. It was noted that this elderly gentleman was much more alert and responsive to his surroundings and appeared to be less depressed. The T'ai Chi routine was expanded to encompass his increasing capabilities and weight shifting postures were started, though one-leg stance T'ai Chi activities were still ommitted from his routine. By the end of the second week, this patient was ambulating to and from all activities with stand-by assistance and no verbal cueing. His extremity pulses had improved to 2+ with no extremity rubor. He still experienced shortness of breath on exertion, but was no longer short of breath at rest and not expectorating blood. He was noted to be spontaneously telling stories and joking with the staff and other residents. He reported amiably "where" his energy was going from time to time and stated that he was "eating everything on my plate."

Mr. K continued to progress in all areas of functional status. By the end of the third week he was ambulating to all activities independently and safely. He was alert and obviously happy. We were able to start one-legged stance postures in his T'ai Chi routine. He was independently taking a shower (which pleased him to no end). He was quite fondly acknowledged by his fellow residents due to his sense of humor, optimism, and compassion for their concerns.

By the end of the fourth week, Mr. K was happily discharged on a home program inclusive of T'ai Chi exercises. Since his discharge, he has enrolled in a T'ai Chi program at a local martial arts facility which he participates in for 2 hours, three times a week, and Mr. K comes back to the nursing home twice a week to assist as an instructor for our T'ai Chi classes.

Perhaps Mr. K's progress sounds too good to be true, but the reality of his improvement has been observed in many of our patients participating in the T'ai Chi classes. Beyond the physical aspects of this exercise form, the most notable improvement appears to be in the area of "outlook." Elderly individuals participating in the T'ai Chi classes express pure enjoyment in the slow, rhythmic movements and the group interaction. They report that they "feel stronger, more balanced" and that they feel as if they are "dancing, not exercising." Also, the insurers are overwhelmed with the functional successes that seem to be inherent in this mode of exercise. T'ai Chi is a low-cost, low-tech group activity.

CONCLUSION

The increasing body of research related to the use of T'ai Chi as a valuable therapeutic intervention substantiates our need as professionals, in a cost-containment arena, to evaluate the merits of this exercise form.[1-11] T'ai Chi is viewed as an "alternative" therapy and often is perceived as "flaky"; however, it has been observed clinically and now scientifically has been shown to enhance function in our elderly patients. Recently, the use of T'ai Chi has been identified by the National Institutes of Health as one of a list of "alternative therapies" that will be targeted for research funding as a legitimate area for investigation. Physical and occupational therapists should seize the opportunity to provide leadership in this emerging area as complementary to rehabilitative techniques. T'ai Chi, although a "non-traditional" approach to therapeutic intervention, merits further traditional scientific analysis to quantify its apparent therapeutic validity.

REFERENCES

1. Wanning T. Healing and the mind/body arts: massage, acupuncture, yoga, t'ai chi, and Feldendrais. *AAOHN Journal.* 1993;41:349-351.

2. Tse SK, Bailey DM. T'ai chi and postural control in the well elderly. *Am J Occup Ther.* 1992;46:295-300.

3. Ng RK. Cardiopulmonary exercise: a recently discovered secret of t'ai chi. *Hawaii Medical Journal.* 1992;51:216-217.

4. Province MA, Hadley EC, Hornbrook MC, et al. The effects of exercise on falls in elderly patients. A preplanned meta-analysis of the FICSIT Trials. Frailty and injuries: cooperative Studies of Intervention Techniques. JAMA. 1995;273:1341-1347.

5. Lai JS, Lan C, Wong MK, Teng SH. Two-year trends in cardiorespiratory function among older t'ai chi chuan practitioners and sedentary subjects. *J Am Geriatric Soc.* 1995;43:1222-1227.

6. Wolfson L, Whipple R, Judge J, Amerman P, Derby C, King M. Training balance and strength in the elderly to improve function. *J Am Geriatric Soc.* 1993;41:341-343.

7. Wolf SL, Kutner NG, Green RC, McNeely E. The Atlanta FICSIT study: two exercise interventions to reduce frailty in elders. *J Am Geriatric Soc.* 1993;41:329-332.

8. Lai JS, Wong MK, Lan C, Chong CK, Lien IN. Cardiorespiratory responses of t'ai chi chaun practitioners and sedentary subjects during cycle ergometer. *J Formosan Med Assoc.* 1993;92:894-899.

9. Judge JO, Lindsey C, Underwood M, Winsemius D. Balance improvements in older women: effects of exercise training. *Phys Ther.* 1993;73:254-262.

10. Jin P. Efficacy of t'ai chi, brisk walking, meditation, and reading in reducing mental and emotional stress. *J Psychosom Res.* 1992;36:361-370.

11. Brown DR, Wang Y, Ward A, et al. Chronic effects of exercise and exercise plus cognitive strategies. *Med Sci Sports Exer.* 1995;27:765-775.

12. Liao W. *T'ai Chi Classics: New Translations of Three Essential Texts of T'ai Chi Chuan.* Boston, Mass: Shambhala Publications, Inc; 1990.

13. Lynoe N. Ethical and professional aspects of the practice of alternative medicine. *Scand J Social Med.* 1992;20:217-225.

14. Wardwell WI. Alternative medicine in the United States. *Soc Sci Med.* 1994;38:1061-1068.

15. Kronenberg F, Mallory B, Downey JA. Rehabilitation medicine and alternative therapies: new words, old practices. *Arch Phys Med Rehab.* 1994;75:928-929.

16. Jou, TH. Shapiro S (trans, ed). *The Tao of T'ai Chi Chuan Way to Rejuvenation.* Warwick, NY: T'ai Chi Foundation; 1988.

17. Blofeld J (trans, ed). *I Ching: The Book of Change.* New York, NY: E.P. Dutton & Co, Inc; 1965.

18. Da L. *T'ai Chi Ch'uan and I Ching.* New York, NY: Harper & Row Publishers; 1987.

19. Da L. *T'ai Chi Ch'uan & Meditation.* New York, NY: Schocken Books, Inc; 1991.

20. Huai-chin N. *Tao and Longevity.* New York, NY: Weiser Publications; 1984:8-12.

21. Legge J. *The Texts of Taoism.* Vol 1. New York, NY: Dover Publications; 1962:256-257.

22. Fung Yu-lan. *A History of Chinese Philosophy.* Vol 2. Princeton, NJ: Princeton University Press; 1953:436-444.

23. Sohn RC. *Tao and T'ai Chi.* Rochester, Vt: Destiny Books; 1989.

24. Kirsta A. *The Book of Stress Survival: Identifying and Reducing Stress in Your Life.* New York, NY: Simon and Schuster, Inc; 1986.

25. Reynolds JP. Profiles in alternatives: "East and West on the information superhighway": t'ai chi. *PT Magazine of Physical Therapy.* 1994;2(9):52-53.

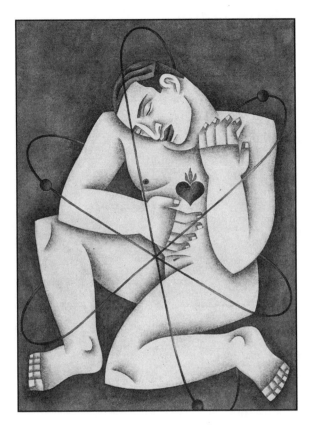

MOVEMENT
AWARENESS

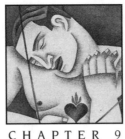

CHAPTER 9

THE ALEXANDER TECHNIQUE

Diane Zuck, MA, PT

INTRODUCTION

Frederick Matthias Alexander (1869-1955) developed The Alexander Technique. On one level, his story is no different from yours or mine. On another, his search for personal healing and self-fulfillment led him down a path that changed his life and the lives of many others. Unlike most people, he possessed the capacity to observe himself and make systematic deductions about his movement and posture that he was then able to correlate with his symptoms.

At the age of 19, Alexander was already renowned as a Shakespearean elocutionist in the British theatre. A recurrent hoarseness and loss of voice threatened his career. His physician recommended rest which, Alexander believed, meant keeping his voice silent or not speaking above a whisper. The prescribed treatment worked and his voice returned for use in daily conversation. Then it was time for him to perform. Again and again, Alexander would experience hoarseness at the moment his voice meant the most to him—during his delivery on stage.

As a result, his physician recommended surgery on the vocal cords. Unwilling, indeed unable to accept this drastic option, Alexander confronted his physician with a condition. He believed "...that it was something I was doing...in using my voice that was the cause of the trouble..."[1] Although the physician agreed with the theory, he was not able to help Alexander with the answer. Thus, Alexander was driven to help himself.

Over the next 3 years, Alexander devoted his time to the systematic observation of himself via mirrors and observing with his most objective mind. He made thousands of observations of the same subject, himself, within the same controlled environment, to prove or disprove his hypothesis that something he was doing was causing the trouble he was having with his voice.

Alexander observed himself in the act of speaking, or during his process of verbal behavior, under two conditions: when he intended to talk in an "everyday way," and when he intended to deliver a performance onstage. The more revealing observation occurred when he intended to perform. As he took in a breath, even before he spoke he heard himself gasp; he saw himself lift his chin and pull the head back and down, which then caused his stature to become short and narrow, to allow his upper chest to expand for air. As he sucked in the air, his larnyx depressed. This action was not present when he spoke in conversation.

Later, Alexander would call the head-neck-back relationship the "primary control," and called the condition of the primary control "use."

He then focused on his actual speaking behavior when he intended to perform. Over and over, he saw himself lift his chin and pull his head back and down at the moment he intended to speak, but before a word was spoken. So then he waited, and before the word was said, he restored his head to a position that was not pulled down and back, and his stature to a place that was not short and narrow. This later became Alexander's "principle of inhibition."

As it turns out, the waiting gave Alexander a second chance, a chance to use himself, his body, in a different way. Regardless of his attempts to change his behavior, over and over he observed the same habit of his head pulled down and back.

In the next series of trials to change his behavior, he eliminated vision. He observed himself breathe in with the intent to perform without speaking, observed his pulled down and back habit, and then closed his eyes. With eyes closed, he tried to undo his habit by moving his head to a position that was not pulled down and back. He intentionally moved his head forward and up.

However, when he opened his eyes, nothing had changed. He found himself in his same habitual pattern of use, with or without visual feedback. This became Alexander's "principle of faulty appreciation."

He went back to his hypothesis that something he was doing was causing the trouble he had with his voice, and began again. Not surprisingly, under the same conditions, the same results appeared. The more he tried *not* to repeat his habit, the more the habit appeared and reappeared. Later, this became the Alexander principle of "end-gaining" and a process called the "means whereby." But the story does not end here.

The result of his research, the 1918 publication of *The Use of Self*, included an introduction by the father of the description of the Scientific Method in America, Professor John Dewey. Alexander's discovery is described in his own words in the first chapter. The chapter, according to Dewey, is an "exemplar of all the major steps that are characteristic of a scientific inquiry."[2] Alexander's self study parallels what we today describe as a single case research design. In addition to proving his hypothesis, Alexander made a number of discoveries about himself that he later developed into the principles of the Alexander Technique named above. Thus the father of the description of the scientific method, John Dewey classified the descriptive research method employed by Alexander as exemplary of valid and reliable research.

Over time, Alexander became able to avoid pulling his head back and down which, he discovered, eliminated the sucking in of air and the depression of the larynx.

"The importance of this discovery cannot be over estimated, for through it I was led on to the further discovery of the primary control of the working of *all* the mechanisms of the human organism, and this marked the first important stage of my investigation."[1]

Alexander did not discover the universal primary control, for it turns out that we each use the structure of our head, neck, and back in unique ways. He did discover his *own* primary control and how it affected his use and function. This is the value of single case research design. By discovering how his primary control affected his function, he could generalize the effect of one's primary control on one's function.

THE PRIMARY CONTROL

The primary control is operationally defined as the organization of the head to the neck to the back. Anatomically, the head is defined as the skull with mandible and hyoid; the neck is defined as the top vertebrae of the spine; and the back is defined as the middle vertebrae of the spine which supports the rib cage with the shoulder girdle and arms. The back also relates with the lower vertebrae of the spine, connecting with the pelvis and legs. The head is a center for receiving sensory input and houses the brain and midbrain until it exits the skull as the spinal cord. Muscles of the hyoid attach to the skull, the larnyx, and the shoulder blade.

The head is delicately balanced on the neck, where cranial and peripheral nerves overlap, and thus the head on neck site is a major locus for reflex and voluntary and involuntary movement. The back supports the rib cage, housing many vital organs, the back supports the movement of the arms, and also supports the autonomic nervous system, which directs the function of our internal organs. The back extends into the lumbar and pelvic areas, where it supports other internal organs and the movement of the legs. The organization of the head-neck-back, the primary control, thus affects the functioning of each part of the organism.

"As the head moves, it imposes an attitude on the body [a dynamic influence] by redistributing muscular tonus."[2] The head houses the brain and is the center for our conscious and unconscious intentions and choices. Thus the presence of consciousness is inseparable from the primary control. Therefore, each choice a person makes reflects the condition of the primary control and affects the dynamic state of the primary control which in turn affects the entire organism and sets the conditions for the next choice. Conscious use of the organization of the head-neck-back (primary control) means consciously integrating the voluntary and involuntary experiences with constructive choice. This then results in the mutual development of the acts of inhibition and volition. This discovery of his own primary control led Alexander to discover the other principles of the Alexander Technique.

INHIBITION

Alexander's principle of inhibition expands the stimulus-response model to a stimulus-process-response model. At the moment Alexander intended to speak, he waited and observed his process. If he saw his habit emerge, he did not speak. He consciously inhibited the desire. During this pause, he reorganized his primary control and intended to speak again. If the habit reappeared, he continued to consciously inhibit it. In Professor Raymond Dart's mind, "The basic discovery Alexander made from 1888...was the practice of deliberate conscious inhibition."[3] Alexander accessed his primary control by conscious inhibition of pulling his head back and down through use of his intention to do just the opposite motion. He did not say to himself, do not pull the head back and down; instead he asked himself to move the head forward and up. In a sense, he gave his nervous system a positive direction, as the nervous system does not respond as well to what not to do. Alexander developed a series of directions, or orders, that he said to himself to sustain his level of inhibition and to maintain access to his primary control. He worked with these directions sequentially until they became a unity of intent with each being a part and the whole in the same moment.

A stimulus-process-response model is supported by the work of Dr. Benjamin Libet, Professor of Physiology at the School of Medicine of the University of California, San Francisco. "Evidence indicates that there are 100 - 150 milliseconds within which a person may either prevent or allow an urge to move to become an action."[4] Frank Pierce Jones remarked "...I found that the paradigm of inhibition...could be applied equally well when the activity would be classed as mental or emotional."[2] Conscious inhibition brings to conscious awareness thought processes and intentions, leaving the individual able to choose a response. The habitual response is still available, but now under the conditions of conscious control. Everyday events, previously thought to be not under our control, suddenly become available to our choice.

Conscious inhibition reveals that, given a stimulus, we are not bound to a habitual, learned response or reaction. Most of one's day is not dependent on life-threatening decisions which, if under true reflex control, we have no choice but to make. Instead the nervous system has time between stimulus and response to process what's occurring before a response reaches the final common pathway. Three options of response are usually available. We can choose to act in our habitual way, to act in a brand new way, or not to act at all. To *not* act, to inhibit, is a valid, active response. To decide not to act is as equal a decision as to decide to act. In 1937, Sir Charles Sherrington wrote:

> I may seem to stress the preoccupation of the brain with muscle. Can we stress too much that preoccupation when any path we trace in the brain leads directly or indirectly to muscle? The brain seems a thoroughfare for nerve action passing on its way to the motor animal. It has been remarked that Life's aim is an act not a thought. Today the dictum must be modified to admit that, often, to refrain from an act is no less an act than to commit one, because inhibition is co-equally with excitation a nervous activity.[5]

Frank Pierce Jones also notes Sherrington's writings on inhibition. "There is no evidence that inhibition is ever accompanied by the slightest damage to the tissue; on the contrary it seems to predispose the tissue to a greater functional activity thereafter."[2]

Professor Jones defines inhibition as,

> In general, any suspension of activity or temporary withholding of a response. In Alexander's usage, inhibition releases, rather than represses spontaneity by suspending habitual responses to stimuli long enough so that intelligent guidance and reasoning can intervene. Alexander saw this ability to inhibit automatic responses to stimuli, and to allow reason to intervene before making responses as "man's supreme inheritance."[2]

In fact, Alexander's first book is entitled *Man's Supreme Inheritance.*

Richard M. Gummere, Jr, past professor at Columbia University, wrote the prologue to the 1988 edition of Alexander's first book, describing it as "...a book of imperial scope."[6] In this book, Alexander quotes Leonardo Da Vinci: "You can have neither a greater nor a less dominion than that over yourself."

FAULTY SENSORY APPRECIATION

In the early stages, when he was working with his eyes closed, Alexander relied on his internal sensory awareness for feedback. But even without visual feedback, his internal senses led to the habitual outcome. Alexander concluded that his kinesthetic awareness, or appreciation, was wrong and unreliable. He continued to work in front of the mirrors with his eyes open for the objective view. He watched himself with the intent to deliver a speech using inhibition to access his primary control until he could open his mouth without tilting his head back and down, could move his head without moving his shoulders, and could take in a breath without shortening and narrowing his stature. The directions became integral at this stage of his learning. With each direction, he became more aware of new sensory information present with each conscious inhibition. Over time, Alexander came to understand that he had retrained his nervous system to new ways of use and function. The newer ways of use and function were available to him when he accepted his sensory assessment as faulty, inhibited his response, gave direction, and chose to respond within less familiar sensory surroundings.

Anatomically, our proprioceptive senses offer internal information about the body's position, direction, and mass. Behaviorally, as we use our self in one way over time, we develop a response that becomes habituated to the sensory information triggering that response.

> In many habitual and much-practised activities, such as those involved in balance and locomotion, sequences of 'elementary motor acts' come to be assembled by the inclusion, in the gestalt to trigger a specific element, of sensory messages that are parts of the kinesthetic re-afference occurring during the consummatory phase of other "elementary motor acts" performed earlier in the sequence....Once a habitual motor sequence has been initiated, the successive stages follow one another as in a chain reaction....in which voluntary intervention can be effective. If this crucial stage is omitted, the most assiduous practice serves merely to reinforce the undesired habit.[7]

Areas in our body also become contracted through use and habit. Habitual responses and contracted areas are deprived of sensory experiences, and new information may feel, and be perceived as, wrong. For example, a person may habitually interlace his or her fingers with the left thumb over the right thumb. It the same person performs the same act with the right thumb over the left, it feels wrong or uncomfortable, so this new act may be excluded from the motor repertoire. This is a very simple experiment. But if that person chose to inhibit the usual response and to go with a new use, the person may find him or her self open to receiving more information. If we are able to free our self from habit, areas open and new information brings a wider range of choices.

Alexander found that he could change his use by not relying on the familiar sensory information he knew to be wrong, by attending to conscious inhibition and direction, and by receiving new sensory feedback from his actions. Alexander was changing his habits by altering his kinesthetic re-afference. In the writings of J.J. Gibson, "We can now suppose that the perceptual systems develop perceptual skills, with some analogy to the way in which behavioral systems develop performatory skills."[8]

END-GAINING AND THE MEANS WHEREBY

Alexander observed himself under two conditions: one, while intending to speak in an everyday way, and the other, while intending to deliver a performance. The latter was the act triggering the habit that caused his loss of voice. He discovered that if he could give up his desire to deliver a commanding performance, his use changed and he was able to speak his lines without any loss of affect or effect. He concluded that being solely attentive on the goal, or "end-gaining," took his awareness away from how he was going to get there, or the "means whereby." He discovered that his thought or intention alone was sufficient stimulus to elicit his undesired use. According to Professor Dart,

> In 1965, a decade after his death and three quarters of a century after F.M. Alexander's self analysis, an arresting neurological fact came to light through its having been recorded electronically in numerous encephalograms. Changes in electric potential take place in the nerve cells in the frontal lobes of human brains before, as well as during and after, voluntary muscular movements. H.H. Kornhuber and L. Deecke, two German neurologists, found that while an individual is thinking about carrying out an action, the action is being preceded by a slow negative wave occurring in the front region of his brain.[9]

Alexander used conscious inhibition to redirect his attention away from his goal, momentarily, and focus on his primary control and how he was using himself toward the goal. He brought his intentions to a level of consciousness that was accessible to a deeper desire to change his use. During this process, Alexander gave himself orders which later became the "directions."

Alexander's principle of end-gaining may seem obvious at first. We all strive for health, wealth, and happiness. We each have an understanding of what health, wealth, and happiness means, along with a plan of how to achieve them. Full understanding of the end-gaining principle is attained when it is applied to the simple, mundane activities of daily living. The everyday tasks of standing, walking, sitting down, standing up, drinking, eating, talking, etc., become actions integral with our goals. Everyday activities bring out typical patterns of use, or what is called "postural set."[10] Even as you pick up a book and prepare to read, muscular tension increases and is enough to alter the relationship of the head, neck, and back. As you continue to read, you may literally be pulled in toward the goal of reading the words. In a short time, the head is pulled back and down as the shoulders become rounded and elevated with the effort of holding the book up against gravity. If you happen to be sitting against the back of a chair, you may easily fall into a slump and end up sitting on the sacrum. After years of this use, this may become the only postural set within which you are able to read a book. Such daily actions are not foremost in our consciousness because we have delegated them to the realm of automatic actions or habit. For example, locomotion can be accomplished on the spinal level and serves to move animals toward food and away from danger. Consciousness of the desire to walk toward a non-food item, or approach a potentially dangerous item, is unique to human behavior. Humans have the ability to be aware of and to contemplate their actions.

"The means whereby" is the integration of awareness and attention. While studying the technique, Professor Jones commented, "It was only after I realized attention can be expanded as well as narrowed that I began to note progress."[2] And, "Movement within an expanded field of attention is the means by which change is effected in the Alexander Technique."[2]

In 1949, C. Judson Herrick wrote a biography of George Ellett Coghill, author of the document, "Appreciation: The Educational Methods of F. Matthias Alexander."[4] Coghill was a biologist and worked in comparative anatomy. While at Brown University, he was influenced by professors trained in the experimental psychology work of William James. Herrick reviewed Coghill's papers over varied topics but stated that all had a central theme "that was to correlate the development of behavior with the development of anatomical structure."[25] This is a more expanded view of the relationship between structure and function.

Professor Jones based this "extended field of consciousness" on the two ways that individuals gain knowledge from experience. One way is through the knowledge gained from within the individual, or "introspection." The other way is through the knowledge gained from outside the individual, or what C. Judson Herrick called "extraspection." However, it is not one or the other focus of attention, but a unity of awareness.

"The attention is focused wherever it is wanted. But it is focused in such a way that when something in the environment is central, consciousness of the environment remains."[2] Consciousness thus has a dual mechanism to gather information.

How is it possible for humans to be conscious of external and internal information in a coherent way that makes each avenue of information equally available? The intermediate relationship between structure, function, and environment is based on internal, interactive connections between the information received from within and without the organism.

A dual mode sensory process model has been applied to the senses that serve behavior. In the visual system, the focal and ambient sub-systems support visual input and perception.[11,12] The focal process provides for detail discrimination, and the ambient process provides for spatial orientation, movement detection, and balance. The functioning and use of each sub-system directly influences learning behavior. In the auditory system, Dr. Alfred Tomatis, developer of the Audio Psycho Therapy Approach, describes the right ear focused on precise sound and the left ear on background sound.[13] A dual process of functioning within a sensory mode, like vision or hearing, is beyond a left-right brain model and goes deeper into the neural networks between the hemispheres, the cerebellum, and the mid-brain. These sensory functions also sub-serve higher cortical functions which, if the whole is greater than the sum of its parts, may even be supra-cortical, and literally out of the body within the realm of the mind. If the sensory systems sub-serve human consciousness, and if these sub-systems work on a dual mode process, it is likely that the consciousness also may function in dual mode. And, like the sensory systems, the consciousness can be accessed through educational and intentional efforts. For example, by utilizing the Alexander Technique, a person accesses intention as he or she chooses how to respond to the sensory information at the moment. We are not bound to every response in our neural networks and can intercept the neural impulses through inhibition, choice, and a conscious change in direction.

Alexander did not *cure* his laryngitis. He did discover a way to integrate his mind and body to access a deeper desire to change his use, while moving toward a goal in such a way that prevented him from a hoarse voice at the time he most needed it. Aldous Huxley offers:

> One has to make the discovery for oneself, starting from scratch, and to find what old F.M. Alexander called *the means where-by*, without which good intentions merely pave hell and the idealist remains an ineffectual, self-destructive and other-destructive *end-gainer*.[2]

This statement may mirror the essence of a controversy in physical therapy practice. Some practitioners are bound to science and use treatment procedures only if they have been firmly substantiated by rigorous, quantitative research. Other practitioners who are more open to the art in physical therapy, can receive information that tells them something has worked to help a client, and place validity on that information as it comes from a valued source.

WHY LEARN THE ALEXANDER TECHNIQUE?

A way to bring the mind and body into harmony seems desirous. Use of the consciousness and use of the body are equal and inseparable aspects of being human. The desire to meet a goal directs our bodily functions and vice versa. Innate awareness of this mind-body/body-mind connection is present in each human at birth, but is lost as we develop within environmental constrictions that limit learning about our self and about the choices we are free to make.

For example, young children exhibit innate use of the body. A child bends, squats, and sits on the ground with ease and poise. At some point, the child is required to sit in a chair and experiences an environmental constriction. Chair sitting is not innate. It is an acquired skill that is imposed upon the body-mind/mind-body process.

The Alexander Technique offers a chance to regain mind-body harmony, and has been called a method of psycho-physical education. Professor Dewey "considered that the Alexander Technique provided a demonstration of the unity of body and mind."[2]

Mr. Thompson[14] tells a revealing story of a 14-year-old boy who took lessons with him. The boy was strong and sturdy, played football, and would frequently beat up the kid next door. After the boy understood the principle of inhibition, Mr. Thompson worked with him through the postural set that accompanied his intent to "beat the kid up." The boy came to understand the kinesthetic difference he felt when he was or was not with his potentially harmful intent. He was sent home to perform an experiment. The next time he saw his target, the boy was asked to work with inhibiting his initial desire to fight, and to decide if the circumstance was going to direct his response or if he could choose the extent to which the circumstance directed his response. The boy gave up fighting, gave up football, and took up music.

Focus on the outcome without attention to process requires being pulled toward that outcome in a way that strengthens habit and limits options. We become stuck in our own actions. The mind becomes stifled and the body eventually rebels. How individuals use their bodies then becomes a factor in many bodily ailments. Most musculoskeletal problems and some neurological problems have been greatly helped by giving the individual a way to control and manage his or her own body. Individuals striving for peak performance apply the technique with success. Musicians and athletes, for example, have taken Alexander lessons to improve physical and artistic performance. Even equestrians working with the technique experience a greater harmony between their self and their mount.

HOW THE ALEXANDER TECHNIQUE IS LEARNED

Alexander thought his discovery was not that unique. It is possible for anyone to do what Alexander did—discover your own primary control. It also is possible to learn about the technique from books, journals, and articles, and to apply what you have learned. Most people choose to find an Alexander teacher or are referred to one by a friend or medical professional.

Alexander used the directions to guide the student through the experience of discovering his own primary control and new use. The directions, or orders, can be an integral part of learning the technique, but do not define the technique. At one point, Alexander stopped using verbal orders/directions while teaching others. He found he could use his hands on the student in a way that elicited the primary control and offered the student a different kinesthetic experience. The Alexander teacher will place his or her hands on the student for the purposes of bringing the student's awareness to areas of tension, assisting the student with inhibition of habitual use, and facilitating redistribution of postural tonus, thus providing the student with a different kinesthetic experience. Because the head, neck, and back area are central to the primary control, the teacher's hands will be in contact with these areas. The teacher's touch can be described as neutral, without effort or intent. The touch is a guide for support and trust. As the student becomes able to trust the support, the ability to let go and open up areas is experienced.

A teacher of the Alexander Technique exemplifies the principles. As Jones states, "You can't teach someone else an improved use of himself until your own manner of use has improved."[2] The teacher imparts his or her understanding of the principles through the use of voice and hands. Some Alexander teachers use their voice more than their hands or vice versa, or use each in balance. Use of voice and hands also is variable within and across lessons. This is a matter of the teacher's teaching and the learner's learning styles. Sometimes it is good to work with several teachers before choosing one you want to work with over time. A teacher will have at least 1600 hours of teacher training over a period of 3 to 4 years.

Alexander lessons are not restricted to one location. For example, people receive lessons in their home, at their work site, or their place of recreation. An Alexander teacher's studio has a few essentials like mirrors, chairs, and possibly a table/plinth. There is no need for the student or client to remove any clothes with the possible exception of shoes, which allow the feet to be more receptive to support from the floor. Chair work is very common. Alexander used sitting and standing from a chair as a typical example of an everyday activity that we are least likely to think about, and which is most likely to elicit our worst habits. Changes in habit are more likely to happen during a non-threatening activity like standing up from a chair or walking across the room than during an activity of high tension like facing your boss. If you play the piano or ride a horse, the teacher may ask you to work with those intentions in mind, and may later work with you sitting at your piano or on your horse. Table work and floor work can be used during lessons for the gravity eliminated experience on the primary control (head, neck, back relationship).

An Alexander lesson is an experience of mutual respect. Each lesson is a recognition of the fine line between teacher and student. The aim of the lesson "...is to bring a pupil to the point of self-discovery that F.M. reached when he was able to translate what he saw in the mirrors into kinesthetic terms and to apply his new knowledge to the solution of his own problems and become in effect his own expert in the use of himself."[2]

RESEARCH AND DOCUMENTED SUPPORT

There is value in remembering that research cannot be limited to the controlled laboratory and must include the life experience.

Many people have found their way to the Alexander Technique. Some are rather well-known figures in the world. Some have written about personal experience with the Technique and others have reported rigorous research that has been conducted on the Technique. This section summarizes the contributions of a few people. The reader is invited to follow along the path of these contributors and to identify his/her own personal interests.

Anatomist and anthropologist Raymond Dart was appointed Chair of Anatomy at the University of Witwatersrand, Johannesburg in 1922. In 1925, he published his findings of the Taung skull, later called Australopithecus africanus. Professor Dart showed the skull to be more man-like than ape-like. But because his conclusions did not support the prevailing theory, they were met with great speculation.[15] Eventually, after new fossils were uncovered, the Tuang skull was recognized for the traits resembling later forms of the genus Homo.[16] Significant to the Alexander Technique, among those traits is the poise of the skull on the spine. In the evolutionary development of uprightness and bipedal locomotion, the downward weight of the cranium center of gravity and the upward support of the articulating cranial condyles became closer in space. The two forces are almost coincident in humans. Along with evolutionary changes in cranial shape and direction of muscle pull, the human uniqueness is the support of the cranium.[17]

Professor Dart recognized that a critical feature of being human is the poise of the head on the neck.[18] In the same article, "The Attainment of Poise," Professor Dart states:

> Terminological failure to distinguish the static symbolism of *posture* from the dynamic plasticity of *poise* has thus been responsible for a great deal of confusion both in the nomenclature of, and medical thought concerning movement, ...a considerable number of *intermediate positions* are necessarily assumed...from the initial posture...to the terminal posture. These intermediate positions should always be positions of *poise* or equilibrium. Every phase of the movement...is in a state of *mobile equipoise* or balance.[18]

Professor Dart met Alexander in 1949, received lessons from him, and later from Miss Irene Tasker, and said:

> ...Alexander was striving to explain...the body misuse and correction...Alexander's work is important because it is based on the fundamental biological fact that the relation of the head to the neck is the primary relationship to be established in all proper positioning and movement of the body.[3]

Alexander's only sibling, Alfred Redden Alexander, was probably Alexander's strongest supporter and can be considered the "first teacher of the Technique." It is common within the Alexander community to refer to the brothers by their initials, F.M. and A.R. Both were born in Wynard, Tasmania. F.M. began taking students in 1894. In 1904, A.R. went to London with his brother to teach.

Ethel Webb was F.M.'s secretary and received lessons from him. She was also well read in the writings of John Dewey. Ms. Webb understood a connection between the Alexander Technique and the work of Maria Montessori, and she went to Rome to study at the Montessori School. While she was there, she met Irene Tasker and Margaret Naumberg. Ms. Naumberg had studied with Professor Dewey at Columbia University and was instrumental in F.M.'s reasons for going to the United States and the eventual meeting with John Dewey. Ms. Naumberg later founded the Walden School. F.M. arrived in New York City in late 1914. Ms. Webb accompanied him and A.R. followed shortly after. In 1916, Ms. Tasker accepted an invitation to teach at Walden School and also enrolled at Columbia University to study with Professor Dewey. Ms. Tasker continued to take Alexander lessons and became F.M.'s assistant in 1918 and worked primarily with children. At this point in time, F.M., A.R., Ms. Webb, and Ms. Tasker were the only teachers of the Technique. As interest in the Technique grew, so did the need for a formal teacher training course. F.M. and A.R. had returned to London and the first teacher training course began in 1931with 7 students. In 1935, A.R. returned to New York and traveled between there and Boston to start other training courses. A.R. died in 1946 after devoting his life to the teachings of his older brother. Ms Webb died shortly before F.M., who died October 10, 1955, without naming a successor to his work. Ms. Tasker would have been the best claimant. A more thorough historical account of the Alexander Technique can be found in Dr. Jones' book, *Body Awareness in Action.*[2]

American philosopher and educator John Dewey met Alexander around the year 1915, and was his first student in America. He took lessons throughout the 1920s and 1930s, the latter part of that time with Alexander's brother. In 1923, Professor Dewey wrote the introduction to Alexander's book, *Constructive Conscious Control of the Individual.* He also described Alexander's discovery "as a new scientific principle with respect to the control of human behavior as important as any principle that has ever been discovered in the domain of external nature,"[2] and as "...comparable to the discoveries that were made in the Renaissance and that caused men to change their ideas..."[2] Dewey wrote several books during the time he was receiving lessons. It has been said that the reader's potential for learning from these books, *Art as Experience, The Quest for Certainty, How We Think, The Theory of Valuation,* and *Experience and Education,* is greater when understood in the light of the Alexander Technique. In *Experience and Education,* Jones quotes Dewey stating, "The crucial educational problem is that of procuring the postponement of immediate action upon desire until observation and judgement have intervened."[2]

Dewey specifically referred to Alexander in *Human Nature and Conduct* and *Experience and Nature,* thus giving a written endorsement of the Technique. *Experience and Nature* is considered Dewey's best work and the one which most clearly and deeply exposes the Alexander principles.[2] Professor Dewey gave moral and intellectual support to Dr. Frank Pierce Jones to pursue research of the Technique. Unfortunately, Dewey died before Jones received sufficient financial support.

As a professor of classic Greek at Brown University, Frank Pierce Jones first heard of the Alexander Technique in 1930 from his colleagues in psychology. He was so drawn to the technique that he took a 3-year leave of absence to work with A.R. Alexander in the Boston training program. F.M. Alexander was at the training program during each of his visits to America. Dr. Jones qualified as an Alexander teacher in 1945. He met Professor Dewey in 1947, and both were greatly concerned by the lack of scientific foundation for the technique. He recognized the need to establish "...the physical equivalents of the great mental experience...to discover a mechanism that would account for the long-term effects on health and well-being."[2] Doctors in the Boston area were impressed by the physical improvements in their patients after Alexander lessons, but distressed because some form of non-scientific method was credited for the positive change. However, Jones knew "...a clinical study of the technique would be of little value until the principle it rested on had been demonstrated experimentally, and it could be shown that the clinical results followed from the means employed and could not be attributed to some other mechanism like suggestion."[2]

After a long search, and with encouragement from Professor Dewey, Jones gained a 7-year grant from the United States Public Health Service to find empirical support for the Alexander Technique in the knowledge base of anatomy and physiology. Another long search gave Jones access to conduct his study at the Tufts University Institute for Applied Experimental Psychology.

Jones used the startle pattern as a model for postural malalignment demonstrating increased muscle tension and displacement of the head. He felt the same malposture was associated with lack of exercise, aging, or disease. In the research lab, he imposed a startle response stimulus to subjects and used photography and electromyography to record the pattern. The startle pattern is a primitive response that stays with the organism for its life span. The startle paradigm is "...appropriate for developmental and comparative studies," showing "...different types of plasticity such as habituation, sensitization, prepulse inhibition, and modification by prior associative learnings."[19]

Jones also studied subjects using multi-image photography (upon advice from Harold Edgerton at MIT), electromyography, x-ray photography, and force platform records during activities like rising from supine position, standing from a chair, and walking up and down stairs. He recorded the changes in a subject's habitual movement compared to guided movements facilitated by an Alexander teacher. Jones' research recorded that least muscle tension, least force, and least head displacement were achieved with guided movement.

Jones also had subjects complete an adjective checklist to describe the kinesthetic effect of guided movement, and compared the subjective response with the objective measure. The descriptions of "lighter," "less familiar," "higher," and "smoother" were most consistent with measurable change. Jones concluded that his findings were consistent with the principles of physiology and psychology. Unfortunately, Jones died in 1975, just before completing the last chapter of his book, *Body Awareness in Action*, which was published the next year.

A lover of music and horse riding, Walter HM Carrington completed his training with Alexander in 1939. He continued on as Alexander's assistant and married a fellow teacher. Walter and his wife, Dilys, continued the teacher training program after Alexander's death in 1955. They continue to teach and are among the few living senior teachers of the Technique.

A London physician, Wilfred Barlow, met Alexander in 1938, and later married Alexander's niece, Marjory. Dr. Barlow's book, *The Alexander Principle*, summarizes 30 years of work and outlines the scientific basis of the technique. His articles on the Technique were published in many medical journals, and he wrote Alexander's obituary for The Times (London). Dr. Barlow died in 1991, and Marjory Barlow continues to teach in London.

Renowned author Aldous Huxley was so crippled with pain he was bedridden, but continued to write with his typewriter on his chest. Huxley was one of F.M.'s students in America. His condition improved greatly with the lessons. In 1936, he wrote *Eyeless in Gaza*.[20] The character of Miller is based upon F.M. Alexander. In 1937, Huxley wrote *Ends and Means*,[21] which endorses the Alexander Technique. In *The Alexander Principle*, Barlow quotes a 1941 article by Huxley:

> It is now possible to conceive of a totally new type of education, affecting the entire range of human activity, from the physiological, through the intellectual, moral and practical, to the spiritual...an education which, by teaching them proper Use, would preserve children and adults from most of the diseases and evil habits that now affect them: an education whose training would provide men and women with the psycho-physical means for behaving rationally.[22]

Musician and film director Laura Archera Huxley addressed the Alexander community in 1991 and described the Technique as "...a window, opening on new and wider horizons...inviting us to apply its principles..." to our personal and professional lives.23

Physician and physiologist Nikolaas Tinbergen took lessons from several Alexander teachers. In 1973, Professor Tinbergen shared the Nobel Prize for Physiology and Medicine with Konrad Lorenz and Karl von Frisch. He devoted half his acceptance speech to the Alexander Technique, and stated "...that many types of under-performance and even ailments, both mental and physical, can be alleviated, sometimes to a surprising extent, by teaching the body musculature to function differently..."[24]

A noted research scientist and university professor in physiology in the United Kingdom, Kathleen J. Ballard, PhD, became certified as an Alexander teacher in 1984. She is a regular contributor to reference journals, and presents her research at local and international meetings within the Alexander community. She is on the faculty at Walter Carrington's Alexander teacher training course in London. With her scientific background, Dr. Ballard helps to establish the validity of the Technique.[25]

Senior lecturer at the School of Physiology & Pharmacology, University of New South Wales, Australia, David George Garlick, MD, PhD, has been a regular contributor to *Direction*, a journal on the the Alexander Technique, and a presenter at international Alexander conferences. He edited *Proprioception, Posture and Emotion*,[26] a compilation of papers and posters at the Symposium on Proprioception, Posture and Emotion, sponsored by the Committee in Postgraduate Medical Education at the University of NSW in February of 1981. Dr. Garlick's support for the Technique included chairing the Fourth International Alexander Congress in Sydney, Australia in 1994.

A student of the Technique since 1969, Christopher Stevens now directs a teacher training program in Aalborg, Denmark. With his background in physics and physiology, he has conducted research on the Technique in the Department of Anatomy and Human Biology at Kings College, London, and in the Department of Anatomy, University of Copenhagen, Denmark. Stevens replicated Jones' study comparing habitual and guided sit to stand movements.[27] The findings of the two studies were consistent. Stevens did further study in postural stability between individuals who had taken Alexander lessons and individuals who had not taken lessons. He found the trained group had significantly less postural sway than the control group when standing with feet together and eyes closed.[27] He concluded that the Alexander-trained subjects had increased awareness of kinesthetic feedback to access for postural stability. Full details of Stevens' work can be found in his book, *Toward a Physiology of the Alexander Technique*.[28-30]

While at Tufts University, Lester "Tommy" Thompson was a colleague of Frank Pierce Jones. Mr. Thompson studied the Technique with Dr. Jones for several years. Shortly before his death in 1975, Dr. Jones gave Thompson full approval and sanction to continue teaching the Technique. Since Dr. Jones' book was published after his death and there were many inquiries about his work and his records, Tufts University agreed to keep the records for a limited time unless further scholarly interest was evident. In 1982, the Frank Pierce Jones archives was established under the administration of Mr. Thompson, Dr. Richard Brown, and Mrs. Helen (Frank) Jones. In 1985, the Wessel Library at Tufts University agreed to keep the Jones Collection on a permanent basis. At the same time, a new collection of the F. Matthias Alexander papers was admitted. These collections include Jones' research papers and the correspondence he held with Alexander, Dewey, and others. Mr. Thompson directed the Archives until 1988. He continues to train Alexander teachers and is one of the 1993 founders and charter members of Alexander Technique International (ATI). The purpose of ATI is to promote and advance the F. Matthias Alexander Technique and to disseminate information among its members and to the public.

This listing is by no means complete and only provides partial notes of a few people. Many individuals have contributed to the advancement of the Alexander Technique through their practice, research, publications, and presentations.

CASE EXAMPLES

Alexander did not approve of the use of case histories to substantiate his theories, believing this was a medical orientation toward research and he saw his work best applied in the field of education. "Case histories are important and do throw light on the mechanisms involved in the Technique. But they confuse by overstressing the medical aspect."[2] However, Alexander did cite "examples" of students who improved using the Technique. In fact, case examples can be found in Alexander's books[1,6] and in almost every other book written on the Alexander Technique.

The first case example must be of Alexander himself. In discussing the authenticity of somatic pioneers, Don Hanlon Johnson states, "Alexander found that his laryngitis was not just a matter of germs infecting mucous membranes; it was also the result of the way in which he muscularly responded to expectant audiences."[31]

Dr. Barlow's book, *The Alexander Principle*, is illustrated with photographs of many subjects. Although photographs are limited, as they depict still moments in movement, the text clearly describes the dynamic aspects of misuse, especially the chapter on "Use and Disease."[22]

Tommy Thompson's presentation at The First International Congress of Teachers of the F.M. Alexander Technique at the State University of New York, Stony Brook, in August, 1986, cites two examples. The case briefly described earlier in this writing of the 14-year-old neigborhood bully demonstrates the moral implications of the Technique. The other tells of an National Football League player with neck and back pain interfering with his performance, and demonstrates the influence of use on action. His body carried the actions of the game even though he was off the field. In other words, the somatic effects of previous games influenced his daily activities and the next game. The player never put his football down. Over the course of lessons, the player realized he could let go of the ball and receive the next play as a unique event. He was soon relieved of his pain and his performance on the field improved.[14]

An Alexander teacher and a physical therapist, Deborah Caplan has specialized her work to people with back problems. She frequently lectures to physical therapists and presents to the Alexander community. Case examples can be found in her writings.[32,33]

Students of F.M. Alexander and the Technique are a diverse group. Students of the technique include Henry Irving, Lily Langtry, Viola Tree, Oscar Asche, Matheson Lang, Paul Newman, Colin Davis, Roald Dahl, Edna O'Brien, Barry Tuckwell, John Cleese, Aldous Huxley, George Bernard Shaw, the Duchess of York, Sting, Sir Stafford Cripps, John Dewey, James Harvey Robinson, Sir Charles Sherrington, Professor G.E. Coghill, Archbishop William Temple, Frederick Perls, Moshe Feldenkrais, John Houseman, Paul McCartney, Mary Steenburgen, Irene Worth, Christopher Reeve, Joel Gray, Julie Andrews, Joanne Woodward, and Patrick Stewart.[2,18,28,34-38]

Some institutions that recommend or offer the Alexander Technique in their curricula are the Julliard School, the Royal Shakespeare Company, the Israeli Airforce Pilots, the

Los Angeles Philharmonic, the University of Wisconsin, the University of Washington, New York University, Boston University, Ohio State University, Southern Methodist University, and the American Conservatory Theatre.[38]

HOW AND WHY I CHOSE THE ALEXANDER TECHNIQUE

In 1982, my life fell into disharmony. I had been practicing physical therapy for 12 years and had just finished a master's degree. I was unhappy that my practice of physical therapy was draining me and I was unhappy with the way I felt. Over the next 5 years, I pursued every alternative approach that could possibly satisfy two basic needs: first, I looked for an approach that could help my aches and pains. Second, a taller order, I looked for an approach that I could believe in to the extent that I would learn it and be able to help others with it, even after I retired from physical therapy, and on until the day I died. Only in retrospect can I describe what my belief in an approach entailed. I wanted something I could do with my hands, one on one with another person, and something that had a scientific foundation I could accept. Essentially, "high touch and high tech." One evening in 1986, I went to an adult education center to hear an introductory lecture about "the" approach I had finally decided on, which was given by a teacher I had learned about in my search. An introduction to the Alexander Technique was also on the agenda. I had never heard of this approach, nor of the person listed to present. Serendipity was with me that night because I found myself in the Alexander Technique lecture given by my future teacher, Tommy Thompson. Within the first 5 minutes, I realized I had found what I was looking for—an approach that met my two criteria.

The Alexander Technique was a hands-on approach based on sound, scientific reasoning and was amenable to research methods. It was also more educational and preventative than medical in orientation, and being more schooled in education than physical therapy, I was quite receptive. I scheduled a lesson but it was 6 months away. In the meantime, I read all of Alexander's books as well as those of Frank Pierce Jones and Edward Maisel. Reading F.M.'s books was like simultaneously stepping backward and forward in time. His style was difficult to read and not easy to comprehend. F.M. wrote about his work within a culture that was restrained. His insights were progressive and offered a solution to the human dilemma. I went to that first lesson with dread, because I'd read that F.M. Alexander

> Would not accept therapists of any kind or teachers of physical education, who, he was sure, wanted merely to pick up a few new ideas to enliven their own teaching and be able to say that they were using the Alexander Technique.[2]

My first degree was in physical education, the next in physical therapy, and the master's didn't matter. I had allowed myself into a situation with a two strike score. If I failed this, I would be out. Tommy started my lesson with the usual hands-on approach. I literally took three steps back and said, "No! I'm just here to talk." We talked, and it was another 6 months before I had a real hands-on lesson.

I immediately understood the connection between the consciousness and body use. I also began to understand the reason for my aches and pains. I had several more lessons from Tommy, and from a visiting teacher from Israel, and entered Tommy's training program in the Fall of 1987. I continued my lessons and training. It took me 5 years, instead of the standard 3, to be certified. That was because of an "adjunct lesson" I took by breaking my leg. After two surgeries and 2 years to heal and process, I call my experience a sledgehammer lesson. I had not been paying attention to the moment-by-moment events affecting my life and I needed information I could not ignore. It took me 5 years to become certified as an Alexander Teacher, but I did it the only way I could. I needed the extra time to learn my lessons my way. I often share my sledgehammer learning technique with my patients and there is immediate understanding.

Learning to be a teacher of the Alexander Technique takes place within an apprentice model. I do not know why I was presented with the teacher I needed, or how I ended up in Tommy's lecture and training course. But over time, I came to understand and to value my teacher's lineage to Alexander himself. Tommy had studied with Frank Pierce Jones. Dr. Jones had studied with F.M. and A.R. Alexander. Thus, my training included the intuitive approach side by side with the anatomy and physiology foundation.

I have only had a handful of my own Alexander students, one of whom I have been seeing for 7 years. I may soon have the opportunity to work with a 15-year-old boy with Wolfram Syndrome, a rare, hereditary disorder causing diabetes mellitus, diabetes insipidus, optic atrophy, and deafness. I have been told the lad has poor posture and poor awareness for the internal signs from his body. His mother had heard of the Alexander Technique and connected with me through the grapevine. I have also worked with colleagues, family, and friends on an intermittent basis.

I was pleased to be able to help my father, a stoic person. As a child, he was plagued with allergies and asthma, which led to several serious bouts of bronchitis in adulthood. Several years ago, when Dad was about 76 years old, I learned he had been suffering from severe headaches almost daily. He was also quite curious about this approach, and eventually asked me to work with him. As I placed my hands on the "right upper quadrant," as physical therapists call it, I felt a subtle, yet powerful release. Although my hands were in contact with specific muscles overlying specific bones, I sensed the release was from deeper areas, closer to the core of his being. My father, who rarely shares his feelings, acknowledged that he too had sensed a change. Following this single session, he was headache-free for about 2 years, and now has an occasional, tolerable sinus-type headache. He also practices a home program I designed for him based on the principles to keep his spine, hips, and shoulders free from the daily build-up of tension.

COMBINING THE ALEXANDER TECHNIQUE WITH PHYSICAL THERAPY

Currently, I do not have a full Alexander practice, but I apply the principles of the Technique to my approach with patients while I am performing the standard tasks of physical therapy treatment. I work primarily in pediatrics with patients with vision and hearing deficits, head trauma sequelae, autism, and developmental delay, and also with adults in orthopedic sub-acute rehabilitation. I am impressed by two major changes in my work; how I use my hands to touch others and how my presence in treatment influences the well-being of each party. My touch is lighter and not directed toward a specific action. I also observe the words I use to reach the person. I talk less about the bones and muscles, and more about effort, grace, and poise. I accept that the individual has an understanding of what I say as I observe his or her use change. My presence in treatment is neutral, giving me room for acceptance of the individual's current position and needs. I no longer see total hip replacements or scoliosis or brain and birth traumas; I see individuals with unique life circumstances and life's imposed conditions. I am then able to work with individuals in a way that empowers them to change, and I do it without the need to carry their medical and emotional burdens on my shoulders. Physical therapy treatment, as with my Alexander lessons, then becomes an energizing experience. I am not drained or depleted of physical and emotional strength by what I should give to, or do for, the individual.

After I provide an Alexander lesson, I actually feel better than I did before the lesson. In an Alexander lesson, I have no intentions in mind (or inhibit my desire to plan a treatment) and allow the individual to lead me down the path he or she needs to explore. I act as a guide to suggest the means whereby the path may be taken. In physical therapy treatment, I have intentions because I have required functional goals and third parties to remind me, but I try to inhibit my desire to meet the needs of parties not present at the moment. Treatment outcome may be the same, and likely even more beneficial, because the individual has been given "unimposed upon space" to change his or her use, and thus to heal.

This is not to say the individual would have accomplished the same without me. I believe my presence, guided by the principles of the Alexander Technique, facilitates a change in the whole person, directly affecting his or her condition in a positive fashion. And with the Alexander Technique, I have a means to manage those moments that "push my buttons" or trigger my "internal tapes," and to be aware of other options available to direct my physical and emotional responses. I am reminded of Dr. Jones' first chapter in *Body Awareness in Action*, entitled "Escape from the Monkey Trap." He opens this section with a quote from C.J. Herrick:

> In an expanding system, such as a growing organism...freedom to change the pattern of performance is one of the intrinsic properties of the organism itself.[2]

F.M. Alexander, through his intense questions and motivation to find answers within himself, defined a new outlook and approach to human development, spanning the space between stimulus and response, therapy and education. Documented scientific studies explain quite clearly how this Technique facilitates the improvement of the whole person by teaching a method where conscious control and freedom of choice is used in preventing and healing habitual causes of pain and discomfort. Thus, the Alexander Technique takes its rightful place, along with physical therapy and other healing approaches, as complementary to the modern search for health and well-being.

RESOURCES

The F. Matthias Alexander Archival Collection, and The Frank Pierce Jones Collection
Archives for Special Collections
Tufts University
Medford, MA 02155
Tel: 617-648-0306

Alexander Foundation
Bruce Fertman
605 W. Phil-Ellena Street
Philadelphia, PA 19119
Tel: 215-844-0670

Alexander Research Trust
18 Lansdowne Road
London, W11 3LL, Great Britain

Alexander Technique Center at Cambridge
Tommy Thompson
1692 Massachusetts Avenue
Cambridge, MA 02138
Tel: 617-497-2242
Fax: 617-876-2709
e-mail: TTATInt@aol.com

Alexander Technique International, Australia
11/11 Stanley Street
Darlinghurst, NSW 2010
Tel: 02-371-6991
Fax: 02-313-8629
e-mail: D.Garlick@unsw.edu.au

Alexander Technique International, France
108 Rue Des Grands-Champs
Paris 75020, France
Tel: (+33) 44-93-59-24

Alexander Technique International, United Kingdom
142 Thorpedale Road
London N4 3BS, UK
Tel: (+44) 0171-281-7639
Fax: 281-9400
e-mail: deegee@alextech.win-uk.net

Alexander Technique International, USA (Head Office)
1692 Massachusetts Avenue
Cambridge, MA 02138
Tel/Fax:617-876-2709
e-mail TTATInt@aol.com

Alexander Workshops, Inc.
William Conable
2841 Calumet Street
Columbus, OH 43201
Tel: 614-447-8258
e-mail: wconable@magnus.acs.ohio-state.edu

Australian Society of Teachers of the Alexander Technique
P.O. Box 529, Milsons Point
Sydney 2061
New South Wales, Australia

Canadian Society of Teachers of the Alexander Technique
460 Palmerston Boulevard
Toronto, Ontario
P7A 4A2, Canada

Direction: A Journal on the Alexander Technique
PO Box 276, Bondi
NSW 2026, Australia
Tel: 02-665-3364; Fax: 02-665-1578
email: jeremy@sydney.dialix.oz.au

International School for the FM Alexander Technique
J. Berthelsensv. 15A
9400 Norresundby, Denmark

North American Society of Teachers of the Alexander Technique (NASTAT)
P.O. Box 3992
Champaign, IL 61826-3992

Society of Teachers of the Alexander Technique (STAT)
10 London House, 266 Fulham Road
London SW10 9EL, United Kingdon

STAT Books
20 London House, 266 Fulham Road
London SW10 9EL, United Kingdom

ACKNOWLEDGMENT

I would like to thank Tommy Thompson for his help in reviewing this manuscript.

REFERENCES

1. Alexander FM. *The Use of Self*. Long Beach, Calif: Centerline Press; 1984.
2. Jones FP. *Body Awareness in Action: A Study of the Alexander Technique*. New York, NY: Schocken Books; 1976.
3. Wheelhouse F. Dart and Alexander. *Direction*. 1988;3:100-105.
4. Sheppard D. Physiology and freedom: a report on Dr. Benjamin Libet's lecture to NASTAT's second annual meeting. *The Alexander Review*. 1989;4:5-17.
5. Alexander FM. *The Universal Constant in Living*. Long Beach, Calif: Centerline Press; 1986.
6. Alexander FM. *Man's Supreme Inheritance*. Long Beach, Calif: Centerline Press; 1988.
7. Roberts TDM. Balance and locomotion. In: Garlick D, ed. *Proprioception, Posture and Emotion*.

Bankstown, Australia: Adept Printing Pty Ltd; 1982.

8. Mixon D, Burton P. Faulty sensory perception. *Direction.* 1989;4:128-134.

9. Dart RA. An anatomist's tribute to F. Matthias Alexander. Memorial lecture before the Society of Teachers of the Alexander Technique in London, England, March 20, 1970. In: *Skill, Poise, and The Alexander Technique.* Long Beach, Calif: Centerline Press.

10. Jones FP. Method for changing stereotyped response patterns by the inhibition of certain postural sets. *Psych Rev.* 1965;3:196-214.

11. Schneider GE. Two visual systems: brain mechanisms for localization and discrimination are dissociated by tectal and cortical lesions. *Science.* 1969:163;895-902.

12. Trevarthen CB, Sperry R. Perceptual unity of the ambient visual field in human commissurotomy patients. *Brain.* 1973;96:547-570.

13. Joudry R. The use of the ear. *Direction.* 1995;3:23-25.

14. Thompson LW. Its practical application in pursuing the possibility of changes in moral and mental attitude and the extension of the range within which free choice and free will can operate. In: *The Scientific and Humanistic Contributions of Frank Pierce Jones on the F. Matthias Alexander Technique.* Long Beach, Calif: Centerline Press; 1988.

15. Falk D. *Braindance.* New York, NY: Henry Holt; 1992.

16. Tobias PV. *Man, The Tottering Biped: The Evolution of His Posture, Poise and Skill.* Bankstown, Australia: Adept Printing Pry Ltd; 1982.

17. Tobias PV. Man, the tottering biped: the evolution of his erect posture. In: Garlick D, ed. *Proprioception, Posture and Emotion.* Bankstown, Australia: Adept Printing Pty Ltd; 1982.

18. Dart RA. The attainment of poise. *So Afr Med J.* 1947;21:74-91. In: Skill, Poise, and The Alexander Technique. Long Beach, CA: Centerline Press.

19. Davis M. The mammalian startle response. In: Eaton RC. *Neural Mechanisms of Startle Behavior.* New York, NY: Plenum Press; 1984:287-351.

20. Huxley A. *Eyeless in Gaza.* New York, NY: Harper & Row; 1936.

21. Huxley A. *Ends and Means.* New York, NY: Harper & Row; 1937.

22. Barlow W. *The Alexander Principle.* London, England: Arrow Books; 1975.

23. Huxley L, Pappas C. Tribalistic thinking: enslavement or freedom? Third International Alexander Congress Papers, Engelberg, Switzerland, 1991. Bondi, Australia: Direction.

24. Tinbergen N. Ethology and stress diseases. *Science.* 1974;185:20-27.

25. Ballard K. The Alexander Technique and Postural Reflexes. In: The Second International Alexander Congress Papers, Brighton, England, 1988. Bondi, Australia: Direction; 35-39.

26. Garlick D, ed. *Proprioception, Posture and Emotion.* Bankstown, Australia: Adept Printing Pty Ltd; 1982.

27. Stevens C. Experimental studies of the Alexander Technique. In: Second International Congress Papers, Brighton, England, 1988. Bondi, Australia: Direction; 136-156.

28. Stevens C. *Alexander Technique.* London, Great Britain: Macdonald & Co; 1987.

29. Stevens C. Scientific research & its role in teaching the Alexander Technique. *The Alexander Review.* 1989;4:171-194.

30. Stevens C. *Toward a Physiology of the Alexander Technique*. 1994.

31. Johnson DH. *Body: Recovering Our Sensual Wisdom*. Berkeley, Calif: North Atlantic Books; 1992.

32. Caplan D. *Back Trouble: A New Approach to Prevention and Recovery*. Gainesville, Fla: Triad Pub Co; 1987.

33. Caplan D. The Alexander Technique and Its Application to Back Problems. In: The Second International Alexander Congress Papers, Brighton, England; 1988. Bondi, Australia: Direction; 73-77.

34. Barlow W. Posture, proprioception and the Alexander Technique. In: Garlick D, ed. *Proprioception, Posture and Emotion*. Bankstown, Australia: Adept Printing Pty Ltd; 1982:228-245.

35. Brennan R. *The Alexander Technique: Natural Poise for Health*. Rockport, Mass: Element Inc; 1991.

36. Brennan R. *The Alexander Technique Workbook: Your Personal Programme for Health, Poise and Fitness*. Rockport, Mass: Element, Inc; 1992.

37. Conable W. Alexander Workshops, Inc. Columbus, Ohio; 1995.

38. Exchange: News Journal of Alexander Technique International. 1996;4(2):20.

SUGGESTED READINGS

Alexander FM. *Constructive Conscious Control of the Individual*. Long Beach, Calif: Centerline Press; 1984.

Austin JHM, Ausubel P. Enhanced respiratory muscular function in normal adults after lessons in proprioceptive musculoskeletal education without exercises. *Chest*. 1992;102:486-490.

Carrington W, Sontag J, ed. *Thinking Aloud: Talks on Teaching the Alexander Technique*. San Francisco, Calif: Mornum Time Press; 1994.

Chance J, ed. The life and work of Raymond Dart. *Direction*. 1988;3:68-86, 96-105.

Dewey J. *Experience and Nature*. New York, NY: W.W. Norton & Co; 1929.

Dewey J. *Human Nature and Conduct*. New York, NY: Modern Library; 1930.

Dewey J. *How We Think*. Boston, Mass: D.C. Heath & Co; 1933.

Dewey J. *Art as Experience*. New York, NY: G.P. Putnam & Sons; 1934.

Dewey J. *Experience and Education*. New York, NY: Macmillan; 1938.

Dewey J. *The Quest for Certainty*. New York, NY: G.P. Putnam & Sons; 1939.

Dewey J. The theory of valuation. *International Encyclopedia of Unified Science*. Chicago, Ill; 1939.

Garlick D, ed. *Proprioception, Posture and Emotion*. Bankstown, Australia: Adept Printing Pty Ltd;1982.

Huxley A. *Eyeless in Gaza*. New York, NY: Harper & Row; 1936.

Huxley A. *Ends and Means*. New York, NY: Harper & Brothers; 1937.

Huxley A. End-Gaining and Means-Whereby. *The Saturday Review of Literature*. October 25, 1941.

Huxley A. *The Doors of Perception and Heaven and Hell*. New York, NY: Harper & Row; 1954.

Huxley LA. *You Are Not the Target*. New York, NY: Farrar, Straus & Company; 1994.

Johnson DH, ed. *Bone, Breath & Gesture: Practices of Embodiment*. Berkeley, Calif: North Atlantic Books; 1995.

Kodish SP, Kodish BI. *Drive Yourself Sane! Using the Uncommon Sense of General Semantics*. Englewood, NJ: Institute of General Semantics; 1993.

Maisel E. *The Alexander Technique: The Essential Writings of F. Matthias Alexander*. New York, NY: Carol Communications; 1989.

Maisel E. *The Resurrection of the Body: The Essential Writings of F. Matthias Alexander*. Boston, Mass: Shambhala Publications Inc; 1986.

Sanfilippo P. *The Reader's Guide to the Alexander Technique: A Selected Annotated Bibliography*. Long Beach, Calif: Centerline Press; 1987.

Tobias PV. A Tribute to Emeritus Professor Raymond Dart. *Direction*. 1988;3:96-99.

Todd ME. *The Thinking Body*. Princeton, NJ: Princeton Book Co.

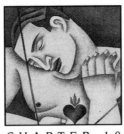

CHAPTER 10

FELDENKRAIS METHOD AND REHABILITATION

A Paradigm Shift Incorporating a Perception of Learning

Osa Jackson-Wyatt, PhD, PT

INTRODUCTION

The Feldenkrais® Method grew from the observations and writings of Moshe Feldenkrais. By background Feldenkrais was a physicist, a judo expert (he wrote the first book in French on judo), and an athlete. As an adult, he faced a knee injury that left him severely limited. When the medical profession offered him only a fusion for his knee problems (pain and instability), he decided to create a different storyline for himself about his life and the choices he wanted.

He realized by observing his own adaptation to the knee problems that human beings have a *choice* about how to move. Choice is defined as the act of choosing and involves people exercising their power to select the option(s) that are most suitable according to their perceptions. As a result, the Feldenkrais approach begins by inviting the individual to choose to participate. The skill or art is to find where to start and what stimulus to choose so that the person will agree to begin to participate in a rehabilitation program. Rehabilitation professionals realize that the first step in leaning how to develop new adaptive skills to deal with an illness or injury is to have the patient believe that rehabilitation is interesting, helpful, and doable.

During the healing process of his knee, Moshe Feldenkrais became an astute observer of his body's responses to injury. When there was pain and discomfort, Feldenkrais carefully noted the predictable response of his central nervous system:

1. At the time of the acute injury, the activation of the limbic system created a localized muscular splinting and other secondary changes throughout the body, for example, changes in breathing.

2. The longer the pain remained, the more alteration occurred from the established natural *habits* of efficient action.

Habit is defined as any activity so well-established that it occurs without conscious effort. Through systematic movement exploration, he discovered that habits of movement can be worked with and alterations can be made in the habitual strategies.[1-3] Why did he care about the habits of action? From the point of view of the physicist, the habits of bony loading through the skeleton and the forces they create are what shape the basic kinesthetic cues that are used by the person to build a strategy for any action. An example of a kinesthetic cue would be that, as you sit in your chair, notice the point of contact on the right heel and note if it feels the same as the point of contact on the other heel. Attending to such kinesthetic cues, Feldenkrais became aware that his knee problems were causing secondary changes in his patterns of loading and in the movement patterns of action throughout his entire body. He also noted changes in his *thoughts* about various actions and the related movements and *feelings* of safety about certain actions and the related movements. He began posing such questions as, "What are the implications of keeping one part of the body stiff or rigid and not allowing natural participation of this segment in the total body action?" He noted that there are endless options for adapting to a particular blockage or restriction in a movement or any aspect of the strategy for action. Based on these insights, he left his chosen profession of physics and studied medicine and movement. He began training himself and exploring the strategies for how an individual can learn to adapt in the most effective manner to life events. In this way he taught himself how to walk again.

If after having read this far you feel confused, then you are at a place where you are ready to examine and explore a new paradigm for how people learn and adapt. The paradigm, or explanatory model for the analytical thinking of Moshe Feldenkrais, presented above is not built on Wolf's Law, as is traditional Western medicine and physical therapy. The Feldenkrais paradigm invites a new look at the theoretical basis for all rehabilitation intervention. There are key differences in the Feldenkrais model for understanding how human beings learn and adapt.

One difference is that there is a recognition that mental and emotional activity can strongly perturb all aspects of human performance. Unlike traditional neurophysiology theory, Feldenkrais Method does not separate the sensory and the motor systems. E.S. Reed,[4] N. Bernstein,[5] and A.R. Luria[6] each emphasize that the traditional neurological and psychological theory that distinguishes between central and peripheral neural processes is no longer functionally relevant. According to Reed, "A review of the relevant psychological research on the control of movement shows that both central-peripheral dichotomy and the distinction between sensory and motor systems derived from that dichotomy are incompatible with what is known about the processes underlying action."[4]

Thus, the Feldenkrais Method is based on a paradigm shift in the theoretical framework for physical therapy and rehabilitation. However, the treatment philosophy behind the therapeutic work of Sister Kenny in her approach to patients with polio contains ideas common to those of Feldenkrais.[7] Avoiding pain or perception of strain, thus causing no limbic recruitment during therapy; treating to avoid splinting of breathing during the learning process; facilitating efficient loading throughout the skeleton during action or movement; finding a pace that is suitable for the patient's functional enjoyment of the moment; and avoiding parasitic movement during specific intended action and self observation are ideas common to both approaches. Individuals who need rehabilitation can benefit from this paradigm shift since they usually present with pain, overuse of one or more components of a functional movement pattern, for example, head forward posture; wrist action; breathholding with any movement effort and/or muscular splinting occurring with the act of listening or thinking; muscle action that substitutes for bony loading, such as a posterior pelvic tilt rather than neutral in sitting or standing; no natural rest-activity cycle; fatigue that is not manageable; and/or discomfort in self-awareness or the act of dissociation from any self-observation, which is revealed when the patient says "It hurts" versus "My leg hurts."

FELDENKRAIS METHOD VS. TRADITIONAL MOVEMENT THERAPY

When the Feldenkrais Method is applied to patients in physical therapy and rehabilitation, the therapist takes on the role of teacher, facilitator and guide. The intention of the therapist is to guide the individual using verbal, visual, and kinesthetic information. Avoiding touch at this point reinforces self-determination and problem solving, which maximizes the patient's current potential for function and his or her ability to adapt. In other words, rather than first evaluating the patient and then treating with massage and strengthening or range of motion exercises, the patient is "invited to learn" using the discovery model. The patient is asked to explore a new focus of movement by attending to altered kinesthetic cues during a desired action. For example, "Pick your foot up off the floor and take a step. Feel what you're doing. Now, can you do that by first lifting your heel?" The patient is carefully guided to compare and observe whether the new focus leads to improved adaptation during the desired functional activity.

Evaluation is not performed separately from the learning process. The therapist constantly observes and adapts stimuli in order for the patient to *maximally explore and adapt* during a particular session; to experience, at best, a sense of success or, at least, the novelty of discovery. The therapist's evaluation records the conditions that facilitate learning for this person, the key cues, auditory, visual, kinesthetic, and/or movements that are observed to maximize functional performance of a desired task, illustrating in each unique case the marvelous plasticity of the central nervous system.

THE IMPORTANCE OF A TRUSTING TEACHER/STUDENT RELATIONSHIP

The essence of the Feldenkrais strategy is to create a personalized learning program for the rehabilitation of each patient.[9] The core ingredient to the Feldenkrais Method is the trust that the therapist purposely fosters as the first and most important goal of interaction with the patient. With this foundation of trust, the therapist begins to set up "learning experiments."[8] Adaptations are made in the learning experiment based on the responses of the patient so that the patient feels safe and can relax as he or she interacts. The starting point for self observation is to help the patient discover his or her current habitual responses in a particular situation. When asked to move, the patient explores the immediate habitual response to identify how they either help or hinder effective functional adaptation. For example, the final focus is to help the patient explore choices for movement and then make new choices for enhancing performance outcome for the desired tasks. In other words, the therapist's role is to help the patient discover new insights, have "Ah-ha" experiences, to celebrate the joy of self-discovered learning and the sense of mastery that this can bring. The therapist's goal is to be perceived by the patient as having the intention of supporting his or her recovery of function by contributing just the right "experiments" that facilitate the patient's discovery of how to maximize his or her abilities. Intervention cues are initially small, gentle, and paced so that the learner's perception is, "This feels doable and worth doing again." The patient is left with a sense that he or she has the ability to adapt effectively: "I can learn new ways to adapt so that I can move more easily in spite of my pain."

Utilizing a learning paradigm during patient interaction, the Feldenkrais Method invites the rehabilitation team to leave the "illness" emphasis behind. The entire patient/therapist interaction is used to discover what movements enhance performance. Therapists still are responsible for adequately documenting patient limitations, but the tone of the treatment process is anchored in supporting patients' exploration of how they can move beyond their current limitations, of which they are often well aware.

CASE EXAMPLE

Mr. G has a history of low back pain that reccurs with the lifting of work-related objects over 30 pounds. He has experienced physical therapy before, which included work hardening exercise and education, yet reinjured himself within 30 days of being on the job full-time. He had been taught the traditional back-strengthening posture exercises and stretching program.

At this time, Mr. G habitually sits in a posterior pelvic tilt and rests his feet primarily on the lateral or outside borders. The x-ray findings show no disc problems. A Feldenkrais treatment begins with an initial conversation to identify what Mr. G is looking for from the therapist. I ask him, "What would you like to learn to be able to do that you have difficulty with at this time?" The typical initial response from the patient contains a long list of complaints and a description of all the limitations he is facing. I then ask the patient to focus on one functional improvement that he would like to work toward today. I support him as he develops a clear "I" statement, which also can be described as a goal statement, or a "script" for the rehabilitation program during this visit.

Sometimes it is not possible for the patient to identify a goal statement within 10 to 15 minutes. Then the session focuses on whatever is on the patient's mind that seems to prevent him from being able to make a goal statement.

The "I" statement represents the patient's cognitive commitment to his or her idea of what is desired. In this case, Mr. G finally states, "I would like to start by being able to sit without pain." Having a goal for today, next I would help Mr. G identify any neuro or orthopedic variables that might be interfering with the effective completion of his desired goal(s). One strategy I might use is to ask Mr. G to do a self-assessment of his kinesthetic status at rest in a significant functional posture, such as sitting.[10] As I ask Mr. G through guided observation to compare the weight on the sole of the right foot to the weight on the sole of his left, his attention is drawn to create a comparison of symptoms, habitual actions, and habitual postures. In this way, I help Mr. G create a discovery about the choices that exist in how he can carry out a particular activity. Mr. G may discover that by placing the soles of his feet flat on the floor and at hip-width apart, he causes a pulling in his right anterior shoulder area and in his neck on the right side. With this simple act, Mr. G may come to realize that what he thought was an "isolated" low back pain problem may really involve several movements he has developed over time to compensate for pain, and that those movements have now become habitual.

I then screen for flexibility with Mr. G by asking him to first place his right hand behind his back with the dorsum of his hand against his body, and then the left hand. This task reveals that the reach and ease on his right is notably easier than on his left. Mr. G is left-handed and he reports that he broke his left collar bone as a child, but has had no local complaints. I then ask Mr. G to sit with support placing his low back in a neutral lumbar curve, and to place his feet flat, shoulder width apart, his hands resting on his stomach, with his palms flat against his body. He can perform this activity pain-free for 1 minute. When I ask him to note what moves when he breathes, without pain, he is aware that his chest is what moves.

After another minute, a feeling of pain and pulling begins in his right low back, which he reports increases the longer he sits. At that time, I invite Mr. G to lie in a comfortable sleep position, and he chooses half-prone, on his left. I ask Mr. G to notice his breathing in this position, but he reports he observes nothing unusual. I note that at rest Mr. G breathes primarily in a shallow apical pattern, at a pace that is 30-50% faster than what is needed to rest in this posture. Mr. G's movement experiment develops as I explore how the breath might match the effort he needs for simple resting in a half prone position. An example of a verbal cue for a movement exploration might be to ask Mr. G to find the most comfortable way to place his hand on his belly just below his belly button. When he finds a satisfactory position, I ask him to direct his breath only into his lower abdomen and let his chest area rest. Mr. G is asked to breathe so that, on inhalation, his abdomen will expand and push slightly against the mat, and on exhalation, his abdomen will shrink, as if a slight pulling in of the belly were occurring to cause a 10% decrease of pressure on the mat. Then I ask, what if the speed of inhale and exhale were slowed a little bit, say by 2%, from the habitual? Can Mr. G find just the amount of air to inhale that feels easy for this activity in this position?

As these movement experiments were explored, I invited Mr. G to proceed at his own pace. I instructed him to pause and observe any urge to move, reposition, or simply take a rest. As the habitual resting tension is altered, there may be a variety of changes that occur, such as the urge to belch, pass gas, scratch, yawn, stretch, and so forth. Mr. G was guided to discover his particular rest/activity cycle that will allow a pleasant learning experience for 30-60 minutes depending on his ability to attend. He then was invited to rest for 1-2 minutes as needed, and then I asked him to return to his starting position (sitting) and feel any changes in how it is to be in this posture after having completed the movement exploration. At rest, Mr. G notes that if he allows the breathing to cause a slight motion of the abdomen, the pain is different than if he holds the abdomen rigid and breathes more in the upper chest area. He also notes that if he breathes 2% slower, that within 1-2 minutes he gets the urge to take a "really good deep breath." He reports that really good free breathing has been difficult for years and gets worse when he is very busy at work. The session ends with Mr. G's identifying the very easy positions where he can perform slow abdominal breathing (2% slower than usual) where the abdomen is moving in a natural excursion in response to the breath, and with a size of breath that matches the level of exertion for resting half prone. Mr. G is invited to explore this at home with the goal of creating practice times for 15-30 minutes twice per day where he is allowing restful abdominal breathing to promote a reflex relaxation in the resting tension in the entire trunk. The outcome was that new data became available to the patient about things that he could explore when fatigue or pre-pain symptoms begin to develop. The clearly identified goal is to practice pain-free movement and to rest and do the breathing experiment whenever pre-pain symptoms such as fatigue, pulling, and/or pressure begin to be noticed.

One important note is that the environment both in the clinic and at home needs to be adapted so that the patient can concentrate and not be distracted, that is, an environment that is acoustically private and supports the intention for clear and small variations in cues and focus (visually appropriate). The environment also needs to take into account the need for utilizing a reasonable rest-activity cycle; thus, space adequate for reclining is provided, plus appropriate help to allow the patient to come for therapy well rested. The environment also needs to support the patient's identity by the therapist's willingness to organize caregiving based on patient preference as much as is possible for scheduling, pace, own clothing, etc.[8]

The Feldenkrais Method has two strategies for exploring with the learner: Functional Integration® (FI) and Awareness Through Movement® (ATM). ATM, the approach illustrated in Mr. G's case, is used to describe the exploration when the therapist/teacher uses primarily verbal and visual stimulus to help the learner discover a strategy that will work best for a particular situation. ATM is the approach of choice as long as the learner is prepared to initiate the movement experiment that will create new awareness and a variety of responses that are different from the habitual actions. FI is used to describe the exploration when the teacher/therapist uses things such as positioning, contact, pressure, and movement combined with verbal and visual stimulus to help the learner discover a strategy that will allow the most effective participation by the patient/learner. Functional Integration is used as a strategy when the individual is not able, for whatever reason, to actively initiate the exploration.

The overall goal is to help the individual discover how to be an efficient learner who can adapt to the ever-changing reality in his or her life. Change grows to be recognized and accepted as a natural situation and the idea is to explore how to maximize the enjoyment in the ongoing learning, and minimize the fear and fatigue.

The Feldenkrais Method allows every physical therapist and assistant to build on the best aspects of their education and training that enhance the effectiveness of patient interaction. If a traditional approach is working with your patient, then don't "fix" it. However, if a patient treatment is not progressing well and the patient is not making progress, that is the time to consider a shift in paradigm. The Feldenkrais Method is a strategy for exploring new and more effective ways to help your patients to achieve maximal functional outcomes in the shortest period of time.

In conclusion, the Feldenkrais Method appears to support the intentions that can be summarized as the general mission of rehabilitation: the actions of the team and of the patients' significant others are designed to promote the self-determination and the maximal functional recovery possible for each patient and help him or her develop the strategies necessary to shape his or her own life.

REFERENCES

1. Feldenkrais M. *Awareness through Movement*. New York, NY: Harper and Row; 1972.
2. Feldenkrais M. *Case of Nora: Body Awareness as Healing Therapy*. New York, NY: Harper and Row; 1977.
3. Feldenkrais M. *Elusive Obvious*. Cupertino, Calif: Meta Publications; 1981.
4. Reed ES. An outline of a theory of action systems. *J Motor Behav.* 1982;14(2):98-134.
5. Bernstein N. *Outline of physiology of movement and physiology of activity* (in Russian). Moscow, Russia: Meditsina; 1966.
6. Luria AR. *The Working Brain*. Harmondsworth: Penguin; 1973.
7. Jackson O. *Natural Ease™ For Work—Can You Move to Get the Job Done?* Rochester, Mich: Physical Therapy Center; 1994.
8. Jackson O. Motivating older adults. In: *Developing Practice in Current Physical Therapy*. Toronto, Ontario: BC Decker; 1988.
9. Jackson O. The Feldenkrais Method: a personalized learning model in contemporary manage-

ment of motor control problems. *Proceedings of the STEP Conference.* Alexandria, Va: Foundation for Physical Therapy; 1991.

10. Murray RB, Huelskoetter MMW. *Psychiatric Mental Health Nursing: Giving Emotional Care.* 2nd ed. Norwalk, Conn: Appleton and Lange; 1987.

11. Rywerant Y. *The Feldenkrais Method-Teaching by Handling.* New Canaan, Conn: Keats Publishing; 1983.

12. Feldenkrais M. *Body and Mature Behavior: A Study of Anxiety, Sex, Gravitation and Learning.* Tel-Aviv, Israel: Alef Ltd; 1980.

13. Pribram KH. *Languages of the Brain: Experimental Paradoxes and Principles in Neuropsychology.* Englewood, NJ: Prentice-Hall; 1971.

14. Jackson O, Gula D, Kreta A, et al. Feldenkrais practitioner training program on motor ability: a videoanalysis. Presented at the American Physical Therapy Association Conference; 1992; Denver, Colorado.

15. Narula M, Jackson O, Kulig K. The effects of a six week Feldenkrais Method on selected functional parameters in a subject with rheumatoid arthritis. Presented at the American Physical Therapy Association Conference; 1992; Denver, Colorado.

16. Ruth S, Kegerreis S. Facilitating cervical flexion using Feldenkrais Method: Awareness Through Movement. *JOSPT.* July 1992;1.

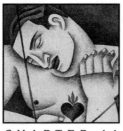

CHAPTER 11

THE TRAGER APPROACH

Adrienne R. Stone, PT

INTRODUCTION

Imagine for a moment that there are no words available for us to use to communicate with our patients. Our language is one of touch. We will communicate tactile feelings with our hands to our patients' tissues. These gestures, offering suggestions and attitudes of softness and freedom of movement, will be picked up through their sensory receptors and interpreted by their minds. This process will require no effort! Concentration, repetition, and refinement are all of extreme importance in this learning. With our most sensitive tools, our hands, our hearts, and our minds, we will feed subtle positive information to our patients to help them relearn what they may have lost along their life path through trauma and illness. At the very least, they will reach a state of profound relaxation which will support their inner healing process.

This process is basic to the understanding of how the *Trager*® Approach accomplishes the things it does. "Every shimmer of the tissue," Dr. Trager has said, "is sending a message to the unconscious mind in the form of a positive feeling experience. It is the accumulation of these positive patterns that can offset the negative patterns to where the positive can take over."[1]

This chapter examines *Trager* Psychophysical Integration, an innovative approach to movement reeducation that has been developed by Milton Trager, MD, over the past 70 years. It is an exciting dimension for us in physical therapy and rehabilitation to explore. This practice, based in feeling not in doing,[1] directs our attention toward reaching the unconscious mind. It is an opportunity to go inside ourselves, not only analytically, but to feel and to find something that will be helpful to our patients. It offers a chance for us to allow our intuition and the sensitive tentacles of our hands to develop their full capacity to feel and to teach, through touch.

GENERAL OVERVIEW

In his work, Dr. Trager stresses the communication of quality feelings to the nervous system. Using a series of gentle, non-invasive movements of joints, muscles, and the entire body, through full available (pain-free) range of motion, this work conveys positive, pleasurable feelings which enter the central nervous system (CNS) and begin to trigger tissue changes by means of many sensory-motor feedback loops between the mind and the muscles. The therapist does not try to fix or change the tissues with his/her hands, but merely feeds the mind with an attitude of how these tissues should feel.[2]

There are several well established neurological routes through which the *Trager* Approach can reach the mind of the patient; and it is these that give us a good, though unproven, physiological model for many of the effects we see in practice. The fluffing, jiggling, lengthening, and shimmering of muscle tissue is communicated to the patient's mind via the type Ia and type II afferent neurons of muscle spindles, resulting in reduction of the tone maintained by the CNS.[3] These neurons are not stimulated to the point that the myotatic reflex is triggered, but subthreshold nerve signals still travel to the CNS. The message created by the manner in which the therapist moves the patient's limbs is carried to the CNS by articular mechanoreceptors.[4] Finally, the rocking of the patient's entire body is sensed by the vestibular mechanism of the inner ear. All of these mechanisms contribute to the message of effortlessness being sent by the therapist.

Additional information that comes out of recent research in the field of psychoneuroimmunology reveals that neuropeptides and their receptors are the biochemical correlates of emotions. They appear to mediate intercellular communication throughout the brain and the body. The limbic system, a key emotional center of the brain, is a central site for neuropeptide action. Theoretically, then, it may be possible for a certain state to affect our immune system in a positive manner.[5,6] This provides a potential mechanism to explain some of the beneficial affects we see in patients treated with the *Trager* Approach.

Beginning at our conception, information is programmed into our vast "computer." Every word, every touch, every thought, from both inner and outer sources, is recorded as patterns in our unconscious. They become part of our being. We have no erase button. The only means we have to change these patterns is to feed in new and improved information. These patterns form the focus of this work. They represent blocks that may have resulted from physical or emotional trauma, disease, or illness. The *Trager* approach provides a safe environment for allowing a release of these holding patterns which have inhibited free movement and have caused a disruption of normal function.[7]

UNIQUE FEATURES OF THE *TRAGER* APPROACH

We are reminded that the word "health" comes from a root that means "whole." "Part of being a healthy person is being well integrated and at peace, with all of the systems acting together."[6]

The system that *Trager* targets is the unconscious mind—the CNS rather than the local tissue. It goes directly to the source of the disturbance.

It is an approach, not a technique. There is the freedom to experience the body in a totally different manner all the time. There is no set recipe, but an attitude about being with the body that can spill over into other treatments and areas of our lives and our patient's lives.

Especially when addressing habitually tight areas, it is the responsibility of the therapist to work even more lightly. Maintaining soft hands is essential. The patient's mind must be reminded of how it feels to be free, moving, and soft. There may be much relearning needed here on the part of the therapist. We have been taught so often to stretch the tightness and massage out the held areas. It is about "not trying" which is the opposite of most of our training as humans. In school and in work we are taught to work hard, do the most we can, push through it. The essence here comes back to "What is nothing?"

The goals of our treatment include: decreased muscular tension, improved body alignment, renewed and greater ease of movement, the experience of total relaxation and peace, and a sense of a functionally integrated body-mind.

DEVELOPMENT OF THE *TRAGER* APPROACH

In a past interview, Dr. Trager cited one of many examples that contributed to his con-clusions regarding his work. He was doing a rotating internship at St. Francis Hospital in Honolulu. His assignment was to do a history and physical exam on a very stiff 75-year-old man who was to have surgery the next day. He was so rigid and tense that in order to turn his head he would have to turn his whole body. During the surgery it became necessary to turn the gentleman to do another small procedure. It took several people to change his position. It wasn't that he was heavy, but he had become extremely limp. Following surgery, Dr. Trager watched the patient while he recovered from the anesthetic. By degrees he slowly came to himself, gradually returning to his original pattern of stiffness. Observing this, he realized that the aging process is not just tissue involvement. The pattern of aging exists more in the unconscious mind than in our tissues. What he witnessed told him that we are the sum total of all the happenings in our lives. He came to the conclusion that one can live in a free, functional manner throughout life. Thus he stated, "I am convinced that for every physical non-yielding condition, there is a psychic counterpart in the uncon-scious mind to the degree of the physical manifestation."[7]

THE *TRAGER* SESSION: COMPONENTS

A session consists of gentle passive movements of the patient while lying on a treat-ment table. The work is subtle and focuses on providing a feeling experience of how it would be to move freely and effortlessly. The table work is often preceded or followed by instruction and practice in a series of active effortless movements called *Mentastics*® Balance, gait, strengthening, etc. may be addressed using Reflex-Response. The effective-ness of all the above is enhanced by working in a state of mindfulness that is central to this approach. This state of mindfulness will be described in the upcoming text.

Each session, viewed not only as a treatment but also a lesson, is modified and adapt-ed to fit the needs of the individual. That is why we call this an *approach* rather than a technique, as there is no set formula. A full session, that may last as long as one to one and a half hours, will often address the entire body. As we have learned, the painful area may not be the most important area on which to focus our work. We must explore the body in order to find from where the holding or compensation is originating. For example, with lower back pain the midthoracic area may be the key region to treat. Patients generally need to be seen less frequently than is traditional in physical therapy. It takes time to inte-

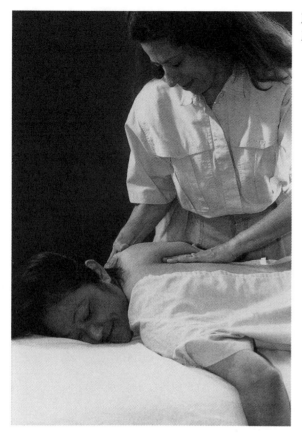

Figure 11-1. *"Going deeply with gentleness."*
Photo by Ninfa Bramble.

grate the information learned in a session. Encouragement is given to the patient to take time following a session to become aware of how he or she feels.

TABLEWORK

Using soft hands, the body of the patient is moved by the therapist, area by area, with curiosity and attention, looking and feeling for involvement of the tissues. (Actually we are looking for holding in the part of the mind that controls the tissue tightness.) We work to bring a feeling of softness and freedom of motion to individual areas and then to unify this feeling throughout the entire body. There is repetition, but each movement is subtly different, with a new message being received by a new mind that is already changed. It is not uncommon for the patient to experience a release of emotions as the tightness softens.

The motions themselves often resemble mobilization techniques with gentle rhythmic oscillations and rocking (Figure 11-1). Traction, elongation, compression, and jiggling of the tissues may be included. The weight of the body is used to help treat itself. For example, to work the lower back, the hips may be set in motion, being softly tossed away by the therapist and allowed to return under their own momentum. Working with the patient's restriction in this noninvasive process is analogous to going up to the door and knocking rather than barging through.

A series of cyclic responses then occurs. As the patients relax, their bodies begin to allow increased movement. A sense of trust is established with the experience of this non-threatening partnership. As trust grows, the subjects are able to allow themselves fuller and greater relaxation, thus allowing greater passive movement of their bodies. And then there will be a breath, a sigh, or some shift, and the tissue will change. A new quality of aliveness and softness will come in. Some surrendering has occurred; the mind has been reached; habitually held patterns are released; and nourishment is provided for healing from within.

Although taking a passive role on the treatment table, it should be noted that the patient is fully responsible for how much their bodies will move and relax. As Dr. Trager has been known to say: "I didn't make it soft, he did. He is the therapist, I am an instigator." The subject picks up the feeling from the therapist.

The benefits of multiple sessions are cumulative. The patient's feeling of profound relaxation is an experience available for him/her to retrieve at a later time. This phenomenon of recall is an extremely valuable benefit. It is enhanced with *Mentastics*.

MENTASTICS MOVEMENTS

Mentastics, a coined word meaning "mental gymnastics," is a very significant component of the *Trager* Approach. This system of active movements is designed to reinforce and enhance the feeling of relaxation, lightness, flexibility, and free flowing movement. This empowering system can be used as an independent modality or as a follow up program to the table work. Resembling, but differing from exercise, these movements are not designed to stretch or strengthen, but to teach people how to release tension from their bodies. All movements are performed in a comfortable range of motion, without effort. Emphasis is on *mindfulness* while moving, with particular attention to any feedback the body may be giving. For instance, pain, tightness, or fatigue would be signals to do less movement, to become lighter, to move with less intensity. *The lesson is in how to feel movement in a manner that is correct for that body*, thus increasing body awareness. The individual experiences how to move in a comfortable free fashion, even though initially it may be through a minimal range. Employing the weight of the body, a person is instructed to initiate a movement and then "let go." This release and allowing the weight of the body part to carry the motion to completion with mindfulness helps separate *Mentastics* movements from exercise. Refinement and deepening of the motions is encouraged by asking "What is lighter

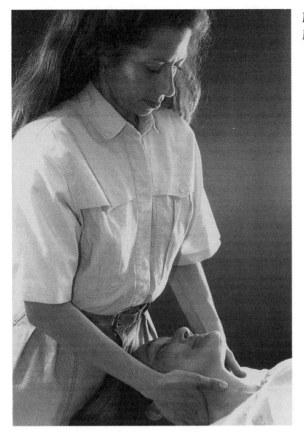

Figure 11-2. *"Hook-up." Photo by Ninfa Bramble.*

than that?" and " What is half of that?" The subject uses the previous repetition as a reference point going for half the amount of effort used on the previous repetition. It is by producing a fine quality movement that we cause the mind to pay attention. Implemented following any task, exercise, static position, etc, *Mentastics* can work for us to release tension on an ongoing basis. Because these gentle movements are done in a comfortable range, feel good, are effective, and are readily available, people are more likely to do them.

HOOK-UP

Mindfulness, an intrinsic component of the *Trager* Approach, is the high level of conscious awareness and focus that the therapist assumes while working. This almost meditative state of alertness, sensitivity, and nonjudgement allows a clear open connection between the therapist and the patient (Figure 11-2). Working in this state, which Dr. Trager calls "hook-up," truly separates this work from other treatments. The session may begin with a moment as simple as the therapist taking a deep breath and becoming totally present in the room with the patient. It is our role as therapist to help bring the patient into this state of being with us. The greater the development of the therapist the better able he/she will be to give a deeper, more integrated treatment.[7] It is through this process that our basic connection with the self, that is so often lost in sickness and disease, can be restored. According to Dr. Trager, without this, the healing process is nearly impossible.

Dr. Trager discusses the essential theory of his approach:

> The success I have had with low back pain is not because the tissues in the lumbo-sacral area were manipulated in a special way. It has come because I have succeeded in reaching the psycho-physiological components. I never tell my hands what to do. I hook up, and I go. My job is to impart to my patient what it is like to be right in the sense of a functionally integrated body-mind. This is transmitted, I feel, through the autonomic nervous system from the therapist's mind, through his hands, to the involved area. This feeling is picked up in the patient's mind because of the manner in which the tissues are worked, creating the feeling of relaxation. In this way, the sensory feedback which maintains the psychic component of muscle spasm is broken. Until this feeling reaches the patient, no lasting results can be expected. It is the manner in which I work, not necessarily the technique that I use, which brings about the change. Every move, every pressure of my hands, every thought, is directed towards bringing new feeling experiences to the unconscious mind of how the affected area should feel. The holding pattern is then broken.[7]

It is the beginning of the shift into a new direction that will continue long after the session.

REFLEX RESPONSE

There is an integral aspect of the *Trager* Approach known as Reflex-Response. In this most sensitive and facilitative aspect of the work, weakness and paralysis are the focus.[8] Reflex-Response aims to induce spontaneous movement where possible and then move to strengthen those sensorimotor pathways. Its additional goals include improved active selective movement, endurance, and balance. Using subtlety of touch and the facilitation of awareness, this portion of the work usually will require active participation from the patient. It is based on the same concept of using the patient's tissues to reach his or her mind.

INCLUSION OF THE *TRAGER* APPROACH INTO PHYSICAL THERAPY PROGRAMS

Although few clinical studies have yet been published, systematic recordings of clinical experience has shown a surprisingly broad applicability of the *Trager* Approach in patients seen by physical therapists. Perhaps the reason for this, as previously mentioned, is the fact that *it is an approach, not a technique*. This approach allows for its effectiveness in a wide variety of situations because it responds to imbalances throughout the body. The following is a discussion taken from reports of the author and colleagues using the *Trager* Approach effectively in patients with varied complaints.

With elderly people, especially those who are frail, the non-intrusiveness and gentleness make *Trager* an effective approach. When verbalization doesn't work and communication is impaired, sensory messages through touch may be all we have to gain their trust. Without that established first, helping them to perform a desired functional task is difficult. Thus, using this approach can improve the quality and functional level of their lives.

In patients with painful joints, such as with rheumatoid and osteoarthritis,[9] and in a variety of patients with myofascial pain syndromes, the lightness of this work reduces the tightness and tension of the joints and surrounding musculature. The relaxation, in combination with significantly reduced pain levels, increases mobility and function. It would be contraindicated, however, in severe flare-ups. The use of a home *Mentastics* program is extremely beneficial.

During pregnancy, at a time when many medications and treatments should be avoided, using the *Trager* Approach for pain and stiffness has been effective, especially in the last trimester. Shorter and more comfortable labor and delivery have been reported. If back pain is present, modified sidelying table work has been most effective.

With chronic lung problems, the *Trager* Approach has been shown to be effective in improving chest wall mobility. This has been exhibited in a study where vital capacity and chest expansion were significantly increased in patients with chronic obstructive lung disease.[10]

In patients with scoliosis and kyphoscoliosis, this work has been helpful in redeveloping muscle balance. The increased sense of body awareness that is established allows old postural habits to come into consciousness, thus providing room for change. Life style habits related to sitting, carrying, etc, can be relearned for improved symmetry. This, combined with a regular program of *Mentastics* movements and exercise, has been successful.

Postoperatively, following procedures such as mastectomies, bunionectomies, shoulder and knee surgeries, and back surgeries, the *Trager* Approach has been helpful in restoring movement and decreasing compensatory actions of the body. Often this type of treatment will be initiated 6 to 8 weeks following surgery. Under physician orders, treatments have been initiated as early as the first postoperative week. The relaxation, restoration of mobility, and decrease in pain levels were remarkable, especially in cases where immobilization has occurred.

When there have been soft tissue injuries, particularly to the neck and back, prompt initiation of treatment with this approach can help defer onset of some holding patterns. In chronic spinal pain, benefits also have been derived.[11]

In patients diagnosed with frozen shoulders, breaking up the cyclic guarding patterns that have contributed to furthering the deficit is essential. As an adjunct to other techniques, incorporating the *Trager* Approach has been effective in making the treatment process more comfortable with faster restoration of range of motion and function.

Trager Mentastics classes have been successfully implemented in the hospital setting in a variety of areas, including: an outpatient pulmonary rehabilitation program, a structured outpatient pain management program, and an inpatient chemical dependency program. In all of these instances, these classes were created to complement an already established program.[12]

There also is an appropriateness of this approach to patients with neurologic pathology including stroke, Parkinson's disease, spinal cord injuries, multiple sclerosis,[13] cerebral palsy,[14] and others. The softening of spasticity and the decreasing of rigidity, combined with awareness of movement as a feeling experience, have facilitated many patients' recoveries. Bringing in the Reflex-Response work here is of great benefit, especially when flaccidity, weak motor connections, or balance are problems.

Finally, this work benefits the generally "healthy" population. It is indicated for those who want to learn to relax, improve posture, prevent pain, reduce tension, or move with greater ease. Athletes have found the *Trager* Approach to offer ways to optimize mental and physical performance.[15] The demand on physical therapists in the future will be to provide services for healthy people who want to remain healthy. This approach will satisfy that demand.

Implemented as an accepted procedure in the physical therapy department of a private hospital, the *Trager* Approach has been used effectively in the outpatient and inpatient departments as both a primary therapy and a complementary therapy in many of the situations listed above. It often provided an alternative positive therapeutic choice when all else had been exhausted.[12] Physician education and successful outcomes resulted in strong support and an active referral base.

CASE EXAMPLE

A 52-year-old female was referred for physical therapy treatment by her rheumatologist with diagnoses of myofascial pain syndrome and low back pain. Prior medical history included: (a) gall bladder surgery 4 years prior, complicated with a 1-month hospitalization for peritonitis, and (b) a fall in the shower, 1 year prior to treatment, hitting her right hip, with progressive difficulty moving since then. She was employed full time as a legal secretary and was barely managing to work and take care of herself, leaving little or no energy for social activities.

Her chief complaints included: generalized stiffness, right hip pain (constant 7/10-8/10) (0=no pain; 10=maximum pain); her abdomen was very sensitive to touch. (She reported being reluctant to touch that area since her surgery.) Functionally, she was unable to do anything physical without becoming exhausted. Walking was limited to one block; lifting, reaching, squatting, and getting up from the floor and out of the car were all difficult. The patient reported a weight gain of 50 pounds over the past few years. She appeared depressed and frustrated about her limited abilities and constant pain. During her evaluation she was also found to have weak abdominals, tightness in her hamstrings and hip flexors, and extreme density and hardness of her right lower extremity. Her posture exhibited a sunken attitude with forward shoulders and head, and an exaggerated lumbar lordosis.

She was seen for ten visits over a 6-week period. The initial visit, including evaluation, was one and a half hours; each additional treatment was an hour. Treatments consisted of *Trager* tablework, including Reflex-Response, with an extensive *Mentastics* and exercise program and instructions in proper body mechanics. Suggestions were given to make her work space more ergonomically correct.

The *Mentastics* she was given included a series of movements performed in different positions.

Lying Supine:

1. bilateral bent knee drops (using pillows as needed for shock absorption)
2. with legs extended (pillow under knees) hip hiking alternately (playfully)
3. legs extended (pillow under knees), create a gentle "waggle" of the hips rolling from internal to external rotation, repetitively
4. pelvic rocking (tilting pelvis posteriorly allowing gravity to return the pelvis to neutral)

Standing:

5. subtle weight shifting (focus on feeling the bottoms of the feet)
6. rapidly shifting weight to create "butt wags" (elbows bent into sides)
7. leg toss out from the back of the hip joint (mule kick)
8. foot rattle (as though repetitively attempting to remove a strapless sandal)
9. rib cage lift (arms overhead, hands clasped, upper trapezius relaxed, using the breath)

Walking:

10. walking kick at the end of swing phase (employing the weight of the leg)

Her exercises, which were introduced gradually after the second week of treatment, included pelvic tilts, abdominal strengthening, double and single knee to chest exercises, and stretches. Later additional exercises were added: moslem prayer, cat-camel, straight leg raising, protected hamstring stretch, and a hip flexor stretch.

The table work she received consisted of movements directed at traction, rotation, softening, compression, and elongation in a *Trager* manner. Work was done first on the legs and back. The entire body was then addressed in other sessions due to the compensations that had developed from so many years of pain.

By the third week of treatment the patient began to report positive changes. Pain levels gradually dropped to intermittent and eventually to less than 2/10 to 3/10. The patient reported an increased sense of body awareness and integration with less fatigue. Abdominal sensitivity was less with reports of feeling more aliveness in that area. (Note: During the third to last session she verbalized during the table work that she had been abused sexually as a child and that at age eight she had been squeezed very hard, resulting in back pain. She stated that the treatments have helped her become aware of how she has been holding her body in protection. She is beginning to recognize and is starting to let go of the protection as she realizes that she doesn't need it anymore.) The patient expressed that her spine felt like a part of her rather than something tight in her back. One Monday she reported that in church she went to genuflect spontaneously, without a problem, something she had avoided for four years. The right lower extremity showed tissue change, with softening, decreased tightness and more aliveness. The patient was able to carry herself more upright with stronger abdominals and improved sense of well-being. She was able to walk several blocks and was excited about the potential of keeping up with her friends.

This report demonstrates a case in which the *Trager* Approach has been used as an effective basis for treatment. Incorporating the *Trager* Approach into our professional tool box is valuable for increasing our own sensitivity, awareness, and ability to focus on the responses and needs of our patients. This artful ability, in combination with our other scientific skills and knowledge, can support our patients in the direction of optimal health with improved function and quality of life.

BENEFITS FOR THE PRACTITIONER

There are benefits to the therapist that include the development of the capacity to feel tissue and see structural relationships change, recognize the difference between normal and pathological states, and develop the ability to begin corrective procedures.[7] Training in this approach teaches us to become mindful, aware of the presence of and to assess unconscious holding patterns. The identification of these patterns, which are palpable manifestations of the mind-body connection, is extremely helpful in providing effective treatment. The gentle rocking motion serves as a constant test of range of motion. The therapist experiences directly the limits of the body. And, as the tension and pain avoidance patterns of the patient disappear, the therapist gets instant feedback on the progress.[16] *Mentastics* can be used for personal health and well-being, especially while working. As therapists, we can learn to maintain a more comfortable body for ourselves and be a role model to our patients.

Both giving and receiving sessions in this work provide an opportunity for our own development. With each new patient, with each moment of treatment, with every movement of our hands on the patient's body, and with each thought, we have a chance to develop as a clinician and as a person. You can only give what you truly have developed for yourself.[7] It is an endlessly rewarding learning process. Once trained in the *Trager* Approach, it is unlikely that one will ever touch a body in the same manner again.

REFERENCES

1. Juhan D. *The Physiology of Hook-Up: How Trager Works.* Mill Valley, Calif: The Trager Institute, 1992/1993.

2. Juhan D. The Trager approach. *The Bodywork Book.* Sherborne, Dorset, England: Prism Alpha; 1984:34-47.

3. Guyton AC. *Textbook of Medical Physiology.* 8th ed. Philadelphia, Pa: W.B. Saunders Company; 1991:591-593.

4. Wyke B. The neurology of joints. *Annals of the Royal College of Surgeons of England.* 1967;4:25.

5. Cousins N. *Head First: The Biology of Hope.* New York, NY: E.P. Dutton;1989:75,276.

6. Moyers B. *Healing and the Mind.* New York, NY: Doubleday; 1993:177-193.

7. Trager M. Psychophysical integration and mentastics. *Trager Journal.* 1982;1(1):3-6.

8. Molatore T, English J. Trager applied to muscular dystrophy. *The Trager Journal.* Fall 1982;1:4.

9. Savage FL. *Osteoarthritis: A Step-by Step Success Story to Show Others They Can Help Themselves.* Barrytown, NY: Station Hill Press; 1988.

10. Witt P. Trager psychophysical integration: a method to improve chest mobility of patients with chronic lung disease. *Phys Ther.* 1986;66:214-217.

11. Witt P. An additional tool in the treatment of chronic spinal pain and dysfunction. *Whirlpool.* Summer 1986:24-26.

12. Stone AR. *The Trager Approach: An Introduction.* Presented at the World Congress of Physical Therapy; 1987.

13. Juhan D. *Multiple Sclerosis: The Trager Approach.* Mill Valley, Calif: The Trager Institute; 1993.

14. Witt P, Parr C. Effectiveness of Trager psychophysical integration in promoting trunk mobility

in a child with cerebral palsy: a case report. *Physical and Occupational Therapy Pediatrics.* 1988;8(4):75-94.

15. Butler M. The Trager Athlete. *The Trager Journal.* 1987:2:6-8.

16. Watrous I. The Trager approach: an effective tool for physical therapy. *Physical Therapy Forum.* April 1992;22-25.

SUGGESTED READINGS

Juhan D. *Job's Body*. Barrytown, NY: Station Hill Press; 1987.

Liskin J. *Moving Medicine: The Life and Work of Milton Trager, MD*. Barrytown, NY: Station Hill Press; 1995.

Trager M, Guadagno C. *Trager Mentastics: Movement as a Way to Agelessness*. Barrytown, NY: Station Hill Press; 1987.

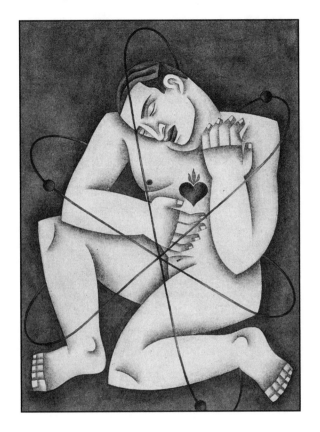

TRADITIONAL
CHINESE MEDICINE

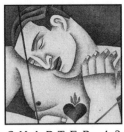

CHAPTER 12

ACUPUNCTURE IN THE PHYSICAL THERAPY CLINIC

Karen Gordon, PT, AP

INTRODUCTION

People often ask why, as a physical therapist, I chose to pursue the study of acupuncture. It was an evolutionary step in professional practice that grew out of observation, which is, as will soon be explained, an inherent aspect of Traditional Chinese Medicine (TCM). My experience of 10 years as a clinician was as an orthopedic manual physical therapist and many of my patients were in chronic pain. As most therapists know, many people with injuries get better on their own without any intervention whatsoever. Of the others, some improve with intervention and some do not. Those who do not often develop chronic pain. Unfortunately, many patients become labeled by their doctors and therapists as "supratentorial" when their symptoms and complaints do not correlate with Western Medicine's neurologic/anatomic/mechanical model. In other words, if the pain or dysfunction does not follow a specific nerve or nerve root pathway, myotome, or dermatome, then "it's all in their head." When we say this, we invalidate the experience of the patient, and I always wondered if there weren't perhaps another model that might better explain the physiologic condition of these patients. Describing two of these histories will help make my point.

CASE EXAMPLE 1— MRS. WHITE

A 53-year-old woman in basically good health was referred to physical therapy with a relatively mild case of Reflex Sympathetic Dystrophy (RSD) of her left arm. She was emotionally distraught, "not herself," and "nothing helped," (as is common with RSD). Finally, electrical stimulation was applied to the affected limb with a neuroprobe to various reactive acupuncture points and her description of her symptoms began to change. She stated that when she went home, her arm began to twitch involuntarily and that she was feeling some relief for the first time. She received another treatment and returned to say that, during the weekend, her arm twitched some more and that she experienced an emotional catharsis of some sort, crying and grieving over something she recognized she had long forgotten. As a result, she said she was feeling significantly better. By the end of the week, she also happily announced that in addition to continuous improvement in her arm, she was no longer constipated, which had been a problem for her for years. This patient's report of the effect of her neuroprobe treatment on acupuncture points illustrates the observation that an acupuncture treatment affects the entire body, not just one system.

CASE EXAMPLE 2 — MR. GREEN

A 48-year-old man complained of severe unremitting pain from his right buttock and hip, along the lateral side of his right leg, and down the lateral compartment of his right calf and foot. He also reported severe lateral headaches, insomnia, tinnitus, indigestion, and belching. He was very angry that "no one seemed to believe him," because all of his neurological tests were normal and that there was "nothing wrong with him." He also complained of a foul body odor that he couldn't seem to get rid of no matter how much he showered, and a bitter taste in his mouth. All previous therapeutic interventions had been without benefit, but when the neuroprobe was used, he was amazed that it picked up hypersensitivity on acupuncture points that correlated exactly along the distribution of pain. This validated his symptoms and he seemed relieved. He said, "At least I'm not crazy—at least this shows something is going on here even if we don't know what it is." Daily treatment with the neuroprobe gave him some, albeit temporary, relief.

Both of these patients had a condition known in Traditional Chinese Medicine as a "painful 'bi' syndrome," or painful blockage. Mrs. White was affected along the lung and large intestine meridian of her left upper extremity and Mr. Green along the gall bladder meridian of his right lower extremity. The significance of this will become more apparent as you read on.

WHAT IS ACUPUNCTURE?

Acupuncture is the insertion of slender, fine, sterile needles into specific anatomical locations at specific angles and depths in order to influence the flow of Qi (pronounced "chi") or a vital force in the body, thereby assisting the body to self-regulate or adjust, promoting circulation and healing and reducing pain. Archaeological findings suggest the possibility that the early roots of acupuncture go as far back as the primitive Stone Age clan society in ancient China, where people used sharpened stones for such medical purposes as minor surgical procedures, blood letting, and regulating Qi circulation. Over the centuries, as Chinese thought and philosophy evolved, so did the medical science of acupuncture. By 500 B.C., metal needles replaced stone instruments, and early written material appeared as physicians began to document their observations and generate early theoretical material. Korea, Japan, and other Asian countries began to embrace acupuncture as a medical treatment (system) as early as the 6th century, but it was not introduced in Europe until the 16th century and not to the United States until shortly after President Nixon visited China in 1971.[1] The impact that the practice of acupuncture will have on the way that Western medicine is practiced is yet to be seen, especially in the realm of prevention.

Acupuncture itself is only a small part of the practice of TCM. The body of knowledge of Traditional Chinese Medicine is complete in its own right regarding such theories as causes of disease, nutrition and lifestyle, diagnosis of symptoms, and the therapeutic effect of herbal medications.

A major difference between Western medicine and TCM is that the Chinese view the human body as an integral part of nature, which, indeed, it is. Many of the traditional clinical medicine diagnoses include such terms as dampness, heat, cold, or wind, and sound somewhat like a weather report of the body's environment. However, it would be an error to think that this approach to understanding the human body is primitive, simplistic, or unsophisticated. One of the main reasons that there is a dearth of scientific research in a Western context is because we have not yet developed the technology sophisticated enough to measure the presence of "Qi," or the effects of blockage in the normal healthy flow of Qi throughout the body along the meridian pathways. No Western medical structure exists that replicates the meridians, and to Western researchers, meridians cannot exist, since they cannot be seen or measured by traditional scientific methods.

RIVERS OF QI

Qi, for which there is no correlate in Western science at this time, is the fundamental basis of TCM and indeed, in Chinese conceptualization, the fundamental basis of the entire universe. It can best be described as the life force or vital energy of an organism. If the quantity and quality of blood and Qi are good, and the blood and Qi are flowing smoothly and freely throughout the body, one enjoys good health. For example, if one were to compare a bowl of fresh picked green beans from a garden and a bowl of the same variety of green beans from a can, a chemist might analyze both and conclude that they are the same in components. However, if offered one or the other, your choice would be clear; most likely, those fresh from the garden would be more appealing. A plant, being a living entity, also contains Qi and, unlike the processed or canned vegetables, the fresh-picked beans still contain Qi or vitality, which when eaten, we take into our bodies along with the nutrients of the bean, and it is transferred into new cells and into energy within us.

SOURCE OF QI

There are two sources of Qi in the human body—prenatal and postnatal.[1-3] Prenatal Qi is acquired from both parents and is indeed the foundation of our constitutional or genetic make-up. One cannot later add to the quantity or quality of his or her own prenatal Qi. After birth, we are dependent upon postnatal Qi to build cells and new tissue and for energy expenditure. Postnatal Qi is derived from the food we eat, the water we drink, and the air we breathe. Choices can be made here regarding the quality and quantity of food, water and air that we take in, and our choices will influence the quality of the Qi in the body and our general vitality. We are accustomed to thinking this way about natural vitamins and minerals, but Qi forms the energy inherent in both. Acupuncture meridians or channels are energy pathways in the body through which Qi flows.

Western scientists have not been able to find specific anatomical structures such as blood vessels or nerves that correlated with meridian channels, because there are none: they are *energetic* pathways that the Chinese have mapped out which flow through the fascia or connective tissue. To help the Western mind to understand this, it is helpful to visualize an air travel route from New York to Paris. This documented route on charts is real and exists; however, one can search the world over, test and examine, and not find any representation in nature that is tangible, thereby causing some to believe it could not exist. Matsumoto and Birch offer a fascinating and detailed presentation of the fascial system including embryologic, bioelectric, and magnetic field theories which explain the anatomy and physiology of meridians in Western terms.[4]

Traditional Chinese Medicine charts 20 pathways: 12 regular meridians (also called channels or vessels), which correlate to and connect with an organ of the body; eight extra meridians, six of which share points with the 12 regular vessels, and two run along the anterior midline and posterior midline of the body. In addition to these 20 major pathways, there are smaller connecting pathways internally and even smaller capillary-like pathways that distribute the Qi to all of the cells and tissues of the body.

Acupuncture points have been demonstrated to be areas of reduced electrical resistance on the surface of the skin.[4] They are in specific anatomical locations on the body and may be compared to subway stations on the surface through which access may be gained (by needles) into the subway line or channel. All acupuncture points are categorized and have specific functions, such as regulating, tonifying, or moving Qi; balancing Yin and Yang; clearing heat; influencing the blood; relieving pain; and balancing, harmonizing, and promoting optimum function of the organs. Point selection is based on the diagnosis according to TCM theory. The acupuncturist is adept at knowing the exact location of each point, the appropriate needling technique, depth and angle for each point, and the therapeutic indication for each point or combination of points.

DIAGNOSTIC METHODS IN TRADITIONAL CHINESE MEDICINE

In modern Western medicine, diagnostics weigh heavily upon technology, such as results of lab tests or radiology, that are designed to examine cells, tissues, or more gross anatomical structures for evidence of disease or pathology. A patient may have various health complaints, receive the appropriate examinations, but find that all the tests were negative, reporting a "clean bill of health." This leaves the patient wondering why he or she doesn't fell well, and still experiences headaches, constipation, insomnia, or palpitations.

TCM includes diagnostic methods that can detect a disharmony at the energetic level, or at the functional level, before it progresses to an organic disease, and also has models for the pathogenesis and treatment of health problems at what are termed the subtle energetic and functional stages. The Four Examinations used by the acupuncture physician are Inspection, Inquiring, Palpation, and Auscultation/Olfaction, or more simply, Looking, Asking, Feeling, and Hearing/Smelling. The physician first observes the patient's function, in addition to posture and gait, but the acupuncture physician observes the complexion, overall vitality, and especially the tongue, observing every detail. To the Chinese physician, the tongue is a map of the body's interior condition and is evaluated by color, coat, shape, moisture or dryness, vitality, and marks or spots. The tongue changes daily to reflect the health status of the patient and provides a wealth of information to the physician. In a healthy patient it should be a strong pink color with a thin, white, even, moist coat[1-3,5-7] (Figure 12-1).

Next, the acupuncture physician conducts a thorough health history interview and gains a wealth of information by inquiring about the bodily functions, such as if the patient tends to feel hot or cold; perspires; has headaches or dizziness; how he or she would describe specific aspects of pain such as location and nature; presence of thirst, appetite, and cravings; sleep patterns; bowel and bladder function; and in women, gynecological functions. These must be answered specifically and in great detail and an answer of "normal" is not sufficient. A patient may believe that having a bowel movement every 2-3 days is normal because that was what he or she has grown accustomed to, or a woman may think that menstrual cramps are normal because she's always had them and so does everyone she knows. However, in the TCM model of health, these conditions are not only not normal, they are not acceptable.

Auscultation and olfaction include listening to various aspects of the patient's voice such as strength or pitch, or if a cough is present, various aspects of the cough. Body odor (not perspiration odor) is a more subtle observation and may be classified according to the five elements and correlated with various organs. Some terms used to describe these odors are burnt, sweet, rancid, rank, and putrid. Odors of the breath and of secretions and excretions also provide a great deal of information regarding the interior landscape of the patient.

PULSE DIAGNOSIS—TCM

The most important aspect of palpation in TCM is a very sophisticated science of pulse diagnosis. In Western medicine, the pulse is usually evaluated for rate, regularity, and overall quality. In TCM, there are 28 designations evaluating the patient based on pulse rate, depth, strength, shape, regularity, fullness or emptiness, and width.[1-3] The acupuncturist uses three fingers on both wrists of the patient at the position of the radial pulse to

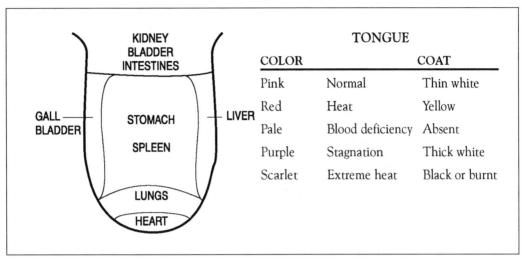

Figure 12-1. *Areas of the tongue for tongue diagnosis.*

evaluate the pulse in six different positions, each of which reflects the relative energy and condition of a different organ. The most distal pulse at the crease of the left wrist reflects the heart, the middle position of the wrist reflects the liver, and the most proximal, the lung aspect of the kidney. On the right wrist, the most distal pulse indicates information about the lungs, the middle position the spleen, and the most proximal, the Yang aspect of the kidneys. A few characteristics of the pulse are: superficial, deep, rapid, slow, thin, wide, empty, full, overflowing, slippery, wiry, choppy, and intermittent. Each characteristic gives a very specific description and interpretation.

Other diagnostic skills using palpation are similar to skills used by physical therapists, such as assessing tissue, muscle tone, and heat/cold sensation, but in TCM, these characteristics are interpreted not only according to anatomical structures such as muscles, tendons, and joints, but also according to distribution of acupuncture meridians and tenderness at specific acupuncture points. It also is important to the acupuncturist if a specific area is better or worse with pressure, or with application of heat or cold, to determine the pattern of disharmony and to formulate treatment strategy.

YIN & YANG

Another concept that is fundamental to the Chinese world view and TCM is the concept of Yin & Yang, which is summarized in Figure 12-2.[1,3,8] Yin and Yang represent the opposites occurring in natural phenomena. Anything can be differentiated and further dif-

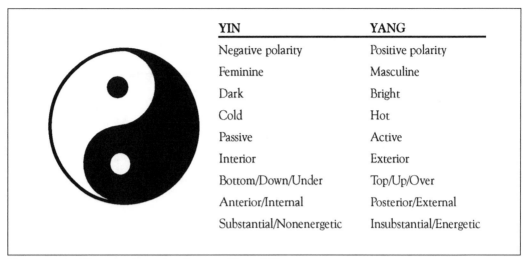

YIN	YANG
Negative polarity	Positive polarity
Feminine	Masculine
Dark	Bright
Cold	Hot
Passive	Active
Interior	Exterior
Bottom/Down/Under	Top/Up/Over
Anterior/Internal	Posterior/External
Substantial/Nonenergetic	Insubstantial/Energetic

Figure 12-2. The interrelationships between Yin and Yang.

ferentiated based on this model, but only in relation to something else. More specifically, the Western mind usually wants to know if something is black or white, good or bad, and tends to be absolute and rigid. Is it this or that? The Chinese however, would say there is no correct answer to an incorrect question and to ask if anything is Yin or Yang is only valid if asked in the sense of Yin or Yang relative to something else.

For example, "Is the abdomen Yin or Yang?" is not a complete question, as it is Yin in relation to the chest above, Yang in relation to the pelvis below, Yin in relation to the back because it is on the anterior surface, and Yang in relation to the organs because they are internal.

The principals of Yin and Yang are:

1. Everything can be differentiated into relative Yin or Yang and further differentiated into Yin and Yang.
2. Yin and Yang mutually control and support each other.
3. Yin and Yang transform into and create each other (night to day, summer to winter).

Applied to TCM, the acupuncturist assesses the dynamic ever-changing balance and harmony of various Yin and Yang aspects of the body. For example, a patient presenting with red eyes, headaches, flushed face, bad temper, insomnia, and palpitations may be exhibiting excessive Yang energy (the above symptoms being heat signs, and heat or Yang energy tends to rise and go up to the head, causing disturbance), and a relative deficiency of Yin (cooling, moistening energy that would control overactive Yang). A patient who is cold, fatigued, and edematous with a slow pulse may be Yang deficient with a relative excess of Yin (cold, edema, excess fluids) and needs warming and tonification of Yang energy to harmonize the condition.

FIVE ELEMENTS AND THE ORGANS

Another concept fundamental to the Chinese world view and thereby applied in TCM is the concept of the Five Elements; Wood, Fire, Earth, Metal, and Water. Each have specific characteristics, attributes, and associations, and anything being evaluated can be classified according to the Five Elements, including behaviors and personality types as well as organs of the body. Table 12-1 provides a sample of some of the associations of the Five Elements.

Notice from the chart that the organs are classified as Yin or Yang and then associated with one of the Five Elements. The solid vital organs are Yin and the hollow organs or bowels are Yang. Organs in TCM not only represent anatomical structures as in Western Medicine, but also represent an entirely different, ingenious model of functions and energetic inter-relationships. This model illustrates how the physiology of the body is governed, and it thereby serves as the foundation of assessing where an energetic disharmony lies, providing the physician with a strategy for treatment to restore harmony and function.

Figure 12-3 illustrates the energetic relationship of the organs according to the Five Elements. There are two co-existing normal cycles: the nurturing, promoting or supporting cycle indicated by the arrows outside the figure, and the control cycle, indicated by the arrows inside the figures. Fire promotes or warms the Earth, Earth promotes Metal (as in mining), Metal promotes Water, Water fosters Wood (as in watering plants), and Wood feeds the Fire. Simultaneously, in this system of checks and balances, Fire controls Metal (can melt Metal), Metal can control Wood (chopping with an ax), Wood controls the Earth (as in conservation, planting on a hillside holds back the soil from landslide and erosion), Earth controls Water (using sandbags in a flood), and Water controls Fire.

A disruption or imbalance in the energy flow in either the nurturing or the control cycle manifests potential health problems.

How does this manifest in the clinical situation? Mr. Green, the patient described earlier, also presented with additional symptoms of red eyes with migraine headaches and insomnia, and had a very wiry, rapid pulse. His tongue was red and dry. Pieces of the puzzle began to fit together for the acupuncturist because:

1. Pain is distributed along the gall bladder channel (Wood element).
2. Wiry pulse indicates liver problems; rapid pulse indicates heat.
3. The bitter taste (usually associated with bile and the gall bladder, but also in TCM is associated with Fire element, the heart).
4. Red eyes (eyes associate with liver, red indicating heat).
5. Lateral headaches indicating liver Yang (heat) rising (as heat rises) to the head.
6. Insomnia indicating that the heart is disturbed by all of this, as one of the func-

TABLE 12-1. THE FIVE ELEMENTS.					
	Fire	Earth	Metal	Water	Wood
Yin Organ	Heart	Spleen	Lung	Kidney	Liver
Yang Organ	Small Intestine	Stomach	Large Intestines	Urinary Bladder	Gall Bladder
Color	Red	Yellow	White	Blue/Black	Green
Emotion	Joy/ Excitement	Worry Anxiety	Sadness Grief	Fear	Anger
Sound	Laughing	Singing	Crying	Groaning	Shouting
Sensory/Organs	Tongue	Lips	Nose	Ears	Eyes
Tissue	Blood Vessels	Muscles/ Flesh	Skin & Body hair	Bones/ Head hair	Nails/Tendons Sinews
Climate	Hot	Damp	Dry	Cold	Windy
Taste	Bitter	Sweet	Pungent	Salty	Sour
Season	Summer	Late Summer	Autumn	Winter	Spring

tions of the heart is to store the Shen or mind at night so that one may have peaceful sleep.

The acupuncturist's goal is to restore harmony to this disharmonious situation. The Liver or Wood element is in an Excess or Replete condition and is affecting or over-feeding the Fire (Heart) causing a disturbance. Other examples of disharmonies that may occur if, for example, Wood is in Excess, would be Wood draining Water, affecting the kidneys, which in turn fail to control the Fire, or Wood invades the Earth, which would result in digestive problems. By using specific acupuncture points to clear heat and calm the liver, calm the heart, and nourish the kidneys, the harmony of the natural cycles would be restored and the symptoms resolved.

PATHOGENESIS

How does all of this happen? What are the causes of disease in the TCM model? Autopsies were not performed and neither microscopes nor microbes were yet discovered when Acupuncture first developed. The causes of disease are very natural and not at all mysterious. They are either internal (emotions), external ("pernicious influences"), or

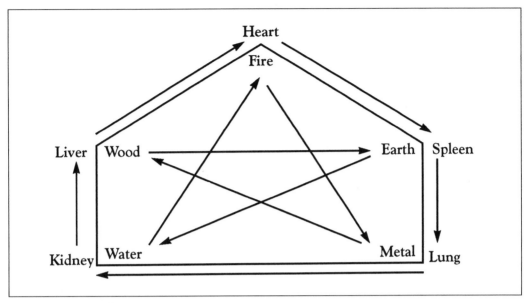

Figure 12-3. Five element associations.

"other," for example, lifestyle, trauma, nosocomial infection, congenital weakness.

EMOTIONAL FACTORS (INTERNAL)

Any given organ may be injured by the long-term negative emotion associated with its element (see Table 12-1). Conversely, if an organ is diseased, it may produce an emotional imbalance in the patient. An example of this has been observed in Western Medicine many times. When a lifelong partner dies, the surviving spouse often dies soon after. Quite often, the surviving spouse dies from pneumonia, affecting the lungs, which are associated in TCM with sadness and grieving. Mr. Green, our example of Wood in disharmony, often expressed how angry he was, especially at his employer, and that he was angry about his working conditions long before the injury.

ENVIRONMENTAL FACTORS (EXTERNAL)

The six Pernicious or Evil influences include the climate or weather conditions that affect the body and cause disease: wind, cold, damp, dryness, fire (or heat), and summer heat, a combination of heat with dampness that is common in late summer. The theory states that if an individual's resistance is weak and he or she is overexposed to any of these conditions, disease results. For example, Bell's Palsy, a paralysis of cranial nerve seven or the facial nerve, is seen as a wind cold invasion of the channels of the face, blocking the flow of Qi to those muscles. Acupuncture points are selected to clear and diminish cold and wind from the face, thus resolving the symptoms.

"OTHER" FACTORS

Of course trauma is neither directly due to emotion or to weather conditions and may cause health problems. But most important in this category of environment is lifestyle; including diet and nutrition, sleep, exercise, overwork or over-exertion, or over-indulgence in sexual activity. There are many suggested guidelines in TCM that, when observed and practiced, significantly influence health and are preventative in nature. For example, too many pregnancies and returning to work too soon after childbirth presents many health risks for a woman, as it depletes her stores of Qi and blood. Too much sexual activity also depletes a person's energetic stores and predisposes him or her to various ailments. Dietary recommendations such as avoiding alcohol, greasy or fried foods, sugar and dairy, spicy or cold foods, and raw foods also are observed for health.

EIGHT PRINCIPLES AND TREATMENT STRATEGIES

Now that the acupuncturist has gathered information from the pulse, tongue, interview, history, and signs and symptoms, he or she must sort it all out and organize a plan. The method of organizing the information is differentiation according to the Eight Principles. Yin/Yang (which actually incorporate the other six), Hot/Cold, Interior/Exterior, and Excess/Deficient provide the framework. If the patient has a "cold disorder," for example, the acupuncturist must determine if it is Interior (are the organs affected?) or exterior, such as a common cold which is known as a "Wind Cold Invasion" attacking the surface. The acupuncturist also must determine if the cold disorder is due to a true Excess of cold, or if it is only a relative Excess due to a relative Deficiency of Yang, which is the energy that warms the body. Patients often present with mixed syndromes, for example, Cold in one area of the body and Heat in another. Treatment strategy is determined according to the Eight Principles of Differentiation. In Mr. Green's case, his condition was Yang/Excess/Interior/Heat. The treatment principle would be to use acupuncture points to clear the Excess and Heat. Generally speaking, an individual with a slow pulse who is pale, weak, and fatigued, feels chilly, has a pale tongue, and shows a lot of signs of deficiency of Qi, Blood, or Yang. The treatment principle would be to use acupuncture points to warm the body and build the energy and blood.

INCORPORATING TRADITIONAL CHINESE MEDICINE INTO PHYSICAL THERAPY PRACTICE

As a physical therapist, I have found the incorporation of both advanced physical therapy techniques such as joint and soft tissue mobilization and aspects of Traditional Chinese Medicine (acupuncture, shiatsu/acupressure, and herbs) to be ideal for most of my patients, a very compatible union. Physical therapy provides the anatomical, physiological, and mechanical model necessary to understand and treat many pain and dysfunction syndromes. The addition of Traditional Chinese Medicine broadens the scope of diagnosis and treatment to include the patient's energy or Qi and a separate perspective on the identical, but equally valid, physiology and pathology. It provides therapeutic tools that exceed the scope of physical therapy, especially in complicated patients, and also is preventative so that chronic patients may experience more holistic responses to their symptoms. In this way, as a practitioner, I am able to move beyond the limitations of purely mechanical intervention.

Take the case of my patient, Sam, a 38-year-old restaurant worker who was injured when pushing a trolley loaded with five folding tables. The tables shifted and began to fall, so he tried to block them with his body and was struck on the lateral aspect of his right neck and back. Magnetic resonance imaging showed disc herniation in both the cervical and lumbar spine. His subjective complaints were pain, stiffness, and limited function. Physical therapy evaluation briefly showed excessive lumbar lordosis, intact bilateral knee jerk reflexes, and on palpation very non-supple, dense/tense lumbar and cervical paraspinals. He was able to heel and toe walk but with pain. Flexing his right hip aggravated his low back and right sacroiliac joint area. He had received physical therapy consisting of massage and exercise (walking) with little benefit, and was on a prescription of a muscle relaxant and anti-inflammatory meds, and pain meds, which he stated caused nervousness, restlessness, and palpitations. Subjective pain level was 7/10 and constant, even with meds. Range of motion of his lumbar and cervical spine was very limited in all planes due to pain, joint dysfunction, and involuntary guarding.

I decided to use acupuncture in addition to a program consisting of manual therapy, craniosacral therapy, myofascial release, gentle muscle energy techniques, shiatsu massage and acupressure, cupping (bell-shaped jars applied to body with suction to invigorate circulation), and finally, a gradually progressive mobility and stretching exercise program. He also received a standard patient education program for correct posture and body mechanics. Sam's symptoms resolved and he made significant progress as his pain diminished and his mobility improved. He stated he could "feel things moving in his body (Qi/energy) and breaking up places where the pain was stuck." He was able to gradually reduce medications to a minimal "as needed" dose for intermittent "bad days."

SUMMARY

Acupuncture, as with all other holistic approaches, is not alternative to conventional Western Medicine, meaning one exclusive of the other, but complementary or adjunctive. Integrating Western and Eastern minds and approaches in health care benefits many patients and actually reduces costs by facilitating a quicker recovery and preventing many other unnecessary health problems that are complications from the incomplete resolution of the original problem.

I hope to see more interest, utilization, research, and education in these areas in the modern practice of physical therapy. Research of Eastern energy techniques, however, does not lend itself to traditional Western quantitative, analytical, double-blind, controlled studies. The Chinese mind is very pragmatic and if something is observed time and time again to work, it is used without questioning or investigating the mechanism by which it works. For example, needling or applying pressure to PC6, a point on the volar aspect of the wrist, is known to relieve nausea and vomiting. The Chinese have found this very useful and have not concerned themselves with justifying its use based on a scientist's official blessing with explanations of the mechanism.

Western research attempts to control all contaminating variables in a person's response in order to specifically measure the effect of just one treatment variable under highly monitored experimental conditions. However, people don't ever respond as machines. Whenever something is "done" to a person, the whole person responds. To measure the treatment outcome as if that outcome were the only response negates what we know about human beings; that is, both the researcher and subject are most often experiencing shifts in energy and biochemistry that seldom are being measured. Because we can't "see" Qi (energy) or meridians we choose not to try to identify them and include them in our results.

What must be done is to accept that holistic responses, affecting much more than one system, will take place, and then commit to a systematic, thorough recording of patient demographics and results that we can see (physiological changes in color, tone) as well as interviewing the subject or patient for his or her description of experienced effects during and after the treatment. In this way we will be able to share comparable information on outcomes and begin to publish our results using complementary therapies as a more complete and thorough approach to patients needing physical therapy.

REFERENCES

1. Xinnong C. *Chinese Acupuncture and Moxibustion.* Beijing, China: Foreign Language Press; 1987.
2. Kaptchuk TJ. *The Web That Has No Weaver.* Chicago, Ill: Congdon & Weed, Inc; 1990.
3. Maciocia G. *The Foundations of Chinese Medicine.* New York, NY: Churchill Livingstone Inc; 1989.
4. Matsumoto K, Birch S. *Hara Diagnosis: Reflections on the Sea.* Brookline, Mass: Paradigm Publications; 1988.
5. Maciocia G. *Tongue Diagnosis in Chinese Medicine.* Seattle, Wash: Eastland Press, Inc: 1987.
6. O'Connor J, Bensky D. *Acupuncture—A Comprehensive Text.* Seattle, Wash: Eastland Press, Inc; 1981.
7. Ross J. *Zang Fu: The Organ Systems of Traditional Chinese Medicine.* New York, NY: Churchill Livingstone Inc; 1985.
8. Ellis A, Wiseman N, Boss R. *Fundamentals of Chinese Acupuncture.* Brookline, Mass: Paradigm Publications; 1988.

SUGGESTED READINGS

Amber R, Babey-Brooke AM. *The Pulse in Occident and Orient.* New York, NY: Aurora Press; 1966.

Becker R, Selden G. *The Body Electric—Electromagnetism and the Foundation of Life.* New York, NY: Quill William Morrow & Co; 1985. Beinfield H, Korngold E. *Between Heaven and Earth—Guide to Chinese Medicine.* New York, NY: Ballantine Books; 1992.

Bischko J. *An Introduction to Acupuncture.* Heidelberg, Germany: Karl F. Haug Publishers; 1985.

Ellis A, Wiseman N, Boss R. *Grasping the Wind.* Brookline, Mass: Paradigm Publications; 1989.

Feit RM, Zmiewski P. *Acumoxa Therapy.* Volumes I and II. Brookline, Mass: Paradigm Publications; 1989.

Firebrace P. *Acupuncture: The Illustrated Guide.* New York, NY: Harmony Books (division of Crown Publishers); 1988.

Hammer L. *Dragon Rises Red Bird Flies.* Barrytown, NY: Station Hill Press, Inc; 1983.

Mann Felix MB. *Acupuncture—The Ancient Chinese Art of Healing and How it Works Scientifically.* New York, NY: Vintage Books (division of Random House); 1972.

Matsumoto K, Birch S. *Extraordinary Vessels.* Brookline, Mass: Paradigm Publications; 1986.

Matsumoto K, Birch S. *Five Elements and Ten Stems.* Brookline, Mass: Paradigm Publications; 1983.

Melzack R, Wall PD. *The Challenge of Pain.* New York, NY: Basic Books, Inc; 1983.

Upledger JE. *Craniosacral Therapy II.* Seattle, Wash: Eastland Press Inc; 1987.

Upledger JE. *Somato Emotional Release and Beyond.* Palm Beach Gardens, Fla: U.I. Publishing; 1990.

Upledger JE, Vredevoogd JD. *Craniosacral Therapy.* Seattle, Wash: Eastland Press Inc; 1987.

Wiseman N, Ellis A, Zmiewski P. *Fundamentals of Chinese Medicine*. Brookline, Mass: Paradigm Publications; 1985.

A *Barefoot Doctors Manual*. Philadelphia, Pa: Running Press; 1990.

"Plum Blossum" Needle Therapy. Hong Kong: Medicine & Health Publishing Co; 1986.

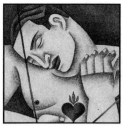

CHAPTER 13

POLARITY, REFLEXOLOGY, AND TOUCH FOR HEALTH

Mable B. Sharp, PT, MS, CM

INTRODUCTION

The techniques described in this chapter are based on the theory that there is a pattern of "energy" in the human body which is invisible and not part of the nervous system. This energy has been used in the healing arts for thousands of years in Eastern cultures and has been well reported in ancient and modern literature.[1-5] It is called "Ch'i" in Chinese Medicine, "Ki" or "Qi" in Japan, and "Prana" in India. This energy is said to be the life force of a person and the Chinese consider good health to be a balance of this energy within the human body. Dolores Krieger[1] and Fritz Smith[2] believe that this energy offers an explanation to phenomena such as spontaneous healing, regeneration and wound healing, mental telepathy, and even fire walking.

This energy varies in quantity and quality, has polarity (yin and yang), and is arranged in specific patterns. The Chinese believe the Ch'i dynamic force of energy is constantly circulating within the body in 12 well-defined channels called Meridians which exist as a series of points following line-like patterns.[3] This energy also relates to organ activity (see

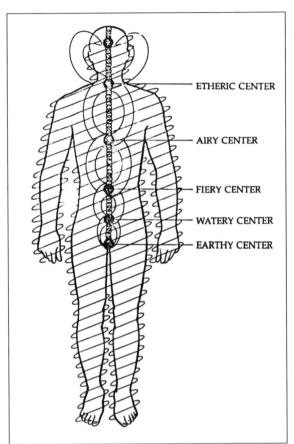

ETHERIC CENTER

AIRY CENTER

FIERY CENTER

WATERY CENTER

EARTHY CENTER

Figure 13-1. Central chakras and caduceus current.

Chapter 12, *Acupuncture in the Physical Therapy Clinic*). In India, Prana, the breath of life, is related to vigor and vitality and is central in the practice of Yoga. Prana manifests itself in a variety of forms including gravity, electricity, and body actions and thoughts; significantly, it can be transmitted from one person to another. From this comes the concept of chakras, which are whirling centers of vortexes of energy. Smith[2] identifies the seven central chakras as coinciding with the normal spinal curves. In polarity therapy[4] the lower five chakras correspond to the basic five elements of ether, air, fire, water, and earth (Figure 13-1). Each chakra relates to the organ and functions located in its area.

Krieger's[4] research has led her to believe that Prana energy is the basis of human energy transfer in the healing act. She states, "The act of healing, then, would entail the channeling of this energy flow by the healer for the well-being of the sick individual." Therefore, we must acknowledge that it is the patient who heals him or herself and that the healer merely acts as a booster for the patient to accelerate the healing process. With this in mind, it is important that the therapist/practitioner, or healer, if you will, becomes aware of his or her own energy and how he or she perceives energy flow through the body.

Some have indicated that energy is perceived as heat, vibration, cold, tingling, pulsation, or an attraction or repelling force.[1,2,4] Because this energy transfer actually takes place during the "laying on of hands, physical therapists must have their own energy in a positive and caring mode prior to approaching a patient in order to provide the most effective care possible.

In order to accomplish this, the therapist must balance his/her own energy through a process called Centering. Krieger[1] defines centering "as a sense of self-relatedness that can be thought of as a place of inner being where one can feel truly integrated, unified, and focused." She describes the following instant centering technique:

1. Sit comfortably, but in postural alignment, while performing this technique.
2. Relax. To assure this, I suggest that you check out your favorite tension spots and relax those areas of your body. If your neck or shoulder muscles are in tension, strongly depress your shoulders—that is, push your shoulders down so that they are not hunched upward toward your neck.
3. Inhale deeply and gently.
4. Slowly exhale.
5. Inhale again—and there you are! It is just here, in this state between breaths which you are now experiencing, that a state similar to that of the centering experience can be simulated. It is this state of balance, equipoise, and quietude that marks the experience of centering.

Another centering technique I have used is to stand or sit, with the feet firmly planted flat on the floor. Relax and imagine a line going through the center of your body to connect you to the earth below and to the universe above. Inhale and exhale deeply and slowly a few times as you visualize the line. This technique balances your energy and connects you to the universal energy needed in the healing process.

The treatment techniques described in the remainder of this chapter and most other chapters are based on the concept of energy and its ability to be transferred from one person to another to enhance the patient's own healing process. Therefore, become aware of this energy and its transfer, use this simple centering technique, and be open to new ways of healing and helping.

POLARITY THERAPY

Polarity therapy was developed in the mid 1900s by Randolph Stone, chiropractor, naturopath, and osteopathic physician. Dr. Stone's study of the relationship of illness or

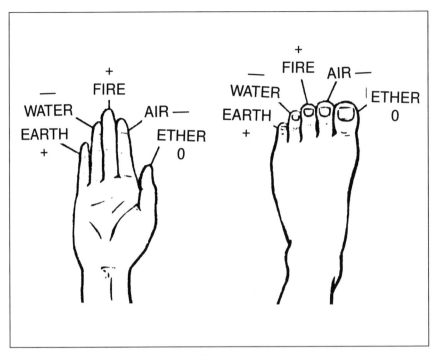

Figure 13-2. *Polarity of each finger and toe.*

disease to energy led him to the belief that there is a subtle form of life energy that permeates the body and gives it health, and that disease is a result of obstruction to that flow of energy. Polarity therapy does not treat disease or illness. Rather it treats the life energy which flows through all the body organs and tissues. The purpose of polarity manipulation is to locate blocked energy and release it. When energy is released, the organs and systems tend to normalize in function and healing can take place naturally.[4]

This therapy is based on the directions in which this life energy flows; longitudinal, horizontal, and diagonal lines of force, chakras, and the five elements (ether, air, fire, water, and earth). Polarity therapy views energy as flowing from positive (+) to negative (-), the feet as - and the head as +, the right side of the body is + and the left is -, and that each element and each finger and toe is + , -, or neutral (Figure 13-2). Each joint is neutral and allows for energy to cross over and charge the polarity which enables the joints to be flexible. The chakras, which are neutral, spin clockwise when received from the back, and give off an energy flow upwards and downwards, forming the longitudinal currents of energy. They are connected by a dual spiral of energy from the head downwards, the caduceus current (see Figure 13-1). These chakras also relate to the organs located in their area.

- Ether chakra governs voice, hearing, and throat
- Air the circulation, heart, and lungs
- Fire, digestion, stomach, and bowel
- Water governs reproductive organs, glandular secretions, and emotional drive
- Earth the elimination of solids and liquids, bladder, and rectum[4,5] (see Figure 13-1).

Structure always reflects the energy. If the structure is disturbed due to illness or injury, the energy pattern becomes distorted. Alan Siegel states, "If a physical correction of some kind is then made without re-balancing the energy pattern, the energetic imbalance will continue to distort the structure, the correction will not hold; complete healing will not take place."[4]

The techniques of Polarity Therapy are very simple and gentle. They involve simple touching using bi-polar contacts (use of two contacts on the patient's body simultaneously). For example, a positive contact (right hand or fire finger) pushes energy and is stimulating while a negative contact (left hand or air finger) is relaxing and receives energy. These contacts balance the chakras to each other and the energy flowing through the longitudinal and horizontal energy currents. Once the appropriate contacts have been made, the therapist should concentrate on feeling energy, which is usually experienced as a tingling or warmth between the hands and the patient's body. Stimulate for a couple of minutes, then hold and feel the energy for 30 seconds to 1 minute and move to another manipulation. If after 2 minutes you do not feel energy, hold for another minute and then move on.

Siegel[14] outlines 20 points to remember when giving a polarity therapy session. While Western science has performed extensive research in the theory of energy or polarity therapy, Tappan identifies subjective indications that some principles not yet recognized by Western medicine are involved. She states:

1. "Subjectively, health is often equated with being full of energy whereas the first sign of impending illness is often its absence.
2. Subjectively, the therapist feels a definite tingling in his or her hands when doing the various mobilizations. The degree and pattern of this tingling vary with the state of health of the area being worked, and they change as the area is treated.
3. Subjectively, the patient and therapist often note simultaneous changes in their sense of energy. The receiver feels freer, lighter, more relaxed; the therapist notes a balancing and strengthening of the tingling in his or her hands, and a sense of an overall increase in energy."[6]

This therapist has noticed that after a few minutes of polarity therapy the autonomic system seems to be affected by this unblocking of energy. Signs of deep relaxation appear, often cheeks flush, blood pressure decreases, pulse slows, eyes may tear, and the intestines may grumble due to a change in peristalsis.

INTEGRATION INTO PRACTICE

When energy is blocked it manifests itself as soreness, tenderness, or pain. I use polarity therapy primarily with patients who have acute musculoskeletal pathology with significant pain, muscle spasm, and movement dysfunction. Such conditions include tendonitis, rotator cuff strains or tears, trauma to muscles or joints, bursitis, spinal nerve root compressions, muscles or ligamentous damage, and often, chronic myofascial pain syndrome. My goal in the use of polarity therapy is to unblock the energy flow which results in reduced pain and spasm and enhancement of the body's own natural processes to facilitate tissue healing and to reduce the inflammatory process. This then allows for more vigorous therapeutic activities such as traction, joint mobilization, myofascial release, therapeutic exercises, and functional activities, which are performed with less pain and increased effectiveness.

A typical treatment session for one of the above problems would be to initiate polarity therapy by placing my left hand over the painful area (ie, anterior right shoulder) and the right hand on the opposite side (ie, posterior side of the right shoulder) of the painful shoulder. Once I have felt with my hands that the energy is flowing through the area, I will apply heat or cold or perform ultrasound treatment to specific structures. During or following this, I perform a specific polarity manipulation for that part of the body.

One example might be working with a patient with a shoulder problem. I stand on the side opposite the painful shoulder (patient is supine) and place finger tips of both hands (one hand on top of the other) inside the pelvic crest nearest me. Slowly and gently I press down and towards the sore shoulder and work along the shape of the pelvic crest, going deeper as the muscles relax. Then I remove my top hand and grasp the sore shoulder with the thumb on the anterior aspect of the joint. This is followed by alternately stimulating (via holding, gentle pressure, or rhythmical rocking of the hand) the pelvis and shoulder until I feel the energy move.

A second example might be treating a patient with back pain. The patient would be supine and I would stand on the side of the pain. With the air finger (see Figure 13-2) of one hand, I locate a sore or tender spot on the back. For each tender spot on the back there is a corresponding tender spot on the front of the body which I locate using the fire finger of the other hand. These spots are alternately stimulated until the soreness disappears; then I continue holding and feel the energy flow. This is repeated for each tender spot in the area where the back is painful.

After the polarity treatment, I then would perform appropriate traditional physical therapy techniques such as joint mobilizations, therapeutic exercises, stretching and/or myofascial release, stabilization exercises and coordination and/or functional activities, such as balance, gait, etc.

The treatment session is concluded by chakra or caduceus current balancing to produce overall relaxation and facilitate deep energy flow. The chakra balance is performed by placing the patient supine, with me standing on the right side of the body. I make loose fists and touch the right thumb to the umbilicus and the left thumb between the eyebrows. I hold for 2 minutes and feel the energy flow through the body.

The caduceus *current balancing* is performed with the patient supine and me standing at the patient's right side. The heel of the right hand is on the inside of the left pelvic crest at the ASIS and the heel of the left hand is on the right shoulder joint. I press down on the shoulder as I rock the pelvis 10-15 times, gradually increasing the rocking movement. Then I reverse the positions and balance the right pelvis to the left shoulder.

Polarity therapy techniques are simple and easy to perform in a short period of time without the need for special equipment or assistance. In his book *Polarity Therapy*,[4] Alan Siegel outlines specific polarity techniques for all joints, the spine, internal organs, lymphatics, the cranium, and various energy current balancing techniques. Once the physical therapist has learned to feel energy with his or her hands, reading the text and applying techniques can produce significant effective changes. However, taking continuing education courses in polarity therapy can enhance the therapist's efficiency of application and problem solving abilities.

CASE EXAMPLE

The patient was a 43-year-old white male policeman with repeated musculoskeletal traumas from falls, motor vehicle accidents, and beatings over the past 2 years. The most recent incident was approximately two months before I first saw him. His complaints were pain and immobility in the rib cage, difficulty breathing, left shoulder pain and reduced ROM, and pain. The patient also had bilateral knee braces provided during previous physical therapy sessions with another therapist. The patient was seen twice a week for heat, joint mobilization, stretching, and visceral manipulation. After a few weeks, it was apparent that the rib cage was not responding to mobilization techniques. He continued to complain of pain, difficulty breathing, and decreased and painful rotation of the trunk.

It was at this time that I decided to use polarity therapy to unblock his rib cage by using the clavicle and diaphragm contacts. In this technique, the patient is supine with the therapist standing at his right side. I placed the pad of my left air finger about one inch below the clavicle starting at the sternoclavicular joint and I palpated for areas of tenderness and worked toward the acromioclavicular joint. For each tender spot located under the clavicle, I placed the pad of the right fire finger on the diaphragm in a direct line inferior to the air finger. Alternately, I stimulated both points until the tenderness at the clavicle was gone or until the flow of energy was felt between the fingers. I worked each tender spot found. Then I repeated this on the left side of the body, while I remained standing at the patient's right.

While performing the techniques on the right side, the patient reported numerous times when the pain completely disappeared within 20 seconds. After the treatment, he indicated that his breathing was easier and that he could rotate the trunk without pain. Objectively his thoracic cage expansion increased 1/2" and the rotation increased by 12° to the left and 16° to the right. Subsequent treatments, which included polarity, joint mobilization and moist heat, resulted in continued reduction of pain, an increase in mobility, and easier breathing.

REFLEXOLOGY

"Reflexology is a science that deals with the principle that there are reflex areas in the feet and hands which correspond to all of the glands, organs and parts of the body (Figures 13-3, 13-4). Reflexology is a unique method of using the thumb and fingers on these reflex areas."[7] Its effects are the relief of stress and tension, improvement of blood supply, restoration of nerve impulses, and to help the body achieve homeostasis naturally. Reflexology has been used as far back as the 6th dynasty, about 2,300 B.C., in Egypt.

More recently, it had its modern beginnings in the technique of Zone Therapy as developed by Dr. William Fitzgerald in the early 1900s. In his 1917 book, *Zone Therapy or Relieving Pain at Home*, Fitzgerald identifies 10 zones that run through the body (Figure 13-5). There are five zones on each side of the body, one for each finger and toe, that run from the top of the head to the tips of the toes. An organ or gland or body part found in a specific zone will have its reflex in the corresponding zone of the foot and hand via nerve endings. Sensitivity of an area on the foot signals that there could be something abnormal taking place in the corresponding body part.

In the early 1930s, a physical therapist, Eunice Ingham, started to develop her Foot Reflexology Therapy method. She studied zone therapy, and through her work in a physician's office began probing the feet and finding tender spots and correlating them with the anatomy of the body and patients' diagnoses. She was able to chart the representation of the zones of the feet to the organs and body parts (see Figures 13-3 and 13-4). Note that single

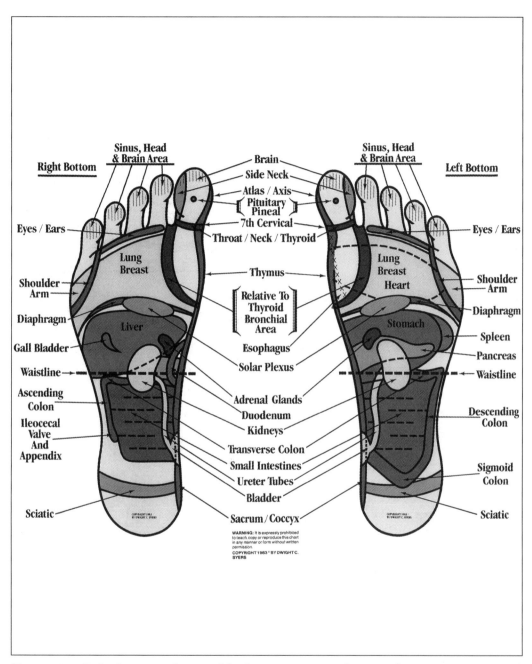

Figure **13-3.** *Reflexology areas, bottom of the feet. By permission from Dwight C. Byers, International Institute of Reflexology & Ingham Publishing, Inc., P.O. Box 12642, St. Petersburg, FL 33733-2646, U.S.A.*

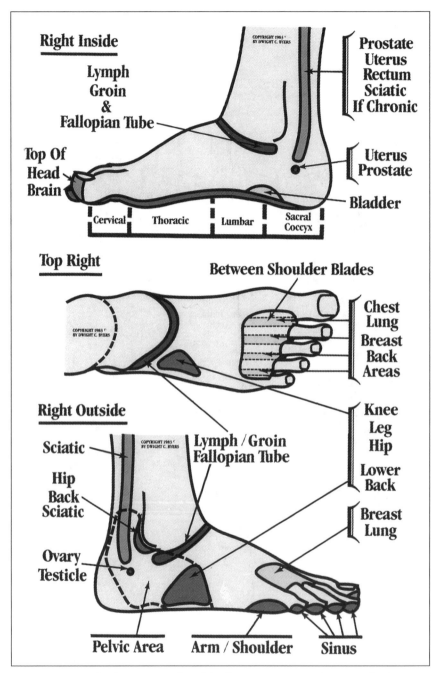

Figure 13-4. Reflexology areas, sides of the feet. By permission from Dwight C. Byers, International Institute of Reflexology & Ingham Publishing, Inc. P.O. Box 12642, St. Petersburg, FL 33733-2646, U.S.A.

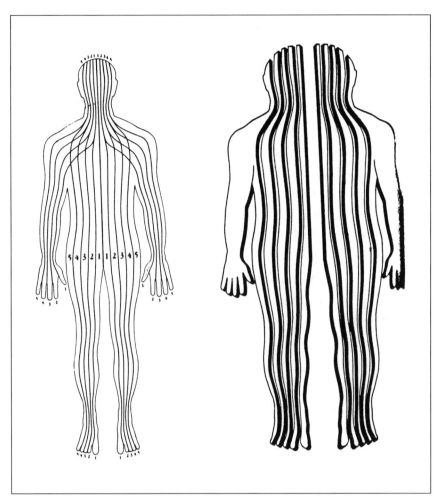

Figure 13-5. *Zones of the body. By permission from Dwight C. Byers, International Institute of Reflexology & Ingham Publishing, Inc. P.O. Box 12642, St. Petersburg, FL 33733-2646, U.S.A.*

organs are represented only on the foot on the side of the body in which they are located, while paired organs, such as the lungs, are represented on both feet. You can see also that the curves along the medial board of the foot, which represents the spine, mirror the natural anatomical curves of the spine. In 1938, she compiled her theory and experiences in a book called *Stories the Feet Can Tell*[8] and then in a sequel, *Stories the Feet Have Told.*[9]

The technique for performing reflexology is very simple. Using the thumbs, fingers, or knuckles, you apply a firm, constant, deep massaging pressure to the sensitive area on the foot for one to two minutes. Working the entire foot affects the entire body; the right foot helps the right half of the body, and the left foot, the left side of the body. Through this technique you are stimulating the circulation, unblocking nerve impulses, raising the vitality of the body, ridding toxins from the system, and thereby assisting the body's own heal-ing mechanisms to attain homeostasis.[8] Because these areas on the feet are sensitive and toxins are released, patients often experience discomfort during the treatment (similar to friction massage) and may develop systemic reactions such as a cold or increased sinus activity. These systemic reactions usually occur if the entire foot is treated and after the second or third treatment session. Patients need to be forewarned that this is a natural out-come of the total treatment process.

Adjuncts to working the specific reflex points of the feet are referral and helper areas.[7] Referral areas are areas that are anatomically related to another area in the body. For instance, the right and left hand are referral areas for the right and left foot, respectively. These areas can be worked instead of, or in conjunction with, the affected area to restore more normal function. They are used primarily in acute conditions where the affected area is too painful to work with, such as with the case of a severely sprained ankle or fractured toe. The referral area, on the other hand, can be worked instead to produce the desired effect in the affected area.

Helper areas are additional areas that have a direct affect on the effected area and hold the reinforcement needed to attain the desired results. For example, a patient with whiplash would naturally have the area between the first and second toes at the top of the feet worked for the whiplash. Because of the anatomical relationship of the neck muscles, vertebrae, nerves, and the shoulder, we also would work the entire cervical spine (medial side of the big toes) and the shoulder (between the 4th & 5th toes) on both feet to attain the maximum effect.

INTEGRATION INTO PRACTICE

In my treatment sessions, I primarily use reflexology for musculoskeletal conditions such as those producing neck and back pain and other joint dysfunctions. For example, a patient presents with lower back pain due to disc or facet joint misalignment. I may place them on a hot pack with pelvic traction and during this treatment I would work the spinal points and helper areas on the feet. I would follow this with joint mobilization, stretching, or stabilization exercises as appropriate.

In another example, a patient presents with a capsulitis of the right shoulder or per-haps a rotator cuff strain. I would give ultrasound to the area, then work the shoulder reflex area of the affected shoulder and follow with joint mobilization, stretching, or appro-priate isotonic or isokinetic exercises.

I also use foot reflexology as part of a home program. Patients are taught the specific reflex area(s) of the feet to stimulate and how to stimulate them. Sometimes patients are not able to reach the feet, for one reason or another. I have given them a marble so they can sit, place the marble on the floor, and step onto the marble at the level of the reflexology point. They can then increase the pressure of the foot against the marble, thus stimulating the point. The patient stimulates the point(s) for 1-2 minutes each, every day, or when an increase in symptoms is experienced.

Reflexology is an excellent tool to use with pregnant women with a musculoskeletal problem. Usually they will not be allowed to take medication, and some physical therapy treatments are contraindicated as well. However, stimulating the appropriate reflexology points on the feet does not produce any ill effects to mother or baby and helps alleviate symptoms.

CASE EXAMPLE

The patient was a 27-year-old white female who had delivered a healthy baby girl just 6 days prior to my seeing her. She presented with right sacroiliac (SI) pain and weak abdominal muscles. She was to be seen for a postpartum exercise program and treatment of the SI joint. However, the patient was very concerned about the severe swelling in both feet and ankles. She indicated that the doctor said, "it would go down eventually and not to worry." My treatment consisted of moist heat to the lower back, postpartum exercises, and muscle energy to the SI joint twice a week. But I also included a reflexology technique for the swelling in her ankles. I worked the reflex area for the groin and lymphatic system on both feet. This point runs across the front of the ankle at the distal end of the tibia and fibula from malleolus to malleolus. First, using the index fingers, I put pressure on this area by "walking" from each malleolus toward the center of the ankle. Next, I grasped the ankle joint area with the web space of one hand and the ball of the foot with my other hand. Then I rotated the foot several times in one direction and then several times in the other direction.

When she returned in 2 days, she stated that the swelling in both feet had completely resolved by next day after the treatment. I also placed her on a home program to work the right SI reflex point on the heel of the right foot.

TOUCH FOR HEALTH

Touch for Health (TFH) "is a practical guide to natural health using acupressure touch and massage to improve postural balance and reduce physical and mental pain and tension."[10] It works with the body's subtle energies at the connection between mind and body using the electromagnetic system, called meridians, which were described previously. TFH's goal is to balance these energies and help to restore structural balance and good health.

The subtle body energies that are used in TFH are beginning to be explained by quantum physics. For more information on quantum physics you may wish to read *Quantum Healing* by Deepak Chopra, MD (see Suggested Readings). Until we have a mechanism for imaging and measuring this energy and its role in the cause and healing of disease, a full explanation of how TFH works will not be possible.

Touch for Health is based in chiropractic. The chiropractor believes that health comes from within and that the goal is to restore the body to a normal position which then restores the relationship of the body parts so that they work together producing good health. Initially, the chiropractor did this by working primarily with the spine, a technique first advocated by D.D. Palmer (the father of Chiropractic Medicine) in the late 1800s. He used the transverse and spinous processes of the spine as levers to adjust the spine and to correct posture.

Later, Drs. Bennett and DeJarnette began working with reflexes to show how deep massage or light touch can get the muscles to move the bones rather than resorting to external manipulation. In the early 1960s, George Goodheart, DC began working with the muscles. He felt that a muscle in spasm may not be causing the problem, but that weak muscles on one side of the body can cause normal opposing muscles to become or seem tight.[10] With this principle in mind, rather than working with the strong, tight or spasmatic muscle, he worked to strengthen the opposite weak muscle. If the tightness persists, he reasoned that you can weaken or calm the tight muscle.

Touch for Health uses the muscles as a biofeedback mechanism. Some muscles are "related to" organs because they share common structures such as a lymphatic vessel, an acupuncture meridian, or a somatic reflex (as with a facilitated segment). The technique tests for specific muscle weaknesses, treats them, and therefore treats the entire body. Touch for Health uses Applied Kinesiology, a form of muscle testing, and muscle activation to determine the need for treatment and the treatment's effectiveness both before and after the treatment. This type of muscle testing, similar to isometric resistance testing used by physical therapists in working with orthopedic patients, tests only for strength or weakness, not to grade the muscle per se. With Applied Kinesiology, a muscle is tested, and if it is graded strong, it's really strong; even the slightest giving way in the muscle is considered "weakness." The muscles are tested within the first few inches of their active range of motion by applying and releasing pressure gradually. When practicing Touch For Health, almost all the muscles are tested with the patient in the supine position and the specific position, of the extremity is one which isolates the specific muscle being tested. The muscle is retested after it has been treated to determine if the treatment was effective and this leads you to the next phase of treatment. In other words, effective treatment helps align and integrate nerve, joint, and muscle for an optimum strength response.

In his book *Touch for Health,*[10] John Thie states that "man is a structural, chemical and psychological/spiritual being and that his problems can be segmented into different systems: structural, neurological, lymphatic, vascular, cerebrospinal, nutritional/chemical and meridian systems." Using these systems, Dr. Thie has developed techniques for strengthening muscles, thus promoting innate healing. His book details each of these areas and provides diagrams as to where these areas can be found on the body (Figure 13-6). However, in this chapter I will simply provide a brief overview of each technique, in the order in which he indicates they should be employed.

SPINAL VERTEBRAE REFLEX TECHNIQUE

To be used first but only if there is bilateral weakness of the same muscle. Thie postulates that the spine and central nervous system have a "reflex" that relates to the restoration of strength to muscles. This external reflex is located in the skin and is activated by moving the skin over the spinal vertebrae which corresponds to the muscle being worked (Figure 13-6). The practitioner is directed to move from superior to inferior over the spinal segment(s) stretching the skin rapidly but gently for 10-30 seconds.

NEURO-LYMPHATIC MASSAGE POINTS

This technique is the first to be used in cases of a unilateral muscle weakness and the second in cases of a bilateral muscle weakness. These points are reflexes located mainly on the chest and back. They vary in size and can occur alone or in groups. Some can be palpated; others cannot, and get turned off when the system becomes overloaded. To work these reflexes, the practitioner is directed to locate the points on the body corresponding to the weak muscle then move around the point with the fingers using a deep, consistent massaging pressure for 20-30 seconds. The tenderness felt will decrease as balance returns to the system.

NEURO-VASCULAR HOLDING POINTS

These points are located mainly on the head and require only light contact with the pads of the fingers and a slight stretching of the skin to activate. Once palpated, these points seem to enhance circulation to the muscle and the related organ. Upon contact a slight pulse of 70-74 beats per minute will be felt; the practitioner allows it to synchronize on both sides and then holds for an additional 20 seconds to 10 minutes, depending on the severity of the problem; the weaker the muscle, the longer you hold.

MERIDIANS

The meridians described by Thie are the acupuncture meridians associated with each specific muscle. Using the hand to trace the meridian line in the appropriate direction on the surface of the body, the practitioner will stimulate the energy flow through the meridian. On retest, if the muscle is not stronger, the practitioner tries tracing in the opposite direction and then retests.

ACUPRESSURE HOLDING POINTS

These points lie on acupuncture meridians and can be used to either strengthen or weaken the meridian, associated muscles, or organ. The practitioner holds the points on the same side of the body as the weak muscle, lightly holding the first arm and leg strengthening points at the same time (see Figure 13-6). One point is held in each hand using the pads of the fingers for about 30 seconds, or until a pulse (70-74 beats per minute) is felt in the leg. Then the practitioner places the hands on the second points and holds, waiting for the pulse in the leg.

ORIGIN/INSERTION TECHNIQUE

These may be used when you have not accomplished strengthening with the previous techniques. The practitioner locates the origin and insertion of the weakened muscle, and places his or her finger on each end and gently juggles the ends of the muscle back and forth. Dr. Thie also has outlined techniques for activating the muscle spindle and the Golgi tendon apparatus. Remember that after each treatment technique has been used, you must retest the muscle to determine if the treatment has been effective in strengthening the muscle.

INTEGRATION INTO PRACTICE

In my practice, I use Touch for Health techniques when I have not been successful at reducing muscle spasm, increasing muscle length, and improving muscle strength with other techniques. I will use the technique to strengthen the weakened opposite muscles of the tight muscles or those in spasm. As an example, a patient presents with tightness in

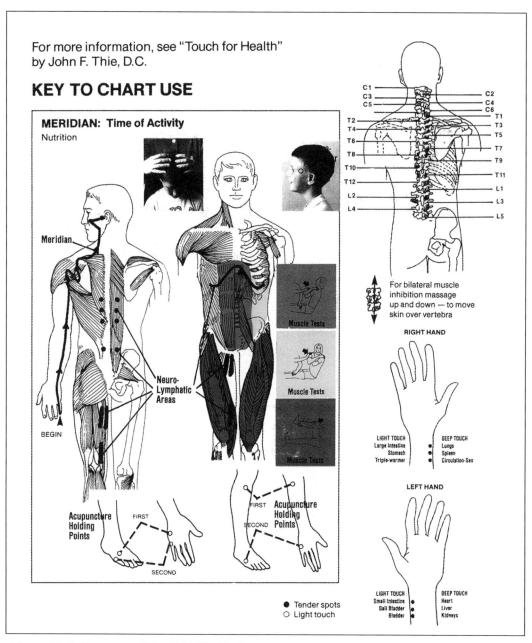

For more information, see "Touch for Health" by John F. Thie, D.C.

KEY TO CHART USE

MERIDIAN: Time of Activity
Nutrition

Meridian

Neuro-Lymphatic Areas

BEGIN

Acupuncture Holding Points

FIRST

SECOND

Muscle Tests

Muscle Tests

Muscle Tests

FIRST Acupuncture Holding Points

SECOND

For bilateral muscle inhibition massage up and down — to move skin over vertebra

RIGHT HAND

LIGHT TOUCH
Large Intestine
Stomach
Triple-warmer

DEEP TOUCH
Lungs
Spleen
Circulation-Sex

LEFT HAND

LIGHT TOUCH
Small Intestine
Gall Bladder
Bladder

DEEP TOUCH
Heart
Liver
Kidneys

● Tender spots
○ Light touch

Figure 13-6. *Key to use of Touch for Health charts.*

the psoas muscle on the right that I have not been able to improve with traditional stretching, myofascial release, or strain counter strain techniques. I will strengthen the opposite muscle, the gluteus maximus (Figure 13-7), beginning with testing the muscle for its strength; it usually will show some weakness. Then I would massage the neuro-lymphatic areas from the top of the thigh to just above the knee on the lateral side of the right leg and the posterior iliac crests at the level of L5. Then I retest the muscle, and if stronger, the treatment is determined to be successful. If not, I proceed to the neuro-vascular holding points at the lambdoidal sutures at the back of the skull. I retest and, if necessary, trace the circulation-sex meridian from the nipple down the middle of the anterior arm to end at the pad of the middle finger. I retest and if necessary use the acupressure holding points of LV1 and CX9, then K10 and CX3. If all else fails, I would weaken the right psoas muscle by using the acupressure holding points for weakening of the right side. These are first K1 (at the metatarsal phalangeal joint, of the big toe) and LV1 (top of the big toe) and secondly, SP3 (on lateral side of big toe just before the metatarsal phalangeal joint) and K3 (between the gastroc tendon and the center of the medial malleoli). This treatment can take from 3-15 minutes and can be done during the application of a hot pack or during pelvic traction or instead of stretching techniques.

CASE EXAMPLE

This patient is a 22-year-old black male with a diagnosis of traumatic brain injury with resultant right side weakness. His injury occurred on the job about two and one-half years earlier. Evaluation revealed minimal spasticity on the right, 3+/5 to 4/5 isolated movement in the right extremities with the exception of the triceps which graded 3, and no active extension in the middle, ring, and little finger of the right hand. The order was for neuromuscular rehabilitation, strengthening, and functional activities twice a week. All of the muscles responded to conventional therapy such as vibration, compression, muscle reeducation techniques, and resistive exercises, with the exception of the triceps. After obtaining no change in the 3 muscle grade, I decided to try Touch for Health specifically to strengthen the right triceps muscle.

First, I tested the muscle and it was weak (3 muscle grade). I then massaged the neuro-lymphatic points at the costal cartilage between the 7-8th ribs on the left and posteriorly between T 7-8 on each side of the spine. The retest showed no increase in strength. Then I held the neuro-vascular holding points on the parietal bones just above and behind the ears. The retest showed minimal improvement in strength.

Next, the spleen meridian was traced from the big toe up the inside of the leg, in front of the abdomen, to the shoulder joint and down to the side of the chest. The retest showed more significant improvement (graded 3+).

I then decided to use the acupressure holding points to strengthen the muscle further. The first points held were SP2 (at the outside of the metatarsal phalangeal joint)

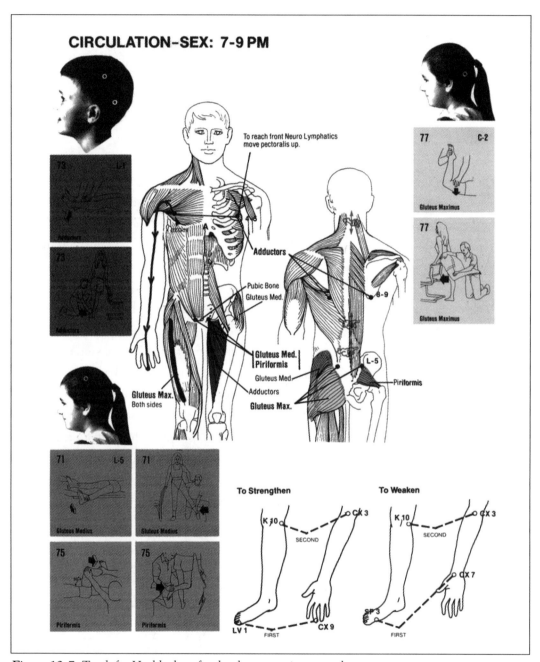

Figure 13-7. *Touch for Health chart for the gluteus maximus muscle.*

and H8 (at the head of the 4th metacarpal in the palm). The second points held were LV1 (on the top of the big toe) and SP1 (on the outside of the top of the big toe). The retest indicated a muscle grade of 4-. I then performed active and resistive exercises to the triceps, vibration to the muscle belly, and compression through the joint. The patient was able to keep the elbow straight while weight bearing on the right upper extremity while sitting. The next treatment session, the triceps muscle tested 4- again. I then added Touch for Health to each of his treatment sessions. In another two weeks the muscle grade was 4+.

CONCLUSIONS

The goal of my approach to patient care is to attain relief of symptoms, improve movement dysfunctions, and restore total body health to the extent possible. These goals have led me to further investigation of a number of alternative techniques which included Polarity, Reflexology, and Touch for Health. In pursuing these methods of healing, an open mind is necessary, a sense of inquisitiveness is helpful, and a desire to treat the whole person is essential.

While many other health care practitioners as well as myself have experienced the effectiveness of these treatment techniques, and patients have reported their effectiveness, the need for systematic validation is critical. Because these techniques have no known or observed contraindications, and require only the use of a pair of skilled hands and an open mind and heart rather than expensive and sophisticated equipment, willing students can easily be taught and implemented. Each of these techniques lends itself to the use of carefully documented studies with patients to measure changes in such parameters as blood flow, nerve conduction velocity, autonomic nervous system function, range of motion and strength, and in pain level and/or the use of pain medication. The research is ready to be done and many practitioners would welcome those interested in investigating and documenting the effectiveness of what they're doing.

Those persons interested in pursuing any of the techniques reviewed should read the references used and the list of suggested readings. The following organizations can be contacted for information about training courses in the techniques:

- The Polarity Therapy Centre of San Francisco, 408-A Lawton St, San Francisco, CA 94122 (415) 753-1298.
- International Institute of Reflexology, P.O. Box 12642, St. Petersburg, FL 33733-2642 (813) 343-4811.
- North American Touch for Health Assn., 6955 Fernhill Ave, Malibu, CA 90265 (310) 457-8342.

REFERENCES

1. Krieger D. *The Therapeutic Touch: How to Use Your Hands to Help or to Heal.* New York, NY: Prentice Hall; 1986.

2. Smith F. *Inner Bridges: A Guide to Energy Movement and Body Structure.* Atlanta, Ga: Humanics New Age; 1990.

3. Manaka Y, Urquhart I. *The Layman's Guide to Acupuncture.* New York, NY: Weatherhill; 1995.

4. Siegel A. *Polarity Therapy: The Power That Heals.* Garden City Park, NY: Avery Publishing Group, Inc; 1987.

5. Brennan B. *Hands of Light: A Guide to Healing Through the Human Energy Field.* New York, NY: Bantam Books; 1988.

6. Tappan F. *Healing Massage Techniques: Holistic, Classic, and Emerging Methods.* 2nd ed. Norwalk, Conn: Appleton & Lange; 1988.

7. Byers D. *Better Health With Foot Reflexology.* St. Petersburg, Fla: Ingham Publishing, Inc; 1987.

8. Ingham E. *Stories the Feet Can Tell Thru Reflexology.* St. Petersburg, Fla: Ingham Publishing, Inc; 1984.

9. Ingham E. *Stories the Feet Have Told Thru Reflexology.* St. Petersburg, Fla: Ingham Publishing, Inc; 1984.

10. Thie J. *Touch for Health.* Sherman Oaks, Calif: T.H. Enterprises, Publishers; 1994.

SUGGESTED READINGS

Becker R, Selden G. *The Body Electric: Electromagnetism and the Foundation of Life.* New York, NY: William Morrow and Co, Inc; 1987.

Chopra D. *Quantum Healing: Exploring the Frontiers of Mind/Body Medicine.* New York, NY: Bantam Books; 1990.

Seidman M. *A Guide to Polarity Therapy: The Gentle Art of Hands-on Healing.* Boulder, Colo: Elan Press; 1991.

Stone R. *Polarity Therapy.* Vol I. Sebastopol, Calif: CRCS Publications; 1986.

Weinman R. *Your Hands Can Heal: Learn to Channel Healing Energy.* New York, NY: Penguin Books; 1992.

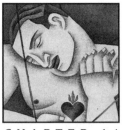

CHAPTER 14

JIN SHIN DO

Gudrun Heyland Mik, PT
Ulrike Treppmann, PT

INTRODUCTION

Jin Shin Do™ (JSD) is a form of acupressure. The English translation would be "way of the compassionate spirit." It was developed in the 1970s by Iona Marsaa Teeguarden,[1] an American psychotherapist, combining Jin Shin Jiutsu, an ancient Japanese self-help technique, Traditional Chinese Medicine (TCM), and Western body-oriented psychology as practiced by Wilhelm Reich and Alexander Lowen.

Reich[2] was the first psychiatrist to touch his patients for assessment. In 1946 he described "psycho-vegetative reactions" and a segmental distribution of chronic muscular tension, which he found correlated with early emotional experiences. He termed these tense segments "armorings." The unbearable excess of an emotion triggers a defense mechanism, like holding one's breath or pulling up the shoulders. Each time the situation reoccurs, we instantaneously repeat the same withholding mechanism until it becomes automatic.

Repetition is the appropriate stimulus for our neurological system to reinforce motor learning as well as emotional learning. Subconscious reaction patterns are developed and feed the original blockages. Thus we keep armorings but constantly aggravate them, until we learn to reprogram our responses.

Releasing tension from the armorings revives the original causal situation, for instance, in a picture in our mind's eye, or any other memory, and triggers the habitual reaction pattern which can be observed by the therapist and/or the recipient. Usual massage technique does not focus on the causes of the tension, that is, the reaction pattern, and thus has little long lasting effect. In a JSD release, the practitioner tries to establish a safe place where the recipient can dare to feel and, with gentle, specific touch, become aware again, and relive the original feeling in slow motion to the intensity that he or she desires. Then access to a choice is gained to modify or continue with a reaction, whichever feels appropriate.

CONTRAST BETWEEN THE APPROACH OF WESTERN MEDICINE TO JIN SHIN DO

Since Descartes, Western medicine practices medical research by reducing the body into the smallest analyzable units, conducts a study of the outcome of a treatment variable, and then puts parts back together. This rather mechanistic approach is somewhat like drawing pictures for an animated cartoon, only the "anima," which actually makes it alive, is left out of the analysis and cannot be captured by it.

The Ancients in China looked at life not as a collection of static images, but as a constant flow of changes. Their research focused on the identification of the dynamics of changes and, as a result, they described various systems or laws which have been collected today under the name of "Traditional Chinese Medicine" (TCM). All systems or laws are thought to be dynamically related, feeding and controlling each other.

One of the systems described in TCM which we use in JSD is the "law of Ying and Yang polarity." Another is the system of five Zang and six Fu organs. The five Zang organs belong to the Yin polarity, the six Fu organs to the Yang polarity. "Organs" imply all functions of an organic system as defined in TCM, which comprises more and sometimes different "alignments" than taught by Western anatomy. Each Zang (Yin) organ forms a functional unit with a Fu (Yang) partner, together with a specific tissue, a sensory organ, and a Yin and a Yang meridian.

In addition to the Yin/Yang polarity, the law of the Five Elements (fire, earth, metal, water, wood) is also of great importance when describing states of transition. The fifth Element, for example, represents a materialization of life and growth, which in nature is associated with *wood;* thus TCM declares that *wood is* linked with the fifth element. No doubt that the season when life and growth become most evident is *springtime,* with wonderful *green* colors, and *wind* as a symbol for fast changes. The emotion which falls within this functional unit is *anger.* Of our internal organs the *liver* belongs to this Element, which even in Western medicine is regarded as the most vital of the glands, irreplaceable in the complexity of coordinating vital functions.

The Ancients didn't study corpses and didn't know about anatomy. They propose that our body is not static, like a machine, but rather dynamic (as was learned later to be due to being composed of atoms and molecules which exhibit the characteristics of both particles and waves). The Ancients described this dynamic quality as due to different interacting energies called "Qi" (chi). One form of Qi we have from birth, other forms we take in through such sources as breath, food, emotions, and surroundings, just to name a few. As Qi is everywhere at once, it cannot be fixed only in material vessels, like veins or nerves, but has to have its own paths throughout the body. TCM calls these paths "meridians" and names six paired Yin-meridians and six paired Yang-meridians, where the Qi travels in a continuum within 24 hours with a maximum flow occurring for 2 hours in each pair.

Eight Strange Flows cross and interlink the main meridians. The energy in the eight strange flows most often runs in opposite direction to meridian flow. Thus, they function as collectors and redistributors of excess energy.

Auto accidents block the flow of traffic in our streets and lead to an accumulation of cars, all stalled (excess), so that at the same time, nobody gets to work (deficiency). In the TCM approach, these two phenomena, excess and deficiency, are regarded as causing main disharmony patterns in the body. Both require balancing.

Along the meridians we can electrically detect specific "points" where the energy flow comes close to the surface, just as the entrance to a subway. The energy continues on deeper internal paths, to which we do not have direct access. All meridians, however, are interlinked. These meridian points on the body surface are treated by acupuncturists with needles and herbs. In JSD we use soft touch or pressure with our fingertips to influence them. As some of the meridians end or begin in the fingertips, these ends are somewhat attracted to points, so no electrical device is needed to locate them. Also, Mann[4] describes fibrocystic nodules as occurring at "the points" in muscles, which can easily be felt. Many times the recipient will tell you, "Yes, there it is!" without being asked. Jin Shin Do™ most often focuses on the parts of the body with an excess of energy with the goal of releasing undesired blocked energy, restoring balance to body, mind, and spirit.

REQUIREMENTS OF PHYSICAL THERAPISTS USING JIN SHIN DO

As traditionally trained physiotherapists, we are conditioned to use our touch to prove what we hypothesize, or carry out what we learned to be "appropriate treatment." The primary perceiving touch is considered to be unmeasurable, irreproducible, non-scientific, and therefore of less value. This belief is very limiting. What makes us want to diminish our capabilities to those of robots, just to get "reproducible" results? Why are we taught to deny or suppress the dimension of human-to-human exchange of warmth, caring, and love in traditional scientifically based physical therapy? The unconditional acceptance of the other and ourselves as we are in the moment would be the starting point for a Jin Shin Do assessment or treatment. Why are we never encouraged to walk the path from this place of mutual regard?

To Western ears this might sound non-scientific, but it just deals with the same problems from a different perspective, accepting that we cannot neglect our own reality. There is no such thing as pure objectivity in a perceiving human being. Perception is unique, subjective and unavoidable in taking in information. Denying this can be highly misleading.

In health care, many professionals tend to burn out because they pour their energy into trying to cure or fix their patients, take too much responsibility for the outcome, and often feel as if they don't get anything back. As JSD therapists, first of all we are required to take good care of ourselves. During the education we learn this. It is important for the therapist to be in a comfortable place, as his/her energy highly affects the state of the recipient and the outcome of a treatment. So both therapist and patient profit as they are equally considered in this approach.

In JSD it is the therapist's compassion and empathy that is required, plus our unique personal companionship, being honestly present with all our qualities and deficits. We don't have to fix anything for anyone. Our role is more that of an amplifying catalyst. We don't channel energy from outside of us, we simply support redistribution of what there is. The recipient and his/her energy do the job, releasing muscular tension and blockages. These impede the free flow of Qi. Free flow opens emotions and the gate to our inner wisdom and knowledge of the natural order, the Tao. From this place, healing as a natural procedure is allowed to occur.

THE APPLICATION OF JIN SHIN DO TREATMENT

As with every comprehensive therapeutic approach, Jin Shin Do therapists start with a history. The recipient tells his or her physical and emotional problems. The therapist listens and applies the criteria of Traditional Chinese Medicine to detect patterns of disharmony. Using Zang/Fu theory, the therapist differentiates somatic problems; the theory of the Five Elements helps to detect possible blockages in the psychic process. Physical problems evolve from emotional problems. Our emotions evolve one from the other. The Ancients associated this evoking of emotions with the Five Elements. Teeguarden[5] described this evolving in the form of an "emotional kaleidoscope."

For the manual examination, the recipient preferably lies supine and the therapist starts from the neck and shoulders. Each person has an individual distribution of tension and armorings. Similar symptoms are not necessarily caused by the same tension patterns. Low back pain, for example, can be a result of various disharmonies. We can assess the individual pattern of tension by touching specific points on the meridians. This gives us the most important information for how to proceed with JSD treatment. The setting for a treatment preferably is interruption-free and designed to create an atmosphere of trust and safety with as little distraction as possible.

The therapist's hands give a foundation (Yin), initiating inner activity (Yang) of the recipient which facilitates a release of tension. We hold one so-called local point of a blockage with one finger, and with the other hand we successively touch two or three energetically connected distal points on other parts of the body to release the tension in the local point. Using the ancient knowledge of the energetic connections between local and far distant parts of the body allows JSD a significantly deeper and longer lasting effect than Western massage techniques.

Both therapist and recipient follow the unfolding of the flow of Qi as it is released by this systematic pattern of light touch. Their attention is always focused on what is happening under the hands and within the body. Thus the therapist can validate the recipient's feeling and awareness by giving feedback on what he or she can feel.

Time devoted to therapy should not exceed one hour per week so that the body and mind are given adequate time to integrate the changes. Chronic diseases are treated in one long session, acute problems in several shorter ones. Finally, time to share the experiences after each session must be factored in.

APPROPRIATE POPULATIONS

Using a holistic approach of energy flow affecting mind, body, and spirit, Jin Shin Do treatments are especially effective in improving disorders of function. Looking for patterns of disharmony, we find that symptoms of low back pain often are accompanied by breathing or digestion problems. All three of these difficulties are affected by JSD energy release. As a gentle relaxation technique, JSD can be used to relieve stress. Another indication for the use of JSD is the presence of the already mentioned "armorings." With a series of treatments, the repressed, locked-in emotions can be released and experienced, thus, the recipient is empowered to decide if the habitual holding of the tension is the desired way to cope with the emotion.

JSD can be applied to recipients in acute care, rehabilitation, or simply to those who want to get more deeply in contact with their body, enabling the body to integrate stimuli by energetic preparation. JSD blends very well with standard Western physical therapy techniques, as the cases below illustrate. It has become a part of our medical approach to patients, allowing a more differentiated diagnosis, which leads to more appropriate therapy.

JSD is contraindicated for patients in radiation therapy. Combining JSD with other energy therapies at the same time might alter the outcome of both.[5] It is safer not to mix energy approaches but apply different approaches after a sufficient treatment-free interval. Further research is needed to document the interrelationship of one energy approach with another and to document the impact one seems to have on the other.

CASE EXAMPLES—USING JIN SHIN DO COMPLEMENTARY TO PHYSIOTHERAPY

Mary (age 72) suffered a subcapital fracture of the humerus with swelling, hematoma, and severe pain, especially at night, which was resistant to the effects of strong medication. The first JSD treatment of neck, shoulder, and arm meridian points significantly reduced the swelling and the pain. Releasing points on the liver and gall bladder meridians, which have their 2-hour energetic high at the time of her pain-maximum, resulted in almost pain-free nights and better sleep. During the day, she started to use her arm to function, and we added PNF patterns to our therapy. With this combination of therapeutic exercise and JSD, she regained full range of motion without pain in a comparatively short time, considering her age and the severity of the lesion. In this case, JSD served as gentle contracture therapy, releasing the tension, facilitating pain relief and mobility of soft tissue, and increasing her range.

Betty (age 55) came to the office with a complaint of severe tension and pain in her neck and shoulder, and the feeling that her back would "break" at the location of her second lumbar vertebra. She often felt dizzy and her back muscles between T4-10 felt like a "string of steel." After the initial neck release, she reported decreased tension and dizziness. In one of the following sessions, she was able to talk about her rather substantial fears.

As already mentioned, the Five Elements also incorporate emotions. In her case, the emotion she experienced in the JSD release led us to focus on kidney and bladder meridians. Special release patterns for them increased her feeling of stability in the lumbar region and she reported that her dizziness disappeared. Becoming aware of, accepting, and integrating her repressed emotions as a result of JSD, she developed increased sensitivity for her body and gained the emotional and physical courage to face her fears. Her body no longer had to repress and "armor" against unwanted emotions. The freed flow could facilitate balance and harmony.

Henry (age 38) came to respiratory therapy because of an allergic asthma. His nose was congested, he was annoyed by constant sneezing, and he used an inhaler continuously because of a feeling of suffocation. His doctor diagnosed a dysfunction in his lung parameters. The pattern of tension showed blockages in the lung and large intestine meridian. In addition to his JSD sessions, he learned combinations of points so that he could treat himself. After only five sessions, the symptoms he had had for years had almost disappeared. He no longer used the inhaler, but between 7:00 and 9:00 at night the feeling of not getting enough air remained. So he was asked to hold a combination of points after 7:00, as this is the energetic high of the pericardium or circulation-sex meridian. After a few evenings of self-treatment, in spite of his prevailing skepticism, he reported his symptoms totally disappeared.

RECIPIENT AND THERAPIST RESPONSE TO JIN SHIN DO

Jin Shin Do supports the natural flow of energy along the meridians, but since we can't actively relocate excess energy from one place to another, we can never totally anticipate the impact released energy will have on the flow inside the recipient's body. We follow the flow with our touch and give verbal feedback to the patient about his or her response as we are perceiving it. For example, we may note the onset of rapid eye movement (REM), a change in breathing, muscle fasciculation, or a tensing up or relaxing under our hands. Recipients may report seeing pictures of colors in their mind's eye, or memories which may arise. When this happens, we help the recipient to direct his or her focus on the body and locate the place of resonance in the body with what is being perceived. Sometimes pain or tension in other parts of the body simultaneously occur. It is important to follow the impulse and together explore what is happening as well as what might help to release the flow again. Being nonjudgementally present to each experience as it happens is the best support a therapist can offer a recipient.

OUR HISTORY OF BECOMING INVOLVED WITH JIN SHIN DO

While working in a neurosurgery unit in Bonn, Germany, as experienced physiotherapists, we were continually confronted with what we perceived to be the limitations of Western medicine. The inadequacies of our mechanistic approach stimulated us to search for a more holistic one. Traditional methods, such as surgery and therapeutic exercise, only had partial impact on the problems of a patient. As physiotherapists, we often were confronted with the odds—therapy-resistant symptoms or remnants after surgery. We had observed many pieces of the puzzle which didn't fit into Western patterns; with the TCM approach the pieces of the puzzle suddenly fell into place. The gentleness of the intervention, the excellent applicability, and the positive results made us continue.

The patients' feedback became an important factor as it determined the individual sequences in therapy. They were much more actively involved, as opposed to traditional physiotherapy, where they carried out or sometimes had to bear what we decided to be good for them.

At the same time, experiencing JSD on ourselves and on others, we, too, became more aware of our selves with our own repressed emotions and armorings, as well as the potential of our empathy. The result of this increased awareness was a noticeable change in our personal and professional attitudes which supported our overall personal growth as clinicians and as people. Thus, JSD did not only help our patients.

BECOMING A JIN SHIN DO THERAPIST

No special training program or advanced certification is required to begin to study Jin Shin Do. For more detailed information, contact the Jin Shin Do Foundation, 366 California Avenue, Suite #16, Palo Alto, California 94306.

SUMMARY

Iona Teeguarden's synthesis of Western psychology, Taoist philosophy, and Traditional Chinese Medicine blend in Jin Shin Do, a simple and gentle therapeutic technique that improves the negative symptoms of everyday tension, as well as the pain and immobility that accompany severe disease and injury leading to diminished function. It is holistic in its approach. It does not apply finger pressure instead of pills to remove symptoms, but looks for connections to get to the root of a problem. Most recipients love it and therapists enjoy applying it.

REFERENCES

1. Teeguarden IM. Accupressure Way of Health, JIN SHIN DO. Tokyo: Japan Publications; 1982.

2. Reich W. *Charakteranalyse*. Koln, Germany: Kiepenheuer and Witsch Verlag; 1989.

3. Kaptchuk TJ, Biller I, trans. *The Web That Has No Weaver. Das Grosse Buch der Chinesischen Medezin*. Munich, Germany: O.W. Barth Verlag; 1992.

4. Mann FB. *Acupuncture, the Ancient Chinese Art of Healing and How it Works Scientifically*. New York, NY: Vintage Books; 1973.

5. Teeguarden IM. *The Joy of Feeling, Body Mind Accupressure, JIN SHIN DO*. Tokyo, Japan: Japan Publications; 1989.

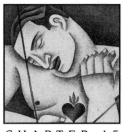

CHAPTER 15

SUBTLE ENERGY MANIPULATION AND PHYSICAL THERAPY

Peter Selby, PT

INTRODUCTION

Qi Gong (Chi Kung') is an ancient Chinese practice dating back more than 5,000 years, involving the regulation of the body's energy through control of the mind and breath, posture and movement, and self massage. Literally, Qi Gong means "manipulation of the breath" or "energy manipulation," and is fundamentally related to acupuncture, Traditional Chinese Medicine, and T'ai Chi and other Chinese martial arts. Qi Gong is practiced by 20 million people in China for its positive effect in both restoring and maintaining health, vitality, and longevity. Not only does Qi Gong relate to self-regulation but also has an external form in which practitioners assess and treat energy disturbances in others. In the discussion that follows, some fundamental principles and practices of Qi Gong will be considered and related to the quest to find a scientific rationale for "Energy Medicine" in general.

The field of energy medicine is a diverse and ancient one, predating our conventional modern Western medicine by thousands of years. It is foundational to Traditional

Chinese Medicine, shamanism, and a great variety of spiritual healing practices. In a sense, the Chinese anticipated the theory of relativity, focusing not on the material aspect of the body but the animating life force that creates and sustains it.

While Western Medicine is primarily oriented toward a biochemical materialist perspective, many practitioners have opted to explore "alternative" approaches based on a broader view, that holds man to be, as William Tiller, Chief of the Material Science Department at Stanford University, wrote:

> A multidimensional Being, functioning on many different levels of Nature simultaneously. He is mostly unaware of these levels of self and cannot grasp the visualization that he has an extended energy structure...if man's energy structure is perturbed at any one of the indicated levels, ripples of effect flow out in all directions to produce corresponding perturbations at all other levels.[1]

But science has yet to quantify or qualify what this energy is. Tiller continues,

> There is a truly great need for reliable experimental devices for monitoring body energies on successively more and more subtle levels. Measurements with such devices will help to forge the bridge between our present chemical medicine and our future energy medicine.[1]

Obviously, the role of science is not to uphold the current dogma, but rather to explore and understand the manifold phenomena of the universe in open-minded inquiry. St. Augustine said, "Miracles do not happen in contradiction to nature, but only in contradiction to that which is known to us in nature."[2] Or as Elmer E. Green, PhD, Director of the Menninger Clinic, put it, "What we have seen and measured in our laboratory (as healers have been tested while healing) is not possible. But it happens anyway!"[3]

Albert Einstein postulated,

> It is possible that there exist human emanations which are still unknown to us. Do you remember how electrical currents and 'unseen waves' were laughed at? The knowledge about man is still in its infancy.

And energy medicine was acknowledged as a potent force by Hippocrates, who wrote,

> It has often appeared, while I have been soothing my patients, as if there was a singular property in my hands to pull and draw away from the affected parts aches and diverse impurities, by laying my hand upon the place and by extending my fingers towards it. Thus it is known to some of the learned that health may be implanted in the sick by certain gestures.

Modern accounts of the efficacy of subtle energy healing methods are so numerous and come from such diverse quarters including all fields of medical endeavor that they beg for deeper consideration by those who hold exclusively to a conventional medical world view. Numerous studies, while not fully establishing the mechanisms, have demonstrated that effects of energy healing modalities are real and measurable. It appears that conventional medicine is neglecting a major element of the physical body and the human being as a totality when it ignores the anatomy and function of the body's energy systems. Imagine practicing medicine without consideration of the circulatory system or the nervous system. The emerging science of energy medicine would hold bioenergetic considerations to be no less important. Perhaps the best known of these new fields of medical science is psychoneuroimmunology.

For many, the incorporation of energy medicine doesn't hinge on doubts as to the legitimacy of the approach but rather on the practical considerations of "what," "when," and "how," not on whether it is effective, but rather, "Can I do it and how will it fit into my practice?" Practically speaking, it is when we can deduce certain fundamental principles that characterize alternative approaches to healing that we possess the key to expanding the boundaries of our practice.

THE NATURE OF QI

The first question, is of course, what is the nature of this energy we are referring to? Many experiments have been designed to determine this, but no definite answer has been articulated. Our ignorance is such that we don't even know enough to design the necessary instruments. The author visited special laboratories in China dedicated to measuring the Qi force manifest by the nation's most famous healers and Qi Gong masters, but, in spite of high tech tools such as "Squid" magnetometers and various electrical monitors being focused on healers inside special electromagnetically shielded chambers, no definitive conclusions were reached. Healers were seen to have specific and unique electromagnetic and infrared signatures when directing "Qi" energy. Photons were also recorded emanating from some of the Qi Gong masters when they were emitting Qi. But it was apparent that some more fundamental force was operating in that the effects did not weaken with distance nor did the electromagnetically shielded chamber wall create a barrier to their emissions.

Qi, in the context of this discussion, is fundamentally the animating force within all life forms, intimately associated with and dependent on the matter it is animating. While the Western concept may attribute "energy" as a byproduct of matter, Qi in the Chinese concept is more original than the matter it animates and provides an organizational field that determines the physical form of the organism. Kirlian photography evidences the presence of this organizational field; for instance, when the top third of a leaf is cut off and then photographed by the Kirlian method, the entire leaf will appear on the photographic plate, including the vein structure of the leaf.[4]

FORMS OF QI

The Chinese distinguish between the Qi, which is this original animating and organizational force, yuanqi (primary ancestral Qi), and another kind of Qi, "acquired" Qi, which is absorbed from food and water (yingqi or nutrient qi), from the air (qingqi), and the physical environment including interactions with the animate world. Thus Ancestral Qi could be thought of as the original deposit of life force at conception, one's "starting balance." In contrast, acquired Qi consists of the deposits which replenish the account amidst ongoing energy withdrawals given the demands of life. This is an important distinction. Some people start out life with a tremendous vitality reflecting a considerable inheritance of ancestral energy. It may be sufficient to compensate for considerable excesses and abuses in their lifestyle, whereas others with less original vitality cannot sustain good health in such a context due to a less vital "constitution." Thus longevity is attributed to more than "good genes" and a healthy lifestyle.

Qi is also classified according to functions within the body. For instance, Zongqi Qi, also known as pectoral qi, is formed from the clean qi of the air combining with the nutrient qi. It is stored in the chest and promotes the circulatory functions of the heart as well as controlling respiration and speech. Weiqi, derived from nutrient qi, serves to protect the surface of the body from exogenous pathogenic factors, controlling the defensive functions of the skin and warming the viscera, an energetic correlate of the cellular immune system. When this qi is deficient, a person will tend to catch colds and flu as well as tend to be easily influenced by other people's energy and moods. The Qi Gong practice of self-massage and skin brushing and rubbing can strengthen this function, helping the Qi to move through specific energy pathways called meridians that have both deep and superficial branches.

Thus the prevention of disease doesn't so much depend on avoiding pathogens as cultivating a healthy vital Qi energy. This echoes Hippocrates' words,

> Disease [is] not an entity, but a fluctuating condition of the patient's body,
> a battle between the substance of disease and the natural self-healing tendency
> of the body.[5]

The Qi energy of the body has fundamental characteristics of polarity—yin, which is more related to the material aspect, is rich in fluid and more internal—whereas yang is more identified with the animating force, being hyper-energetic, radiant, and superficial. Yin and Yang correlate with negative and positive, internal/external, cold/hot oppositions, respectively. These opposing forces are interdependent, inter-consuming, inter-supporting, and inter-transforming. Either polarity can be deficient or excessive and, while equilibrium is ideal, an excess of one can "consume" and thus create a deficiency of the other or a deficiency of one might create a relative excess of the other.

The concepts of yin/yang equilibrium, deficiency, or excess are applied to the body's various organs and their meridian pathways.

Without getting technical, each organ is paired to another and associated with one of five elements: earth, metal, water, wood, and fire. Organ pairs (eg, the kidney which is yin, is paired with the bladder which is yang) interact with specific other organ pairs to enhance/promote energy or control/counteract energy. For instance, the kidney/urinary bladder pair (water element) promotes the liver/gall bladder complex (wood element) but controls/counteracts the heart/pericardial pair (fire element).

Certain "extra-meridial" pathways serve to regulate and promote the organ energies and their pathways. Thus the Governor Vessel, an extra meridian rising in the dural tissue of the spine and along the mid-line of the skull, regulates all the hollow organs, for example, the large intestine, the bladder, etc, while also governing the function of the spine.

GATING THE FLOW OF ENERGY

A key concept relates to the "gating" of energy, which might be understood as a door being open to or shut against the natural flow of energy. When the gate is relatively closed, Western practitioners might call this a blockage. Practically, this equates with specific changes in the physical qualities of body tissue, affecting both the vitality of a given tissue and the physical tensions in the three dimensional connective grid of that tissue and diversely related tissues. Thus, abnormal myofascial tension results from an energy blockage. Written at the turn of the century by the founder of osteopathy, the words of Andrew Taylor Still as quoted by Cottingham echo this insight:

> ...fascia is... a foundation on which to stand. By its action we live and by its failure we shrink or swell or die. The soul of man with all the streams of pure, living water seems to dwell in the fascia of his body.[6]

The meridians and deep energy pathways apparently lie in fascial and collagen-rich tissue, for example, the aforementioned Governor Vessel running in the spinal Dura Mater. Myofascial and collagenous structures which are not being perfused with energy due to a blockage tend to exhibit a "hard" unyielding resistance to stretch, and extremities deficient in energy generally feel heavy and tethered. A blockage in the perineum or at the coccyx may prevent energy from flowing into the Governor Vessel, which originates just anterior to the coccyx. This could result in a positive dural stress test and/or restricted mobility in the spine and cranium. A visceral blockage might manifest as a swollen or congested devitalized feeling on palpation of the organ directly, or as the Visceral Osteopaths such as Barral or Gehain might perceive it, in a loss of normal visceral motility and mobility.

Not only can energy be blocked, but it can also be deficient or excessive. When there is an outright deficiency, the tissue might lack tonus altogether, for example, organ ptosis or sagging flesh in the elderly. When it is excessive, there may be hypermobility or tissue inflammation. Excessive yang energy rising from the liver to the head is said in Traditional Chinese Medicine to be related to the occurrence of stroke. Thus a key aspect in the treatment of stroke is the regulation of the energetic functions of the viscera including the liver, gall bladder, stomach, spleen, and the kidneys that serve to metabolize these energies.

Underlying this phenomena is the relation between blood and Qi. Traditional Chinese medical theory holds that Qi is the commander of blood and blood is the mother of Qi. Thus, a deficiency or imbalance of Qi may lead to a deficiency of blood, poor circulation, blood stagnation, or extravasation. Likewise, excess Qi may cause inflammation or hypertension by "commanding" too much blood to accumulate in a given area.

Qi can be seen to be a vital force where irregularities can manifest in many disease states, including cancer, which the Chinese often attribute to congested Qi and blood. Obviously a healthy circulation of Qi promotes good health and rapid thorough healing of body structures that have experienced injury. Unfortunately, injury of body tissues usually results in impaired Qi flow through those structures which can lead to excess swelling, impaired vascular perfusion, and venous lymphatic drainage and neurological compromise.

Vessels and nerves lie in a three dimensional (often tunnel-like) fascial matrix that can impede neurological function and circulation when this grid becomes constricted due to energy blockage. For instance, a patient who had dropped a computer on her foot 36 hours prior to presenting for treatment reported pain in the foot generally, paraesthesia in her toes, and showed gross swelling and redness/bruising over the entire dorsum, especially the first and second rays. By holding my hands approximately 3 inches away from the foot and sending energy, the patient reported a throbbing exaggeration of her symptom within thirty seconds of commencing the technique. Upon needling Liver 3 (between the first and second ray) on the opposite foot, the intolerant reaction subsided immediately and the swelling diminished rapidly as I continued "sending energy" back and forth between my hands. Apparently the radiation of Qi energy induced more blood flow and thereby stressed the grossly swollen tissues. In fact, Qi Gong is specifically contraindicated in cases of internal bleeding, especially with intra-cranial hemorrhage, and acute infectious diseases.

Since energy systems are interdependent, it is easy to understand how excesses, deficiencies, or blockages in one system or structure may result in energy disturbances in one or more secondary structures. Thus, one must assess and treat the primary deficiency or blockage. In Traditional Chinese Medicine, assessment might involve tongue, pulse, or auricular diagnosis, whereas in Western osteopathic approaches, techniques such as off-body scanning, "arcing" and various listening techniques might be utilized.

DISTANCE PRACTICE

Qi Gong practitioners routinely assess the body from some distance away. An organ not able to conduct energy through itself can usually be palpated off the body from inches to many feet away. This may in part involve the detection of thermal irregularities associated with entropy or energy loss. The Chinese concept of entropy is "geui," which is "the depolarizing, de-energizing and dematerializing force."[7] In visceral osteopathy, this phenomenon is well recognized and students are routinely taught how to feel these energies. Various sensitive infrared devices have been developed which can corroborate these palpatory findings, although they may be only detecting one of many different kinds of simultaneously occurring entropic or dissonant energies.

Bones, which have a three-dimensional collagenous matrix, also are important conduits for energy. Blockages in bone or in adjacent visceral structures give bone a hard feeling. This can contribute to spinal deformities and curvatures (and may also potentiate fractures). For instance, a kidney energy blockage will often reveal itself with a specific paravertebral fullness overlying it on the back. A blockage in the pericardium typically manifests as a hard armored feeling in the sternum and anterior chest and usually can be easily palpated.

LEARNING TO FEEL OR IDENTIFY QI

One of the primary tasks in Qi Gong is to learn the feeling of Qi, an evident a priori in the quest of learning to actively manipulate and direct Qi energy. One common exercise is to rub the hands together and then position them three or so inches apart and feel the pulsating magnetic-like force of fullness, repulsion, or attraction. Note that these phenomena can be altered at will. A variant is to have another person put their hand in the middle of the space between the hands and feel the field intensity. This exercise will usually produce a few "wow"-like exclamations as the sensations are easily felt.

Energy often is perceived by the examiner as a cool breeze, a tingling feeling, a pulsation, a vibration, heat, or an expanding force. On occasion, one's hand will be drawn in, or conversely, repulsed. Acupuncture points typically feel sticky due to increased skin drag and altered electrical impedance, which can be measured with simple instruments. More subtle sensations include feelings of fullness, discharge, or drawing energy into itself. Energy might initially discharge from a point only to be followed by a sensation of energy flowing into the tissue, implying the exchange of negative and positive forces.

On the receiving end, people may experience a variety of effects—tingling, electric shock-like sensations, floating, spontaneous movements, altered states of consciousness, and profound relaxation. Often the movement of Qi through a blockage creates or exaggerates pain. Needling techniques in acupuncture include producing "deQi" (literally, the sensation of the arrival of Qi), which is felt as a deep full penetrating ache which often will radiate down a meridian along the length of an entire extremity. Qi Gong masters can impart sensations of spirals and energy bullets in sensitive people by pointing their hands from across a room.

A fundamental concept in energy work is that the body commonly "knows" what it needs to do; it may just lack the means to accomplish it. Therapies employing large forces may generate a defensive reaction that minimizes and isolates the effect. In contrast, mere observation through gentle palpation and respectful listening to the tissues can impart an energy which may sufficiently augment the body/mind's awareness, intention, and focal energy to successfully surmount an energy blockage and generate a specific release or a broad shift of energy.

In Qi Gong, activating one's energy circulation through regulating the breath and the mind may result in "spontaneous movement,"[6] which is viewed as highly therapeutic and is essentially a swinging motion of the extremities or even a whole body energy "dance," also valued in certain yoga practices. This insight may help to understand the phenomenon of "unwinding" that is integral to the practice of Craniosacral therapy and myofascial release. These energy activations can affect blockages in the emotional, mental, and spiritual arenas as well.

RESONANCE AND INDUCTION

A discussion of Qi Gong would not be complete without reference to the principles of resonance and induction. An example of a resonant system is a container filled with just enough water so that a standing wave form is created when a specific frequency of vibration is placed under the container. By offsetting the source of the vibration from the center, the standing wave will change and create mirror image wave patterns. The body itself is a resonant system with the specific organs and tissues generating and reinforcing the overall resonant field through interactions of their specific fields. The vegetative functions of the brain maintain the efficiency of the overall system through controlling the individual organs and their fields.

However, the limbic system and cortex can generate dissonate wave patterns that distort the overall field in the presence of negative thoughts, feelings (for instance, fear and worry), and excess stress generally. Thus, a fundamental practice in Qi Gong involves "the Inner Smile," which reflectively focuses its positive energy form. In this technique, one focuses upon an event, place, or person that powerfully brings a smile "to mind," which is then gathered in the vicinity of the pineal gland and focused onto the viscera, central nervous system, spine, and extremities. Once again, this technique facilitates and is facilitated by an ability to feel the presence and movement of Qi. Western medical research in the field of psychoneuroimmunology has confirmed the effects of specific thought patterns on the immune system and specific organ systems.

USING QI THERAPEUTICALLY WITH CLIENTS/PATIENTS

Through meditation and quieting the mind, Qi Gong reestablishes healthy resonant dynamics within the organism by resolving the dissonant patterns of the mind and invigorating the devitalized resonant structure. Similarly, through augmenting one's own relatively healthy field, the Qi Gong master can, through resonance and induction, reinforce the overall resonant field of his or her patient by identifying diseased resonant patterns of specific organs and "harmonizing" the energy by "sending" healthy Qi. Thus Becker writes,

> If some people can detect fields from other organisms, why shouldn't some people be able to affect other beings by means of their linked fields? Since the cellular functions of our bodies are controlled by our own DC fields, there's reason to believe that gifted healers generate supportive electromagnetic effects, which they convey to their patients or manipulate to change the sufferer's internal currents directly, without limiting themselves to the placebo effect of trust and hope.[5]

QI GONG AND PHYSICAL THERAPY

Qi Gong has been seen to be useful in treating a large number of medical conditions including asthma, cancer, and heart disease. The concepts and practices can easily be shared with patients, empowering them and providing a tool for maintaining their own health.

Hopefully some of the concepts that have been presented in the above paragraphs will inspire specific applications within the broad field of physical therapy practice. For instance, the fact that improving the quantity and quality of energy flow will tend to result in decreased tension in connective tissue structures has profound applications, specifically in orthopedics and physical therapy in general. Thus some patients with contractures such as occur in subacute and chronic adhesive capsulitis of the shoulder have demonstrated remarkable pain resolution and immediate improvement of range of motion when Qi is "projected" from across the treatment room.

Similarly, this method of energy projection can rebalance movement in patients demonstrating grossly asymmetrical hamstring tensions or painfully restricted range of motion of the neck. Opening the "energy gate" at the base of the Governor Vessel might well enhance dural mobility, range of motion in the spine, and cranial motion, which might prove of special benefit to whiplash patients and those suffering from migraines. Menstrual cramping and irregularity may normalize after releasing energy blockages in the pelvis. Correcting energy imbalances and blocks in visceral structures such as the bladder, kidneys, or colon can result in immediate improvement of range in the lumbar spine and the pelvic and hip articulations. Modulating energy disturbances in the lungs or the liver frequently results in improved range of motion in the neck and thorax.

In physical therapy with athletes, releasing the energy blockages associated with acute injuries can immediately reduce pain and swelling and improve function. In China, athletes practice Qi Gong to improve their performance and focus.

CASE EXAMPLE

A 34-year-old man came for assessment and treatment of an acutely painful right shoulder following an injury the previous day while playing Ultimate Frisbee. He explained that he had fallen onto his shoulder many times previously and had suffered from chronic low grade shoulder pain for which he had consulted an orthopedic surgeon. However, he stated he had never experienced such severe pain as this, having been unable to sleep most of the night in spite of codeine pain medications.

On examination, he was only able to raise his arm to approximately 30 degrees of flexion and abduction and was generally unwilling to move it because of pain. The shoulder was hot on palpation and tender over the lateral and especially the anterior aspect. Off-body thermal diagnosis revealed a blockage of energy in the gleno-humeral area. An impedance was evident when directing energy through the shoulder tissue. Induction of energy along the meridians of the arm revealed a blockage of energy flow at the shoulder.

Treatment consisted of off-body recoil and inductive techniques resulting in the restoration of energy flow along the various meridians of the upper extremity. Energy was then vectored across the shoulder until the blockage was perceived to dissipate and normal flow of energy was restored in the meridians of the extremity. The patient was asked at this point to move his arm and demonstrated a pain-free range until approximately 110 degrees of elevation. The shoulder was then allowed to spontaneously move about in an unwinding type motion while being supported after which the patient was able to fully elevate his arm with little pain. The patient returned the following day to report that approximately two hours after his treatment his symptoms had all but disappeared and that he had slept without problems that night. Follow-up assessment and treatment confirmed a remarkable recovery given the acute pain and limitation the patient had presented with the day before.

Upon reflection, it would appear this patient had acquired an energy "cyst" or blockage in the shoulder joint due to the accumulated trauma to his shoulder. Irregularities of Qi associated with this blockade generated an inflammatory response including abnormal blood and lymphatic flow (recall that Qi commands the blood, regulating such functions as keeping the blood in the vessels). Acute blockages of energy flow often associate with acute pain. Restoration of the movement of the Qi resulted in almost immediate diminution of pain, and shortly thereafter, resolution of the inflammatory response. Healing was therefore very rapid and gratifying without the use of anti-inflammatory medication. To date, there has been no recurrence of chronic symptoms in this patient.

SUMMARY

The listing of specific techniques and their applications is beyond the scope of this chapter but it is hoped that the reader may be inspired to learn more about the field of energy medicine and Qi Gong, creatively exploring and developing further applications within one's area of expertise. Given a thorough grounding in conventional practice, common sense applications of the principles of energy medicine will serve to round out one's practice and potentially fill in a few blanks in the endeavor to treat the multi-dimensional being we call man. It is an exciting field begging for exploration.

Elmer Green, well known author on biofeedback and director of the Menninger Foundation quotes Robert MacCloud,

> The essence of science, it seems to me, is an attitude—an attitude of disciplined curiosity...There is always the lure of the unexplored and the challenge to develop methods that will make further exploration possible.[8]

There seems to be a genuine interest among lay people and health professionals alike in the principles, applications and benefits of subtle energy medicine. If indeed the body's energy system stands beside—or perhaps in—some aspects underlying other major systems, such as the immune system or the circulatory system, then competence in this arena is not a luxury professionally or individually, but rather a necessity. Beyond this, subtle energy medicine provides a tantalizing opportunity to draw on ancient wisdom and the excitement of discovering new knowledge.

REFERENCES

1. Motoyama H, Brown R. *Science and the Evolution of Consciousness Chakras, Ki and Psi.* Brookline, Mass: Autumn Press, Inc; 1978:16,19.

2. Meek GW. *Healers and the Healing Process.* Wheaton, Ill: Theosophical Publishing House; 1977:115.

3. Harpur T. *The Uncommon Touch.* Toronto, Ontario: McClelland & Stewart Inc; 1994:159.

4. Gerber R. *Vibrational Medicine.* Santa Fe, NM: Bear & Co; 1988:55.

5. Becker RO, Selden G. *The Body Electric.* New York, NY: Morrow; 1985:161,269.

6. Cottingham JT. *Healing Through Touch.* Champaign, Ill: Stipes; 1985:47.

7. Dong P, Esser AE. *Chi Gong.* New York, NY: Paragon House; 1990:125-142,23.

8. Green E, Green A. *Beyond BioFeedback.* Ft. Wayne, Ind: Knoll Publishing Co, Inc; 1977:276.

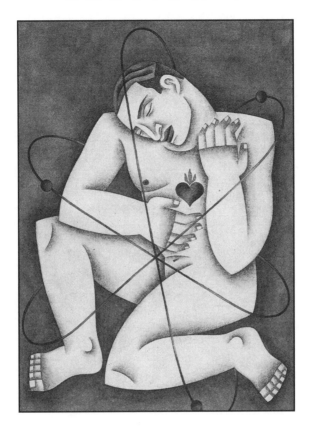

HERBAL
TREATMENT

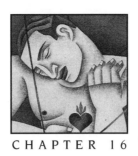

CHAPTER 16

INTEGRATING ELEMENTS OF HOMEOPATHY AND PHYSICAL THERAPY

IMPLICATIONS FOR MAINSTREAM THERAPISTS

Steve Heinrich, PT

INTRODUCTION

As *non-physician* rehabilitation professionals, we do not prescribe medications, herbs, vitamins, or supplements to our patients. However, we recognize on a daily basis the importance of the role medications, vitamins, and mineral supplements play in the health of our patients and ourselves. This chapter presents the role of homeopathy as an alternative pharmacological and energetic discipline which is compatible with both physical therapy and medicine.

HOMEOPATHIC THEORY

Microdosing? Potentizing? Water memory? At first glance, homeopathy may appear irrational, but as one studies the implications of treating somatic and emotional dysfunctions with homeopathy's subtle energy, one cannot help being intrigued.

The practice of homeopathy is based on the principle of "like treats like," first reported in ancient Greek medicine. This philosophy was later developed into the practice of homeopathy by Samuel Hahnemann (1755-1843), a medical physician who became disenchanted with the medical practices of the day and began studying the remedies of nature as an alternative to the treatments of the era.[1]

Hahnemann began experimenting with this new theory as a result of observing the effects of cinchona bark on patients with malaria. Cinchona was malaria's treatment of choice at the time, and when taken internally, the symptoms of fever, chills, etc, were controlled. Hahnemann, in the tradition of nineteenth century physicians, gave himself doses of cinchona to study its effect on the non symptomatic. To his surprise, the symptoms of malaria appeared: chills, fever, nausea, etc.[1]

Intrigued, Hahnemann postulated that cinchona bark was effective because it set up a disease process similar to malaria within the patient, thus mobilizing the body's own defenses to eradicate the malaria and the cinchona-induced condition. In a way, Hahnemann envisioned the introduction of vaccines, even though the system Hahnemann fancied turned out later to be fundamentally different from the vaccination process.

By ingesting controlled doses of natural substances (mostly from plants, but not limited to organic materials), Hahnemann and his associates began to formulate their findings. Meticulously documenting the physical and emotional effects of these substances on themselves and others, Hahnemann produced the original Materia Medica; a compendium of *provings*, or reactions to natural substances that could then be used to treat disease. This *proving* method has continued for more than two centuries, and now a vast number of *proven* remedies are available to the homeopathic physician.

Dr. Hahnemann continued to develop natural remedies, and in ensuing years discovered that diluted tinctures of the remedies seemed to work even better than full strength solutions.[2] This finding was to be the true beginning of homeopathy as a philosophy of treatment and remains one of the biggest sticking points with allopathic physicians.

In order to understand the foundation of homeopathic remedies, one must first understand how herbal materials are transformed into water-based solutions. Remedies are prepared by soaking the plant or other material in pure alcohol. A drop of this solution is then placed into either a 1:10 ratio or 1:100 ratio of distilled water, designated 1x or 1c. Successive dilutions of one drop of each proceeding solution are then placed into a fresh container of either 1:10 or 1:100 distilled water. When the progression of dilutions has reached twelve cycles, for example, the atomic concentration of the original preparation would be less than 10^{24}. Since the number of atoms in a similar amount of fluid is approximately 6×10^{23}, there is little chance that even a single atom of the original substance remains in the dilution.[2] Many observers trying to validate homeopathy have found this difficult to believe.

OBSERVATIONS OF WATER

In an effort to explain this phenomenon, scientific inquiry has recently focused on the water molecule itself. Some researchers have explained the effectiveness of homeopathic dilutions by attributing special properties to water molecules which maintain the essence of the preparation in a constant state. In the intriguing book, *Dreams of Dragons: Riddles of Natural History*, Lyall Watson, a well-known marine biologist and doctor of anthropology, explores the extraordinary properties of water.[3]

Noting research done at the Institute of Physical Chemistry in Florence, Italy, Dr. Watson cites Georgio Piccardi's work with chemical reactions. In a carefully controlled study over 10 years in length, Dr. Piccardi poured identical amounts of bismuth oxchloride—a colloid solution—into containers of distilled water and recorded the time it took to form a cloudy precipitate.[4] The chemical reaction that *should* have been predictable was not. In fact, the times varied widely, and in a pattern that seemed to correlate with disturbances of the earth's electromagnetic field and the frequency of sun spot activity.

His research concluded that the differences in chemical reaction were not related to variables in methodology or chemical composition, but to changes in the very nature of water. To quote Dr. Piccardi: "water is sensitive to extremely delicate influences and is capable of adapting itself to the most varying circumstances to a degree attained by no other liquid."[4] And Dr. Watson, speaking of water, notes: "Its flexibility and its sensitivity around normal body temperature make it an ideal go-between. A point of contact between ourselves and the cosmos."[3]

The ability of water to hold on to and then transmit the vibrational essence of plant and mineral preparations to a living organism is one of the founding principles of homeopathy, and the point most distrusted by traditional science.

In 1976, Theodore Schwenk, a German engineer, conducted an elaborate series of experiments to demonstrate the impressionable nature of water.[5] He took several identical containers of water and mechanically shook them every 15 minutes during, after, and preceding a total eclipse of the sun. Then, after the eclipse, he placed an identical number of wheat grains into each container and left them alone. The grain that sprouted in water shaken during the eclipse grew quite poorly, while water obtained and shaken before and after the eclipse grew well. He concluded that water must pass on impressions gained by its experience, which may then be utilized by plants, animals, and humans.[3] Clearly for this theory to be correct, quantum physics must be at work at the heart of the process. Some form of imprinting appears to be taking place, but whether it is at a subatomic level or somewhere else is still unknown.

In effect, homeopathic practitioners believe they are preserving and magnifying the energetic signature or frequency of the plant or substance by this progression of plant-preparation—dilution process. Thus, when an homeopathic practitioner dispenses a "remedy," he or she is matching the vibrational properties of the remedy to the vibrational properties of the symptom complex.

To counter claims that homeopathy is nothing more than placebo, researchers at the University of Glasgow, Scotland, made a detailed study of homeopathy in a 1991 meta-analysis[6] under the direction of Dr. David Reilly. The study analyzed two groups of allergic asthmatics who were given diluted doses of allergens to induce symptoms. The entire study group received the allergens, but half the group was given homeopathic remedies while the other half was given an identical appearing placebo.

The results were dramatic: 80% of those taking homeopathic remedies improved over a 4-week period, more than twice the improvement rate of the control group. These findings led Dr. Reilly and his researchers to report: "Our results lead us to conclude that homeopathy differs from placebo in an inexplicable but reproducible way."

PUTTING HOMEOPATHY INTO PRACTICE

My own interest in homeopathy started several years ago with a bad case of tennis elbow. I was renting space for a satellite physical therapy office from a homeopathic physician, and while I had been curious about his work, I had also expressed a healthy skepticism.

After treating my elbow with ice, cross friction massage, pressure sleeves, iontophoresis, and electric stimulation in a long frustrating succession with absolutely no results, I agreed to try homeopathy.

Dr. Todd asked me a series of questions about my life, emotional state, physical health and stress level. After a few minutes of reflection and a quick check of his Materia Medica, he gave me a remedy that according to his evaluation, matched not only the pain, but the other holistic factors we had discussed. I was disbelieving, but after six weeks of pain and no relief from my own physical therapy treatment I was ready to try homeopathy.

Much to Dr. Todd's delight, 80% of the pain and swelling was gone the next morning, and by nightfall, none of my symptoms remained. I was very pleased with this result, but still mystified as to how these changes had occurred. He explained to me that physical or structural pain, as well as illness and disease, often result from imbalances in our lives.

Stress, overuse, poor nutrition, lack of exercise, and fatigue all take a toll on the body's energy reserves and its ability to stay balanced. Homeopathy seeks to assist the restoration of that balance through the physical properties of the remedy and its energetic nature as well. A remedy that in small doses reproduces our symptoms appears to have the power to influence our healing as well. Like cures like.

I have since treated dozens of patients who successfully combine homeopathic remedies and physical therapy. This has been especially effective with fibromyalgia and other soft tissue pain syndromes. Others have been very successful in combining physical therapy with homeopathic treatment for joint pain, back pain, sciatica, and many other conditions.

In the end, I suspect that the real struggle with homeopathy centers not so much on the how, but on the why. Why does homeopathy seem to produce tangible, positive results? Why do craniosacral therapy, myofascial release, and therapeutic touch seem to do the same? We like answers that we can write down and look at. Answers that look like proof.

Certainly there are elements in all the methods mentioned that can be measured, quantified, and proven. But not all of it is measurable, in anything. There always will be some unknown element to healing. That's what makes it interesting!

SUMMARY

My observations convince me that physical therapy and homeopathy can be used concurrently with positive results that are both replicable and beneficial to our patients. Homeopathy has gained a great deal of acceptance with the public through celebrity endorsements, infomercials, and patients' positive experiences with their practitioners. Disenchantment with traditional medical treatment is at an all-time high and many of the patients we see already are receiving treatment from alternative health practitioners. Bridge building between ourselves and these professionals can benefit the art of physical therapy through mutual education, generating rapport, and, in many cases, gaining additional referral sources.

For too many years, physical therapists have stood by while other professions have eroded our place in public perception. It's time to forge a stronger identity of our own, one that can accept and embrace consistent alternatives while maintaining our reliance on good science, proven methodology, and practice that is consistent with our professional ideals.

REFERENCES

1. Schapfler T. Interviews. March 1995.
2. Gerber R. *Vibrational Medicine*. Santa Fe, NM: Bear & Co.; 1988.
3. Watson L. *The Dreams of Dragons: Riddles of Natural History*. New York, NY: William Morrow Co, Inc.
4. Piccardi G. *The Chemical Basis of Medical Climatology*. Springfield, Ill: Thomas; 1962.
5. Schwenk T. *Sensitive Chaos*. New York, NY: Schocken; 1976.
6. The Lancet 344: 1610-1606, Reilly: University Dept. of Medicine, Glasgow Royal Infirmary, Glasgow G31 2ER, Scotland.

INDEX